Conquer Chiari: A Patient's Guide to the Chiari Malformation

Rick Labuda

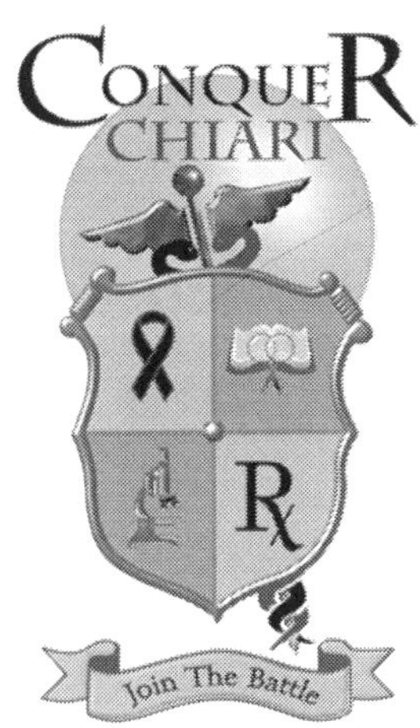

C&S Patient Education Foundation - Wexford, PA

Conquer Chiari: A Patient's Guide to the Chiari Malformation
By Rick Labuda

ISBN: 1-43484-700-4

Cover Design by Melissa S. Neff
Chapter 2 Illustrations by Melissa S. Neff
Chapter 4 Illustrations courtesy of Dr. Ghassan Bejjani
Icons-Title Pages designed by Melissa S. Neff

Conquer Chiari
320 Osprey Court
Wexford, PA 15090
Phone: 724-940-0116
Fax: 724-940-0172
Email: director@conquerchiari.org
Website: www.conquerchiari.org

Disclaimer: This publication is intended for informational purposes only and may or may not apply to you. The author, editor, and publisher are not doctors and are not engaged in providing medical advice. Always consult a qualified professional for medical care. This publication does not endorse any doctors, procedures, or products. While care was taken to ensure the accuracy of the information herein, the author, editor, and publisher are not responsible for any errors or omissions and make no warranty, express or implied, with respect to the accuracy or completeness of the contents of this publication.

Printed in the United States of America.

Acknowledgements

With a book of this size and scope there are many people to thank for their contributions and efforts: first, Melissa Neff for her wonderful graphics, for making the book visually appealing, and for her tireless work ethic; Ray D'Alonzo for his insightful comments and for being a great sounding board in discussing ideas about Chiari and the strength of various research studies; Ed Labuda for taking on the dirty work of proofreading a 300 page book; the Board of Directors of Conquer Chiari for volunteering their time and expertise for a cause they mostly knew nothing about when they started; the many doctors and scientists who have made themselves available to answer questions and sit down for interviews; the loyal readers of Chiari & Syringomyelia News whose feedback is so uplifting; and of course the hundreds of patients and others affected by Chiari who have so generously shared their stories. Finally, I would also like to express my deep gratitude to my wife and family for their unwavering support of my efforts.

This book is dedicated to those who fight…..
We Will Win!

Contents

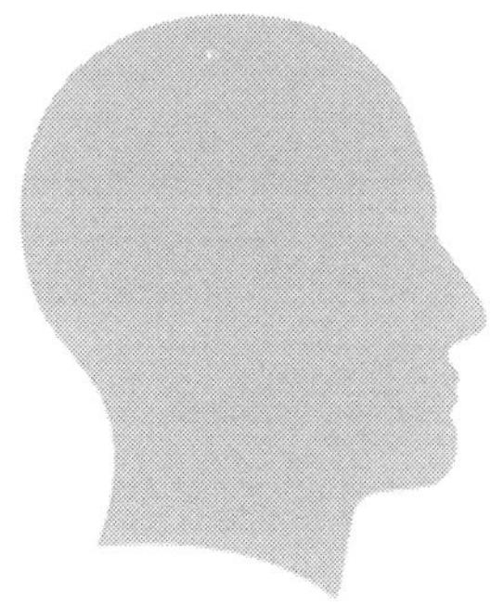

Introduction

"If you know the enemy and know yourself, your victory will not stand in doubt"

~Sun Tzu, The Art of War~

Why A Patient's Guide?

I remember it, literally, as if it happened only yesterday. Of course it didn't happen yesterday, and the ups and the downs, and the false alarms and the false hopes, between then and now could fill a book – just not this one.

It was more than six years ago, but it doesn't take much for me to go back to that moment. I had met with the neurosurgeon briefly a week or so before. He was curious, and quite frankly skeptical, about why I was there. I didn't focus on the symptoms, I was still pretty much in denial about those, instead I passed my reason for being there off on the radiologist.

After years of neck pain, I had finally brought it up to a physician's assistant I had an appointment with for sinus problems. It was at the end of the visit and he quickly said, let's just get an X-ray. I thought he was hustling me out the door; I didn't realize that his off-the-cuff order would end up catching what many others, including myself, had missed for years.

The X-ray showed a congenital anomaly. My top two vertebrae were fused together. The radiologist's report recommended a follow-up MRI to check for other problems. I called an orthopedic surgeon's office and was told they didn't work on the neck and spine and that I should go to a neurosurgeon. Thus, the skeptical look on the surgeon's face as I described some neck pain and headaches. Nevertheless, he ordered the MRI.

When I saw him the second time, he wasn't skeptical anymore, he was more matter of fact than anything. He slapped the scans on the lightbox and said, "Well, you have something called Arnold-Chiari."

After a brief moment of shock, I naturally started firing off questions: What is it? What's going to happen? What do we do about it? What is happening to me?

Maybe he's the best doctor in the world, maybe he patiently answered all my questions and allayed my fears, maybe I was in shock and don't remember clearly. Maybe, but what I remember most from that moment is that he cut me short with, "Look, it's not a life altering event."

Not a life altering event. It's probably the biggest lie I've ever been told, and even then I had a vague feeling he was wrong. Of course, I should probably give him the benefit of the doubt. For some, Chiari isn't a life altering event, but for many it is. It affects every single aspect of their life: their physical well-being, their mental well-being, their emotional state, their spiritual outlook, their economic viability, and perhaps most hurtfully their relationships with friends, family, and loved ones.

"My experience with Chiari challenged me physically, emotionally and spiritually, from when we first found out to the patience required in the healing process after surgery." *~Anne C.~*

So yes, for many, Chiari is a life altering event. Being diagnosed, and trying to come to grips with what is happening can be an overwhelming experience. The analogies are easy and plentiful:

"I felt like I was hit by a [insert one: Mack truck, train, bus, etc.]

"It was like I was drowning and kept having to work hard just to breathe."

"It was like a punch in the gut which doubles you up and knocks the wind out of you."

Although easily available and colorful, as anyone who has gone through it will tell you, they do not do the experience justice. Being diagnosed with Chiari is like being dropped in a whirlpool. You get tossed around, you're disoriented, you don't know what is happening, and just when you think you're able to keep your head above water, another wave comes crashing down on you and you get sucked under again.

I went home that day like so many others have, disoriented, angry, confused, wondering what to tell my family. I didn't even know what was wrong with me. At the time, there was some basic information on the web, but not enough to really understand what was happening or what was to come down the road. The icing on the cake of course, is that no one has ever heard of it and has no idea what to say: *Chiari, what's that? Your brain's what? Syringomyelia, how do you say that? Oh, well, they're doing wonderful things these days in medicine. Gee that's too bad, so are we still doing such and such on Friday?*

Lack of information and awareness are two big reasons why dealing with Chiari can be overwhelming. Since most people have never heard of it before, they don't have a mental picture of what is going on. If a person gets cancer, as awful as that is, they pretty much know what to expect as soon as they hear it. Surgery, radiation, chemo, remission, the mind quickly generates a mental picture, or schematic, of the possibilities. Many of the terms are familiar and talking about the specifics of the disease, and treatment options, is easier because of it. This is by no means meant to minimize what cancer patients and their families go through, but rather to highlight what Chiari patients face.

Most people who are diagnosed with Chiari have no idea what it is. Their spouses don't know, their parents don't know. The mind struggles to create a mental map of the neurosurgical jargon that is thrown around: cerebellar tonsils, CSF flow, syrinxes, decompression, dura. Symptoms are given fancy names, double vision becomes diplopia; can't find the right words, aphasia; trouble walking, ataxia. Even simple words are transformed, front becomes anterior; back becomes posterior…step through the looking glass, Alice, into the Chiari wonderland.

So how do you explain what is happening to your spouse, or your children, or your friends, when you barely understand what is going on yourself? *What is it you have again? Well, you don't look sick. Oh, I'm sure you'll be fine.* Because people don't have a feel for what Chiari is, inappropriate statements fly almost as fast as the medical jargon. What follows is a sense of being alone, and being scared; fear of the unknown, of what will happen; no one understands what you are going through, perhaps least of all yourself.

Feeling alone and overwhelmed, newly diagnosed patients are put in the position of placing blind faith in their doctors. Unfortunately, while the vast majority of doctors are skilled, compassionate, and dedicated, many physicians have never heard of, or really understand, Chiari and syringomyelia. Patients often go years before being diagnosed and are told, ironically, that it is all in their head. This leads to a schism in the doctor-patient relationship and patients become cynical and suspicious of the medical community. To make matters worse, even the experts disagree on important issues, such as when to have surgery and what surgical technique to use.

The result of this situation, for far too many, is a very negative patient experience, and often, a negative outcome as well. Consider the following:

- Chiari causes a wide ranging, diverse set of symptoms, and research has shown that 95% of patients experience at least 5 symptoms.
- There is no single, objective test to diagnose or determine the severity of Chiari; because of this, patients often go 5 years or more before being properly diagnosed.
- A study of over 300 patients found that 57% had at one time been told by a doctor they were suffering from a mental or emotional problem.
- A world-wide survey of neurosurgeons found there is little agreement on how best to treat Chiari.
- Many physicians, including neurosurgeons, are not familiar with the latest findings, so treatment plans are often based on old and inaccurate data.
- For unknown reasons, surgery fails to stop symptom progression about 20% of the time; these patients end up undergoing multiple surgeries.
- While precise data is not available, at least 50% of patients continue to suffer from symptoms such as chronic pain and nerve damage, even after surgery; and many patients end up on disability, socially withdrawn, and depressed.

A couple of years after my surgery, I began thinking back about my experiences. I had learned a lot since those early few months, and I began to realize I had been lucky. I found a different surgeon, underwent a decompression, and began a long, slow recovery. Overall, for someone who had had Chiari and syringomyelia symptoms for years, my outcome was pretty good; but it was also, in a sense, pure luck. As I was going through it, I knew nothing about the critical issues. I didn't even know what questions to ask the doctor; I had no idea what to expect after surgery. The realization that my experience, and outcome, had been a matter of chance did not sit well with me. As I studied the published medical literature, I realized that there was a wealth of information which patients should be made aware of. Unfortunately, this information was locked away in expensive and difficult to understand medical journals, inaccessible to most people.

The answer became clear, because of the lack of awareness and understanding – even in the medical community – patient education was critical. If a disease is well understood, and every doctor knows exactly how to treat it, a person doesn't really need to get into the details of what is going on. However, when there are fundamental questions unanswered, and physicians have varying opinions on what to do, it becomes incumbent upon the patient to educate themselves and make informed, intelligent decisions about their future.

Thus, in August, 2003, Chiari & Syringomyelia News was born. The idea was to give patients access to the latest information by writing about research in plain English, from a patient's point of view. The response to the newsletter was overwhelming and led to the formation of the C&S Patient Education Foundation, and more recently the Conquer Chiari campaign and website.

The Foundation, a 501(c)(3) non-profit, is dedicated to improving the experiences and outcomes of Chiari and syringomyelia patients through education, awareness, and research. Conquer Chiari is a multi-faceted, comprehensive strategy, to do what its name says, and the first step in Conquering Chiari is to understand it. The Conquer Chiari website (www.conquerchiari.org) is intended to be a one-stop shop for patients, families, and medical professionals to learn about, and understand, Chiari and syringomyelia. The site contains extensive background information, over 200 articles in the newsletter archives, and is expanded regularly.

This book is a natural extension of the website and is written, as its name implies, as a guide for patients. It is intended to provide patients with the information they need to:

- Learn the basics about Chiari and syringomyelia, including terminology, definitions, how it is diagnosed, and treatment options;
- Understand what is known and not known, and the key issues they will be facing as they deal with their condition;
- Find a doctor they are comfortable with and communicate with them in an effective and proactive manner;
- Get a feeling for what to expect, during every phase of their experience with Chiari;
- Be able to explain to others, such as family, friends, and coworkers, both what Chiari is, and how it affects them personally;

While its primary purpose is as a Patient's Guide, others may also find the book useful:

- Friends and family can learn about what their loved one is going through and use this knowledge to provide support.
- Non-medical professionals, such as teachers and therapists, can gain valuable insight into how to work with a client who has Chiari.
- Medical professionals will find a concise, accurate, and up-to-date resource.

The Patient's Guide is written in the same easy to understand style as the newsletter and the website, and most importantly, it is written from a patient's perspective. I have experienced the lows and the highs of living with Chiari for the past 9 years. I have felt the shock of diagnosis, the realization that something is wrong, the sudden understanding as past signs and symptoms fall into place, the dread of having brain surgery, the agonizing ride home from the hospital, the hard work of rebuilding strength and endurance, the heart wrenching setbacks, and the incredible joy of doing things that for a time seemed impossible.

The patient's perspective is important, for while doctors are hard-working, dedicated, and compassionate, they inherently have a different perspective on Chiari. Doctors are trained to think deductively, analyze a situation, and develop solutions to problems. Traditionally, they are not trained to educate patients (although this is beginning to change) and they tend to speak a language all their own. Some doctors have a wonderful bedside manner, will take all the time necessary to answer questions, and have a gift for explaining and comforting, but the reality is that not all doctors are like this. The even harsher reality, when it comes to Chiari, is that not all doctors even understand it, or are aware of the latest research.

It is important to note, however, that simply having Chiari is not enough, above all this book is based on science. As with Chiari and Syringomyelia News, I have strived to maintain the highest level of credibility and accuracy. This book does not advocate or endorse any doctor, hospital, or product. It presents the information which is available in as accurate and balanced way as possible, but it will not tell you what to do. It will not say whether you, individually, should have surgery, or which doctor you should see. It will, hopefully, provide you with the information you need to make your own decisions in an informed and intelligent manner.

This approach has proven very successful with the newsletter and website. Since their inception, not a single member of the medical community has complained about any of the information on the site. Rather, the site attracts positive feedback, not only from patients and families, but from doctors, surgeons, nurses, radiologists, and other medical professionals.

In listening to the hundreds of stories of those touched by Chiari, it has become clear that many people tend to humanize their disease. Whether it is because it is named after a person, or for some other reason, some people tend to talk about Chiari almost as if it is alive and has a personality. Another tendency is for people to use military terms in describing their experience; they speak of their ongoing battle with Chiari, and defeating the enemy.

Within this framework, with the patient as a warrior, knowledge becomes their primary weapon. Sun Tzu a Chinese general who lived around 500 B.C., was and is considered a master of military strategy. His book, The Art of War, is often cited as the most comprehensive analysis of the subject, even today.

In it, he states:

"If you know the enemy and know yourself, your victory will not stand in doubt."

Knowing yourself is the easy part, you just need to be honest about the type of person you are so you make the appropriate decisions for your own situation. In this case, knowing the enemy can be difficult. Chiari is a complex condition with many different aspects. Researchers are just beginning to peel back the layers of mystery and reveal its true nature. However, information and research is out there, and it is incumbent upon us to make the most of it and to educate ourselves as best we can.

In the end, you are the one dealing with Chiari, whether as a patient, spouse, parent, friend, or professional. Consider this book, and the knowledge it contains, a weapon in your battle against Chiari.

So, why a Patient's Guide? Because it is necessary and long overdue. It is hard to believe but even with upwards of 300,000 people in the US. directly affected by Chiari, not a single book exists like this one; a comprehensive, up-to-date review, focused on patients, and written in an easy to understand way. I hope you find the book as educational and useful as it is intended to be, and I hope it helps to guide you to a positive experience and outcome.

How To Use This Book

This book is the first in what is intended to be a series of books on Chiari, syringomyelia, and related topics. As such, the focus is primarily on Chiari, but in a broad sense. Syringomyelia is discussed, as are issues such as chronic pain, and pediatric considerations, but these topics are not covered comprehensively. Rather, the book attempts to present a broad and detailed picture of Chiari, and highlight the key issues associated with peripheral topics.

The book is organized, with the exception of the first and last chapters, to flow in a manner similar to most people's experience with Chiari:

Chapter 1: This chapter provides a quick overview of Chiari including definitions, symptoms, diagnosis, treatment, and outcomes. It is modeled after the very popular overview presentation on the website, and presents concise facts in bullet format. It is useful for someone who doesn't have time to read the whole book (such as a friend who wants to know more) or to quickly come up to speed on the basics.

Chapter 2-7: This is the heart of the book and covers a range of topics, including: The Basics, Diagnosis, Treatment, Outcomes, Recovery, and Living With Chiari. It can be read straight through to gain a thorough understanding of

Chiari, or used as a reference to look up specific topics or facts.

Chapter 8: Looking To The Future is not focused so much on an individual's experience with Chiari, but rather takes a broad look at different research fronts and reasons for hope.

Chapter 9: Conquering Chiari is a more personal chapter. While the majority of this book is based on published research, this chapter focuses on my philosophy, developed from my personal experiences with Chiari, on how to overcome and conquer this disease.

As stated earlier, the information in the book is based primarily on published, scientific and medical papers from peer-reviewed journals. Additional sources include interviews with experts in various fields of study and practice, on-line resources, and discussions with hundreds of patients, family members, and professionals. If a topic is introduced which has not been researched, or for which controversy exists, it is noted as such.

While the book is intended to be a fact-based resource, to make the book easier to read, and to present a complete picture of Chiari, a number of features are included throughout the book. These items are likely to include personal opinions and should be evaluated separately from the research based portions of the book. It is hoped that the combination of fact-based information, along with practical tips and personal stories, will present a thorough and balanced picture of the Chiari experience.

These features are clearly denoted with icons, so that they may be easily recognized:

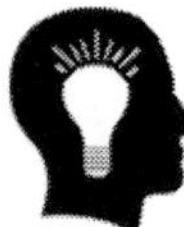

Practical Tips: Exactly as the name implies, tips drawn from both my own experience as a patient, plus tips gathered from talking with other patients and families. Please realize that not every tip will apply to every person, and what worked for one person may not work for someone else.

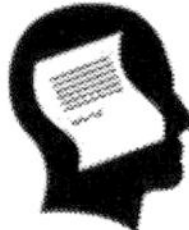

Personal Experience: Anecdotes from my own Chiari experience. Some are humorous, some not so much; but they are intended to provide real examples for what is being discussed and give people an idea of what they might expect.

Did You Know: These are interesting facts which are not critical in understanding Chiari, but which are interesting and help provide a more complete and rich picture of the condition.

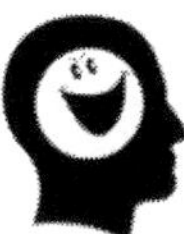

You Gotta Laugh: Humor is a touchy subject when it comes to something as serious as Chiari. Some people use humor as a way to cope, others think that humor is out of place in this situation. While I tend to use humor to help cope, I also respect the other point of view. That is why, while humorous anecdotes are included in the book, they are clearly noted and can be skipped if so desired.

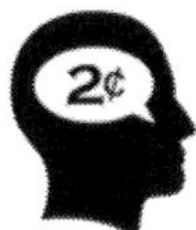

Editorial Comment: Most of the book is based upon published research and a discussion of other people's opionions on a given subject; however at various points I do weigh in with my own opinion. These are clearly marked with the 2 cents symbol.

Most of all, the Patient's Guide is intended to offer something for just about everyone, so no matter how you use the book, hopefully you will find what you are looking for.

Three Keys to Understanding & Dealing with Chiari

As the Executive Director, and founder, of the C&S Patient Education Foundation, and the Editor and primary writer of Chiari & Syringomyelia News, I have had the opportunity to communicate with thousands of patients, doctors, parents, spouses, nurses, teachers, and concerned individuals from around the world. As I listened to people's stories and answered their questions as best I could, I realized that beyond dealing with the physical symptoms of the disease, people have trouble with three specific things.

1. "No one understands what I'm going through."
2. "I don't understand this; why won't someone answer my questions?"
3. "I feel like Chiari has taken over my life."

While these sentiments are perfectly understandable given the overwhelming nature of Chiari, they are also, in my opinion, the key to understanding and dealing with Chiari. Each of the above statements reflects an underlying truth about the Chiari experience which, if accepted and dealt with head on, will better equip people to face what they must face.

Key 1: Each Person's Chiari Experience Is Unique

It can be difficult to accept, but the reality is that no one does understand what you are going through. People can empathize to different degrees; some will be helpful and supportive, others will seem like they are completely clueless, but each person's Chiari experience is unique to themselves.

Chiari is difficult for people to understand for a number of reasons. First, as discussed before, in general people are not aware of what it is. This makes it difficult for someone to really understand what a patient is going through. They will listen to the description, but not realize how it can affect a person's life.

Second, many Chiari symptoms are invisible and hidden. Headaches, fatigue, weakness in the legs, blurred vision, ringing in the ears. A Chiari patient can look perfectly healthy. This is a difficult obstacle for people to overcome. *Why can't you do this? Why can't you go here and there?* For most people, seeing something makes it real, otherwise, it is always open to interpretation. So, when symptoms are invisible, many people will have doubts about the reality of the illness and these doubts will come out in things they say. If someone has a visible disability, it is easy for people to picture some of the hardships they face; when the disability is hidden, however, this is not the case.

Third, even among Chiari patients, everyone is different. Chiari involves an incredibly wide range of symptoms and severity. While there may be two patients with the exact same symptoms, it is more likely that each patient's manifestation is different. So while one Chiari person may struggle with headaches from bright lights and loud sounds, another may struggle with balance problems and walking. Together, they share a bond, yet each person's battle is unique.

Finally, pain and illness are, by their very nature, subjective. No one can tell how much pain someone else is in, or what they are feeling. It's just not possible. Yet, a common reaction people have to someone in pain is to feel that they are exaggerating their plight. For whatever reason, many people feel they would handle the situation better and that the person in pain should be tougher.

This does not mean that patients are by themselves in their battles. Rather, they should seek out the support of friends and loved ones. It does mean, however, that that support, and empathy, has limits. It is often futile for patients to look outward for validation of their experience. In the end, the Chiari road is walked alone, and patients must find it in themselves to validate what they are experiencing. If you are a patient, what you are feeling and experiencing IS real, precisely because you are feeling it.

Key 2: Not Every Question Has an Answer

Unfortunately with Chiari, many questions do not yet have an answer. It is important to realize and accept this. There is no objective, definitive diagnostic criteria for Chiari. Treatments are controversial. There is no way to know how much surgery will help an individual person and which symptoms will go away. There is no way to predict if symptoms will come back years down the road.

The reality is that we are at the early stages of understanding Chiari and key issues remain unsolved. Does this mean patients should just throw up their hands? No, it means the opposite. It means it is even more important that patients take the time to educate themselves and understand what the issues are. For while there may not be definitive answers, there is data and information out there (albeit on a small scale relative to other diseases), and in the void of knowledge, there are an abundance of opinions. It is vital for patients to be able to communicate with their doctors, understand what their doctors are recommending and the reasons behind them, be able to sort through different opinions, and be comfortable with what they are hearing.

Everyone wants answers; that is understandable. But when answers are not available, it is just as important to seek out what is known, what is not known, and what is suspected.

Key 3: There Are Two Options, Take Control Or Be Controlled

When confronting the Chiari reality – lack of knowledge and awareness, feeling isolated, physical and mental strain of symptoms – patients are really faced with two choices. They can either let Chiari take control of them, go with the flow of the medical system, and place their entire trust in their doctors; or they can take control, educate themselves and those around them, and make informed, intelligent decisions.

While I strongly favor the take control option, I am not judging those who choose not to do this. Some people would prefer not to make their own choices and find sifting through the information more disturbing than anything. That's fine, but for others, those in the take control camp, this book can be your starting point.

I believe that educating yourself offers a number of benefits, both external and internal. Externally, an educated patient is able to find a doctor appropriate for their situation, bring critical items to the attention of their medical team, and solicit support from others by being able to explain what is happening. After treatment, an educated patient is also better equipped to deal with any residual symptoms or chronic issues. Research has shown that patient education improves outcomes when dealing with chronic diseases, and I suspect Chiari is no different.

Internally, many Chiari patients report feeling depressed, anxious, and overwhelmed. Being proactive and taking back some measure of control can provide a mental and emotional boost. Keeping the mind busy prevents thinking about negative thoughts, and some people even find themselves transformed in a positive way by their experience.

As I talked about earlier, everyone's Chiari experience is unique and no one should judge how someone handles a situation like this. But if you want to arm yourself with knowledge, take control of your own path, and fight back, then I hope you find what you need in this book.

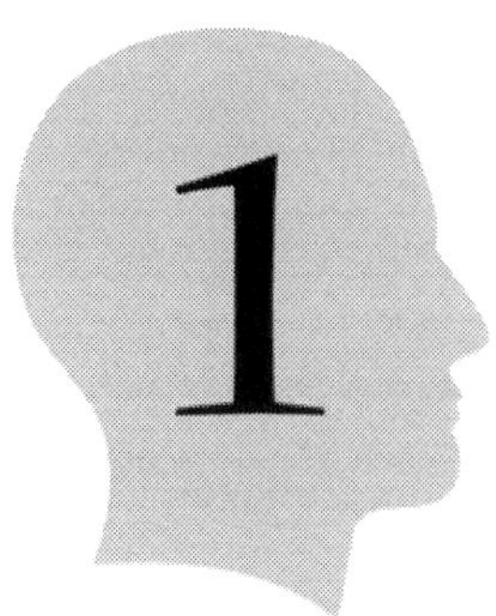

A Quick Overview

"Chiari...Who or what is that?"

~Uttered by thousands of people each year~

This chapter is based on the very popular Overview Presentation on the Conquer Chiari website and is intended to provide just that, a quick overview of what Chiari is, how it is diagnosed, and how it is treated. The information is presented in short bullets and focuses only on the most important items.

The overview is useful for people who want to learn about Chiari but don't have time to read an entire book or spend hours on-line. It is also a great starting point for a more detailed analysis of the disorder. Because Chiari is so complex, and involves a large amount of medical terms, it can take a good deal of time and study to truly understand it. The overview is a way to create an initial mental picture of Chiari, with the details and implications to be filled in later.

What Is Chiari?

- Chiari Malformation is a serious neurological condition. The problem is at the base of the skull, where the spine comes in.
- Part of the brain, the cerebellum, descends out of the skull, into the spinal area.
- This results in compression of parts of the brain and spinal cord, and disrupts the normal flow of cerebrospinal fluid (a clear fluid which bathes the brain and spinal cord).
- Chiari is also referred to as: Arnold-Chiari, ACM, ACM I, ACM II, CM, tonsillar ectopia, and hindbrain herniation.
- Exact numbers are not known, but it is estimated that Chiari affects as many as 1 in 1,000 people, or 300,000 people in the United States.

Figure 1-1

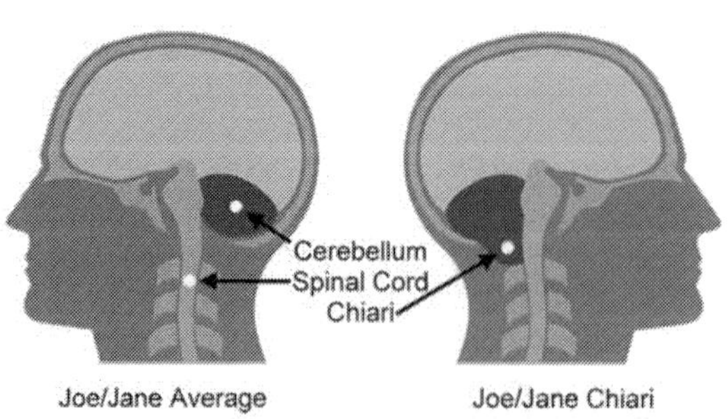

- Most people suffer from Chiari Type I (Figure 1-1), however 30% of children born with Spina Bifida also are born with a Chiari Malformation. This is a more serious form of the condition, known as Type II, and involves more of the brain being located outside the skull.

- It is believed that most cases of Chiari are congenital, meaning people are born with it; however, there are documented cases of acquired Chiari as well.
- There is evidence that people with Chiari have too small of a skull, not too big of a brain.
- Chiari does tend to run in some families, meaning there is a genetic component. However, it is not known what percent of cases have a genetic basis, the responsible genes have not been identified, and there is currently no genetic test.
- Chiari was first identified in the 1800's by Hans Chiari (thus the name), but was very difficult to diagnose until Magnetic Resonance Imaging (MRI) machines became common.

Symptoms

Figure 1-2

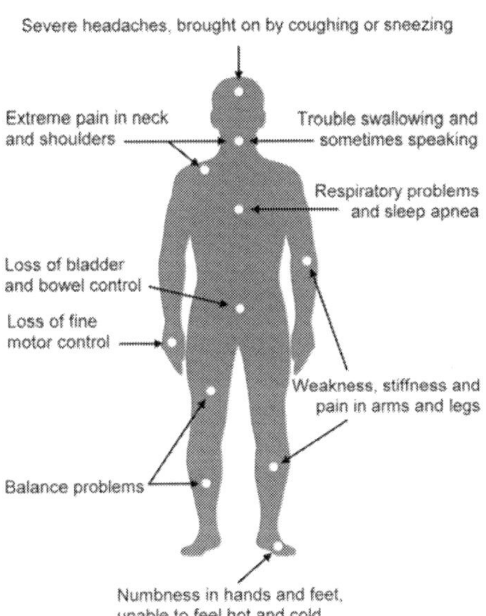

- Causes many different kinds of symptoms (Figure 1-2) and affects everyone differently.
- 95% of patients experience at least 5 symptoms.
- One study of 265 Chiari adults identified 13 symptoms which were reported by at least 50% of the group, 49 symptoms were reported by 2 or more people.
- Most common symptom among adults is a severe, pressure type headache in the back of the head, which is brought on (or made worse) by straining, coughing, sneezing, bending over, exercising, yelling, etc.

- Other common symptoms (to name a few) include balance problems, visual problems, weakness and abnormal sensations in the arms and legs, respiratory problems, neck pain, and fatigue.
- There is a poorly understood link between scoliosis and Chiari. Scoliosis is a common symptom among older children with Chiari.
- Among young children, symptoms related to the mouth and throat, such as reflux, trouble eating, gagging, and chronic cough are the most common.
- Symptoms can be caused by compression of brain and nerve tissue, disruption of the flow of cerebrospinal fluid, and elevated cerebrospinal fluid pressure.
- There are indications that Chiari can also affect mood and intellectual processes.

Syringomyelia

- In some people (estimates range from 20%-70%), Chiari leads to the development of a fluid-filled cyst, or syrinx, in the spinal cord itself. This is known as syringomyelia. (Figure 1-3)
- How or why a syrinx forms is not well understood, but most theories focus on the disruption of the normal flow of cerebrospinal fluid caused by a Chiari malformation.
- One current theory is that the cerebellar tonsils drive down into the spinal area, like a piston, with each heartbeat, and force CSF into the spinal cord.
- Common symptoms associated with syringomyelia include pain and weakness in the arms and legs, abnormal sensations, inability to feel hot and cold, abnormal sweating, and bladder/bowel problems.
- As a syrinx expands, it can stretch and damage nerve tissue in the spinal cord; this can lead to permanent nerve damage and even paralysis.

Figure 1-3

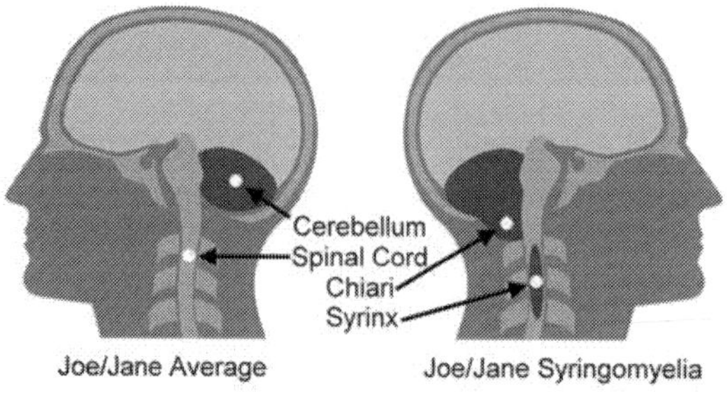

- Syringomyelia can also be caused by trauma (such as a spinal cord injury) or tumors.
- When there is no apparent underlying cause, it is referred to as idiopathic Syringomyelia.

Diagnosis

- Magnetic Resonance Imaging (MRI) is the main test used to diagnose Chiari.
- An MRI uses magnetic fields to generate a picture of structures inside the body; in this case it can show whether the cerebellar tonsils are out of position.
- Originally, based on an MRI, Chiari was defined as the tonsils descending greater than 3mm-5mm out of the skull.
- However, research has shown there is little to no connection between the size of a malformation and clinical symptoms or outcomes. Some healthy people actually have cerebellar tonsils that are out of position; and some people have severe symptoms with very small herniations (1mm-2mm). *There is still a lot of confusion and controversy in the medical community regarding how Chiari should be defined.*
- Because of this, an MRI by itself, while very useful, is not sufficient to diagnose a symptomatic Chiari. Rather, diagnosis is made through a combination of MRI, neurological exam, other tests, and a physician's experience and judgment.
- Cine-MRI is a type of MRI which can show the flow of cerebrospinal fluid (CSF) and is often used to evaluate whether the cerebellar tonsils are blocking the normal flow of CSF, and can contribute to a Chiari diagnosis.
- The lack of a single, objective test to diagnose Chiari contributes to delays in proper diagnosis, and often misdiagnosis. Chiari patients often go 5 years or more with active symptoms before being properly diagnosed.
- Because Chiari symptoms can be so varied, and because there is an overall lack of awareness regarding Chiari, many patients struggle with being believed by their doctors and are often told, ironically, the problem is "in their head". One study of over 300 patients found that 57% had at one time been told by a doctor they were suffering from a mental or emotional problem.
- Being diagnosed with Chiari can be an overwhelming experience. The physical strain of symptoms, combined with the stress of not knowing what will happen, can be difficult to cope with. In addition, due to lack of awareness and understanding, support can be hard to find.

Treatment

- After diagnosis, most patients end up seeing either a neurologist or neurosurgeon.
- There are not a lot of treatment options for Chiari, and treatment plans tend to center around whether the patient should have surgery.
- If symptoms are mild and/or not progressing, sometimes doctors will recommend waiting, observing with regularly scheduled MRIs, and treating individual symptoms. For example, some headaches respond to different medications.
- If symptoms are severe, progressing, or if the nervous system shows signs of being compromised (by a syrinx for example), doctors may recommend surgery.
- Unfortunately, there is little agreement among the medical community about how best to treat Chiari. Patients are likely to get conflicting opinions from different doctors. In the end, the decision to have surgery or not, must be made by each individual in consultation with their doctors.
- The goal of the surgery, called *posterior fossa decompression* and performed by a neurosurgeon, is to create more room around the cerebellar tonsils and restore the normal flow of spinal fluid.
- There are many different variations of the surgery, and no one technique has been proven conclusively to be the best.
- A decompression surgery may include any of the following: removing a piece of the skull in the back at the base of the head (craniectomy), removing part of one or more vertebrae (laminectomy), enlarging the covering of the brain/spinal cord with a patch (duraplasty), removing scars and adhesions, and removing part of the cerebellar tonsils themselves (tonsillectomy).
- The surgery typically lasts 3-4 hours. Patients usually spend the first night in Intensive Care and then an additional 2-3 days in the hospital.

Outcomes

- In general, there is not a lot of good outcome data. In addition, there is no generally accepted definition of a "successful" surgery. Physicians often base their definition of success on MRIs or whether the primary symptom has been relieved. It should also be noted that most published reports only follow patients for a couple years at most. There are almost no studies which show outcomes over a 10 or 20 year period.

- However, it appears that for people with Chiari only, about 50% will have good outcomes with few or no symptoms. An additional 30% will experience a significant improvement. 20% will not benefit from the surgery, and will remain the same or continue to get worse.
- For people with Chiari and syringomyelia, while there is even less data available, it is generally believed that the outcomes are not as good. Syringomyelia patients often continue to suffer from symptoms, especially pain, even after surgery.
- Currently, it is difficult to predict who will benefit by how much from surgery, and whether individual symptoms will go away. Research has indicated that the length of time someone has symptoms before surgery may be related to outcomes. Specifically, the longer someone has symptoms, the worse their outcome tends to be. Additionally, research has shown that people with severe or total blockage of CSF flow, actually experience greater improvements than people with mild blockage.
- Other factors which may influence the outcome include a person's individual anatomy and the existence of other problems in addition to the Chiari.
- The natural history of Chiari, meaning what happens to people who don't have surgery, is not well documented or understood.
- Long-term recurrence of symptoms, meaning that symptoms come back years after surgery, has been identified as a problem, but again has not been thoroughly researched.

Recovery

- How quickly someone recovers from Chiari surgery varies greatly among individuals.
- Factors that influence recovery time include (but are not limited to): how long symptoms were present, physical condition before surgery, presence of other health problems, time to devote to recovery, surgical complications, and perhaps most importantly, how successful the surgery was.
- Each patient should discuss recovery issues in detail with their doctor: when to drive, when to return to work, when to engage in physical activities, whether to go to a physical therapist, and how hard to push.
- A quick recovery may involve resting at home for 4-6 weeks; a gradual return to normal activities, and full recovery in 3-4 months.
- For many people recovery will take longer, and may involve a long sequence of gains and setbacks.
- For people with syringomyelia, it is important to realize that the syrinx may take up to a year to collapse or shrink and that the nerves which were stretched by the syrinx can take years to recover (if they do).

- There is no published research involving physical therapy after Chiari surgery, so it is not known if physical therapy is beneficial, or what specific types of therapy work the best.
- Many patients have reported experiencing new symptoms, which may come and go, during the months immediately after surgery.

Living with Chiari

- Some people will continue to suffer from residual symptoms even after surgery (or choose not to have surgery in the first place), and for them, Chiari is a chronic condition that must be dealt with on a daily basis.
- The most common residual symptom is pain, which is often multi-dimensional and difficult to treat. Chiari patients can suffer from several types of pain, such as neuropathic pain due to nerve damage, and musculo-skeletal problems due to muscle weakness and atrophy. It is important for patients suffering from chronic pain to see a pain specialist for evaluation and treatment.
- Although not well understood, Chiari also appears to affect mood and cognitive functioning and there is evidence that there is a high rate of depression among Chiari patients.
- Like other chronic diseases, especially ones involving chronic pain, Chiari can have an adverse effect on employment, finances, and family relationships. Unfortunately, there is little direct research on how Chiari affects family dynamics.
- Patients with residual symptoms often have to modify their lifestyle in an effort to manage their health. This can include changing work, going on disability, reducing physical, recreational, and social activities, etc. Many patients will learn over time what they can and can't do, and when to push and when to rest.
- Chronic pain has been shown to have a wide-ranging negative impact on health, including increased blood pressure, increased risk of additional chronic diseases, and even a reduction in the size of the brain.
- It is important for someone living with Chiari to be as healthy as possible, eat a balanced diet, get as much exercise as possible, and get plenty of sleep each night.

The Chiari Experience

- Everyone's Chiari experience is unique. One person may have mild symptoms which do not respond to treatment, while another may have severe symptoms, which come on quickly, but also resolve quickly after surgery. Some people are diagnosed in a matter of weeks, others struggle for years to be believed. Some people end up with no residual problems, others are severely disabled and unable to work.

- This variability makes it difficult to help people understand what to expect, because as of now, there is no good way to predict what an individual patient's experience and outcome will be.
- However, one way to get a better feel for the experience is to look at the different stages – or phases – which most patients go through, and understand the extremes of each. In other words, what is a mild or best case situation, what is a severe or worst case situation, and what is a moderate or middle of the road case. Please keep in mind the diagrams which follow are only meant to impart a general feel for the experience; the descriptions are by no means complete and there is no way to represent all the different possible experiences someone may have. It is also important to realize that people do not necessarily travel a straight line through the Chiari experience. In other words, someone may have severe symptoms, but their surgery and recovery may go extremely well.

Symptoms

Mild Case	incidental diagnosis or occasional headaches; some tingling in extremities; fullness in ears
Moderate Case	gradually worsening headaches which begin to interfere with daily activities; some visual problems; progressive weakness in arms/legs; stiff neck
Severe Case	crippling headaches; muscle atrophy in arms/legs; trouble walking; trouble swallowing; cognitive and/or emotional impairment

Diagnosis

Mild Case	MRI ordered quickly; Chiari identified in 3 months or less
Moderate Case	years of slowly progressing symptoms; see 2-3 doctors/specialists; MRI finally ordered after neurological exam reveals problem
Severe Case	years of debilitating symptoms; not believed by doctors; bounced around the medical system; when finally diagnosed seen as vindication

Anatomy/Condition

Mild Case	Chiari only; no complex bony structures; no other health problems
Moderate Case	Chiari with mild/moderate scoliosis; mild unrelated medical condition
Severe Case	Chiari with expansive syrinx; complex bony anatomy (such as basilar invagination); kinked brainstem; other health problems

Treatment

Mild Case	monitor with regularly scheduled MRIs; tolerate any symptoms or treat with medication
Moderate Case	Standard decompression surgery with no complications; 5 days or less in hospital
Severe Case	Decompression surgery requiring neck stabilization; surgical complications such as infection or CSF leak; extensive hospital stay or return visits; possible additional procedures

Recovery

Mild Case	4-6 weeks resting at home; return to work/school, back to full activities in 3-4 months
Moderate Case	Slowly improve over the course of 1-2 years; return to work/school is hard but doable; some setbacks
Severe Case	Years of ongoing struggle marked by many ups and downs; return to work/school is very difficult

Outcome

Mild Case	Few or no symptoms; no permanent deficits; no restrictions or lifestyle changes
Moderate Case	Some symptoms and deficits; feel good sometimes, not so good other times; some lifestyle changes required to improve quality of life; may have to change type of job, modify physical activities, etc.
Severe Case	Symptoms continue to progress; severe debilitating pain; permanent deficits develop; unable to work; become socially isolated and withdrawn; depressed at times; each and every day is a struggle

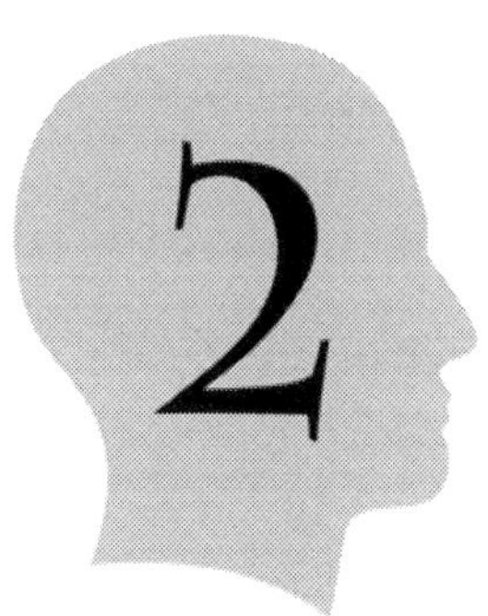

The Basics

" Chiari is the duck-billed platypus of diseases"

~Ray D'Alonzo, PhD...Chiari Patient & Advocate~

What Is Chiari ?

Chiari can mean different things to different people. To a neurosurgeon, Chiari is a structural defect which can be corrected with surgery; to a patient, Chiari is a difficult to understand disease with many symptoms and manifestations; to an uninformed physician, Chiari might be considered a harmless defect and nothing to worry about; to a family member, Chiari is often an invisible affliction hurting their loved one; and to a researcher, Chiari is a twisted, tangled puzzle waiting to be solved.

Saying what Chiari is exactly is not easy, because research has shown that how Chiari was originally defined is probably not accurate. In addition, the anatomy of many Chiari patients is complicated – with more than one structural abnormality - which means that Chiari is also used as an umbrella term to encompass a number of different problems.

To really understand Chiari requires some basic knowledge of human anatomy, the introduction of a few key medical terms, and a look back at how the definition of Chiari has evolved over the last 10-20 years. While this might sound like a lot of work, taking the time to understand the fundamentals is critical to understanding the more subtle aspects of how to deal with Chiari and where modern treatments and research are headed.

However, before diving directly into the anatomy and medical jargon, it might be helpful to begin the definition process by stating what Chiari is in general terms:

Chiari is a serious neurological disorder which involves abnormalities of the cranio-vertebral junction.

So what does this mean? The term neurological refers to the nervous system, which is comprised of the brain, spinal cord, and the many nerve fibers which run through our body. Chiari is often referred to as a disorder (or malformation, or condition) rather than a disease, because it is not a disease in the sense that many people think of, like a virus or infection (see the adjacent Practical Tips for more on this subject). The cranio-vertebral junction is where the skull, or cranium, meets the spine. And in this case, abnormalities refer to anatomical structures which aren't normal. In the broadest terms, Chiari patients have an unusual anatomy at the base of the skull and brain and the top of the spinal cord, which can cause serious problems.

Since Chiari is inherently an anatomical malformation, to gain a true understanding of Chiari, requires at least a basic familiarity with anatomy of parts of the brain, spine, and cerebrospinal fluid (CSF) system. While it may be a dry way to start a book, without this knowledge, what Chiari is, and its implication for patients, is almost impossible to understand.

Practical Tip: The terms disease, disorder, condition, and malformation have become a source of conflict between doctors and patients. In particular, some physicians choose to be very precise in saying that Chiari is not a disease per se, because it is considered more a structural malformation than the type of disease which can be treated with drugs. Whether Chiari is a disease or not is open to semantic debate, but given what is at stake, it hardly seems worth arguing about, especially as such arguments poison the doctor-patient relationship.

If as a patient (or parent, spouse, etc.), you encounter a doctor who insists on correcting the use of the word disease, it is best to keep in mind the purpose of the visit and not react, or get into an argument. Although, you may want to consider whether a doctor who focuses on such a trivial item when dealing with a patient facing a serious health concern is the type of doctor you want.

If as a physician you encounter a patient or family member who repeatedly refers to Chiari as a disease, it is best to let it go. From the point of view of the patient and their family members, they are dealing with a disease, which may end up being a chronic one at that. Correcting a patient's use of the term disease is extremely counterproductive.

Chiari & Human Anatomy

The reason that understanding the anatomy of the skull, brain, and spine is so important is that fundamentally Chiari is about abnormal anatomy. Chiari patients tend to have skulls which geometrically are not like the average person's. This in turn, leads to parts of the brain pushing out of the skull into the spine region, which disrupts the normal workings of the cerebrospinal fluid system. In addition, many Chiari patients are born with, or develop, structural problems of the spine, such as abnormal curves. That is why a basic understanding of these anatomical systems is critical to understanding what Chiari is.

The Skull & Brain

The skull, or cranium, is comprised of the bones of the head which enclose and protect the brain. As mentioned above, Chiari involves problems where the skull meets the spine, more specifically the back of the skull. (Figure 2-1) shows the occipital bone located in the back of the head and the bony spinal column. In this diagram, the region of interest is the lower part of the occipital area and the top of the spinal column.

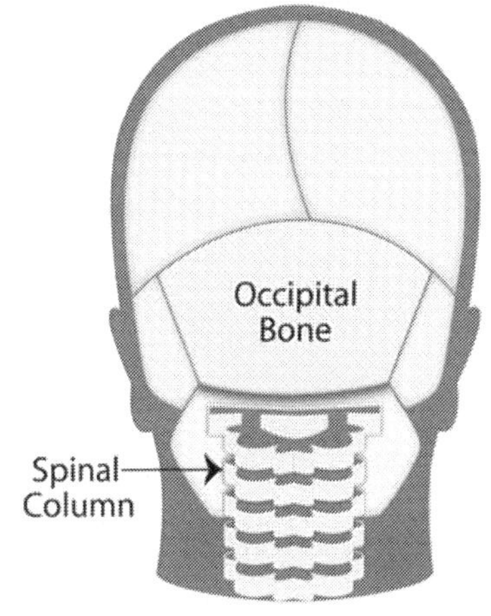

Figure 2-1

Removing the occipital bone and the bones of the spine (and rotating to a side view) shows the cerebellum (C), the brainstem (BS), and the spinal cord (SC). (Figure 2-2) The brain is comprised of several lobes, the cerebellum, and the brainstem.

The cerebellum is situated in the back, lower part of the brain and rests in the curved depression of the skull known as posterior fossa. (Figure 2-3)

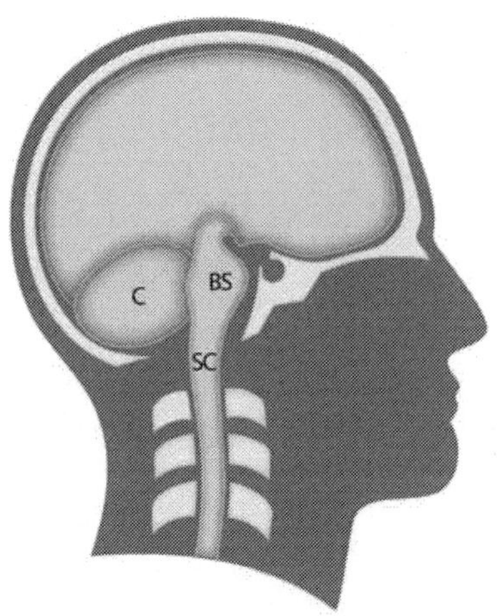

Figure 2-2

The cerebellum is believed to be important in controlling movement and balance, although recent research has shown that it may play a role in higher order thinking as well. Of particular interest to Chiari patients are the cerebellar tonsils, which are two structures which hang down from the bottom of the cerebellum. Normally the cerebellar tonsils are contained completely in the skull and have a rounded shape. As we will find out later, in Chiari the cerebellar tonsils extend out of the skull into the spinal area (like a cork in a bottle), and become pointed in shape from the pressure.

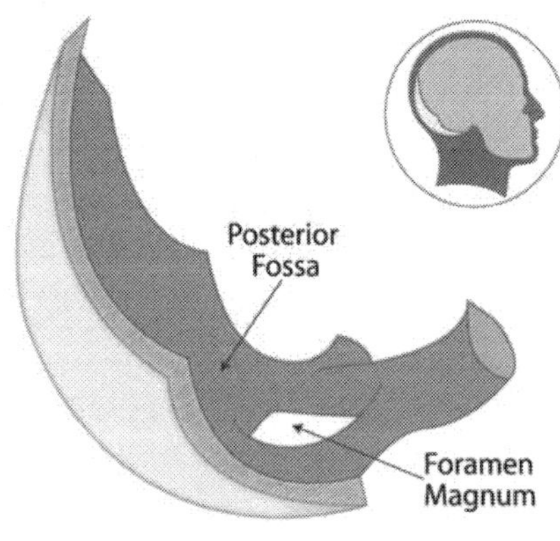

Figure 2-3

The brainstem, which is essentially the bottom of the brain, is the place where the brain meets the spinal cord. These two structures join through the opening in the base of the skull known as the foramen magnum (foramen is Latin for opening). The brain stem, in addition to passing on signals from the spine, controls many critical bodily functions, such as breathing. Damage to the brainstem can be very serious.

The cerebellar tonsils extend out of the skull into the spinal area.

The Spine

(Note: Parts of the following are taken from an article written by Kathryn Quintana)

Moving down the spine, like the brain, is nerve tissue protected by bones. The spine is a strong, flexible, and curved column composed of thirty-three bones called vertebrae. These vertebrae are grouped into five regions: cervical, thoracic, lumbar, sacral, and coccygeal. (Figure 2-4) The top of the spine, also known as the cervical region, contains seven vertebrae. Below that are the twelve vertebrae of the thoracic region, and the five vertebrae of the lumbar region. The vertebrae in the cervical, thoracic, and lumbar regions are flexible; however the vertebrae in the two regions below them, the sacral and coccygeal, are fused together in adults and form the sacrum and coccyx bones.

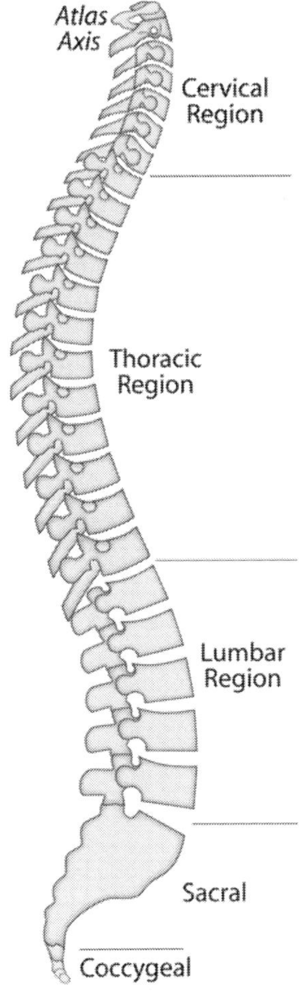

Figure 2-4

When properly aligned, the vertebral column acts as a central axis for the body. A healthy spine seen from a side view will have four curves, including two inward curves and two outward curves, which support the structures above them and act as shock absorbers. It is important to note that a healthy spine does not have any pronounced lateral curves. Abnormal curves to the right or left is known as scoliosis and will be discussed later.

Of particular significance to Chiari patients are the first two vertebrae at the top of the cervical spine, the atlas and the axis. The first cervical vertebra carries the weight of the head and is named the atlas after the mythological Greek figure, Atlas, who was sentenced to carry the weight of the Earth on his shoulders. This vertebra does not have a body. The atlas is ring-like with two bulky structures that support the head which moves forward and backwards on this vertebra. The second vertebra is called the axis and forms the pivot upon which the atlas, carrying the weight of the head, rotates. The two are linked by the odontoid process which protrudes up from the axis and forms a joint with the atlas. Interestingly, the odontoid process is not aligned properly in some people with Chiari and in others the atlas and axis are fused together.

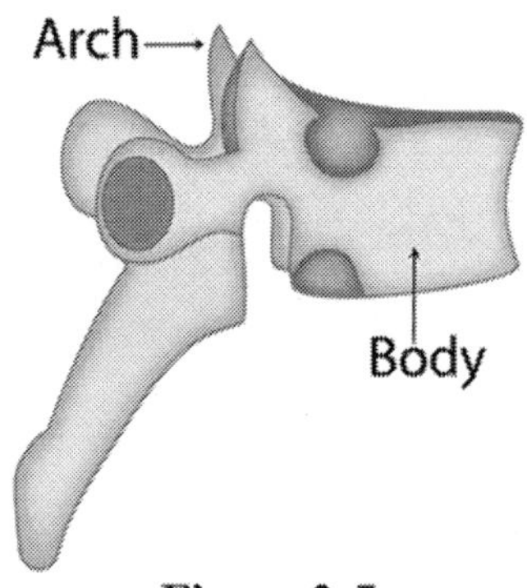

Figure 2-5

With the exception of the first two cervical vertebrae, all of the flexible vertebrae have certain characteristics in common. (Figure 2-5) Each vertebra has two parts, the body and the arch which come together to form an opening for the spinal cord to pass through, known as the vertebral foramen. The body is the largest part of the vertebra and is positioned along the front side of the body. When the vertebrae are joined together, the bodies form a strong pillar of support for the head and torso while maintaining flexibility and protecting the spinal cord. The vertebral arch is important for the attachment of muscles and ligaments responsible for giving the spine its integrity as a mobile structure.

The bodies of the vertebrae are separated by discs which absorb shock and act as spacers keeping the bones apart. Each disc contains a central core of gel-like substance, encircled by a series of fibrous rings. The central position of the gelatinous cores, together with the ligaments, holds the vertebrae in alignment.

Spinal Cord

Within the vertebral column is the long, cylinder shaped spinal cord. As mentioned previously, the spinal cord, which is essentially a bundle of nerves, exits the brain and extends downward through the center of the vertebral column to the level of the first or second lumbar vertebra. At each vertebral level of the spine, nerve bundles branch out and spread throughout the body like roads. (Figure 2-6)

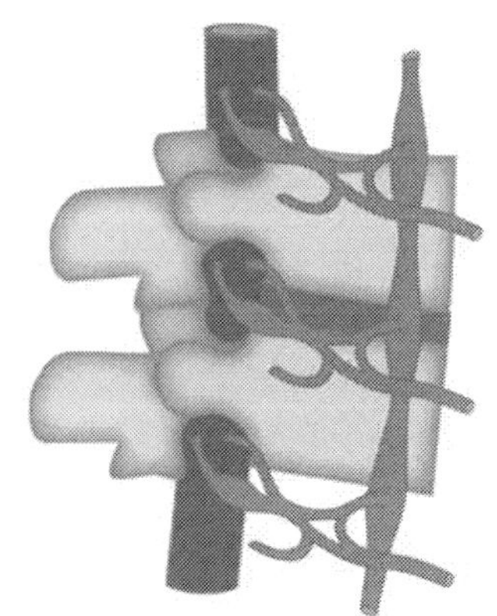

Figure 2-6

It is also important to note that the spinal cord, like most other part of the body, has a blood supply with arteries and veins passing through it. The small spaces around where these blood vessels penetrate the spinal cord are known as perivascular spaces and may play a role in the development of syringomyelia.

The tissue of the spinal cord itself, and the brain for that matter, is covered with several protective layers which are known collectively as the meninges. (Figure 2-7) Lying directly on the tissue of the spine is the very thin, innermost layer, the pia mater. Working out from the pia mater is actually a fluid filled area known as the sub-arachnoid space (SAS). Obviously, the arachnoid, or middle layer, is above the SAS and encloses the space. Finally, the thicker, outermost layer of the meninges is the dura, which as will be discussed in great detail in later chapters lies at the heart of an ongoing debate regarding Chiari surgery.

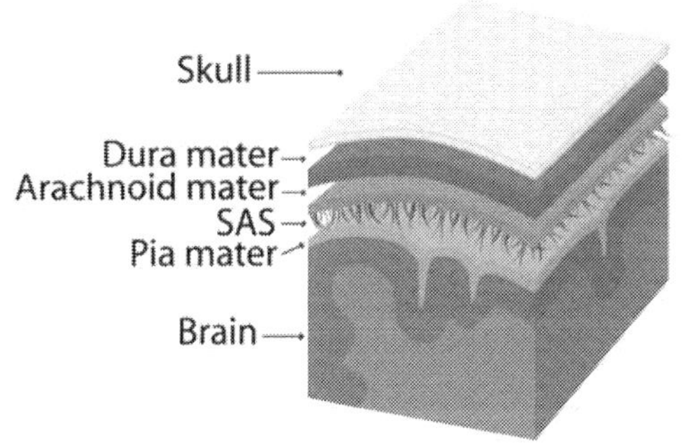

Figure 2-7

CSF System

Cerebral spinal fluid (CSF) is a clear fluid which circulates around the brain and spine in the sub-arachnoid space, bathing and cushioning the tissue underneath. It is produced in the choroid plexus of the brain and its movement is driven by the natural rhythm of the heart. Basically, with each heartbeat blood rushes into the brain which in effect pushes some amount of CSF out of the brain and into the spinal region. During the second phase of the cardiac cycle, this process is reversed and CSF flows back into the brain. With each heartbeat, CSF continues to flow back and forth in this fashion.

This concept is important because with Chiari the natural flow of CSF between the brain and spine is disrupted and can even be blocked completely.

Medical Jargon

Medical terminology is one reason that being diagnosed with Chiari can be an overwhelming experience, and why Chiari can be tough to understand. During a short session with a neurosurgeon, it can seem like they are speaking a different language; and in fact, they are. While some doctors are very good at explaining things to patients, many are not. They are so immersed in the medical world that they constantly use medical terms and jargon, rather than simple, plain English. To make matters worse, oftentimes different doctors use different terms when talking about the same thing. This is especially true with Chiari (and syringomyelia).

There are two things a patient can do to improve this situation. First, speak up if you don't understand something. It is easy to feel rushed during a doctor's appointment, but it is also critically important to understand what is being said. If a doctor uses a word or phrase you are not familiar with, don't be embarrassed, just say, "I don't understand what you are saying, because I am not familiar with that word. Is there another way you can explain it?"

Having said this, the second way to improve the situation is to learn some of the most commonly used medical terminology related to Chiari. Understanding some basic words will go a long way in deciphering the medical speak that can seem so confusing. The reason that doctor's visits can be so confusing is precisely because of the jargon that is used. While it is reasonable to ask a doctor to communicate without using jargon, it is also useful for patients to come up to speed on the terms they will be hearing over and over in order to improve both their understanding, and their ability to effectively communicate with their medical team.

With this in mind, following are thirty of the most common medical terms – listed alphabetically - associated with Chiari, and their definitions. Taken as a set, they constitute the minimum that an informed patient should have an awareness and understanding of. It is by no means a complete list of the terms a patient is likely to come across. Rather, they serve as a starting point for those who want to begin deciphering the medical jargon necessary to gain a true understanding of Chiari.

1. **brainstem -** part of the brain which connects to the spinal cord; controls critical functions such as breathing and swallowing -
2. **central canal** - very center of the spinal cord, so named because it starts as a hollow tube which closes in most people as they age -
3. **cerebellar tonsils -** portion of the cerebellum located at the bottom, so named because of their shape -
4. **cerebellum -** part of the brain located at the bottom of the skull, near the opening to the spinal area; important for muscle control, movement, and balance -
5. **cerebrospinal fluid (CSF)** - clear liquid in the brain and spinal cord, acts as a shock absorber -
6. **cervical** - the upper part of the spine; the neck area -
7. **Chiari malformation** - condition where the cerebellar tonsils are displaced out of the skull area into the spinal area, causing compression of brain tissue and disruption of CSF flow -
8. **Chiari II** - more severe form of malformation which involves descent of parts of the brainstem and is usually associated with Spina Bifida -
9. **cine MRI -** type of MRI which can measure CSF flow -

10. **cranio-vertebral junction** - the area where the skull and spine meet -
11. **cranium** - the skull -
12. **craniectomy -** surgical technique where part of the skull is removed -
13. **decompression surgery -** general term used for any of several surgical techniques employed to create more space around a Chiari malformation and to relieve compression -
14. **dura -** tough, outer covering of the brain and spinal cord -
15. **duraplasty** - surgical technique where the dura is opened and expanded by sewing a patch into it -
16. **foramen magnum -** opening at the base of the skull, through which the brain and spinal cord connect -
17. **graft** - material, or tissue, surgically implanted into a body part to replace or repair a defect -
18. **herniate** - to protrude through an opening abnormally -
19. **hydrocephalus -** a condition where there is an unusually large amount of CSF in the brain, resulting in swollen ventricles -
20. **ICP** - intracranial pressure; pressure of the CSF inside the skull -
21. **laminectomy -** surgical technique where part of a vertebra is removed
22. **lumbar** - the lower part of the spine -
23. **magnetic resonance imaging (MRI) -** diagnostic device which uses a strong magnetic field to create images of the body's internal parts -
24. **posterior fossa -** depression on the inside of the back of the skull, near the base, where the cerebellum is normally situated -
25. **syringomyelia (SM)** - neurological condition where a fluid filled cyst forms in the spinal cord -
26. **syrinx** - fluid filled cyst in the spinal cord -
27. **thoracic** - relating to the middle part of the spine, or chest area -
28. **tonsillar herniation** - descent of the cerebellar tonsils into the spinal area; often measured in mm -
29. **Valsalva manuever** - a straining activity which in Chiari patients often causes an immediate headache -
30. **vertebra -** one of the individual bones of the spinal column -

The Traditional Definition of Chiari

Having established a basic knowledge of the relevant anatomy and key medical terms, the next step in understanding Chiari is to look at how the definition of Chiari has evolved over the years. It may be surprising to some to learn that Chiari was first described by its namesake, Hans Chiari, more than 100 years ago. A German pathologist, Chiari made note of people during autopsy whose cerebellums' were displaced out of their skull, into the spinal area. Based on his work, he classified his findings into 3 types, which serve as the basis for the classic definition of Chiari:

Chiari I: When the cerebellar tonsil(s) are elongated and herniated through the foramen magnum by at least 3mm-5mm. The size of the malformation is measured from the foramen magnum to the tip of the tonsil(s).

Chiari II: Considered more severe than Type I, when more brain structures, such as the brainstem or cerebellum proper are herniated out of position. Most people refer to Chiari II as coinciding with Spina Bifida. In fact, up to 30% of children born with Spina Bifida also have Chiari II.

Chiari III: A very rare, severe form of the malformation.

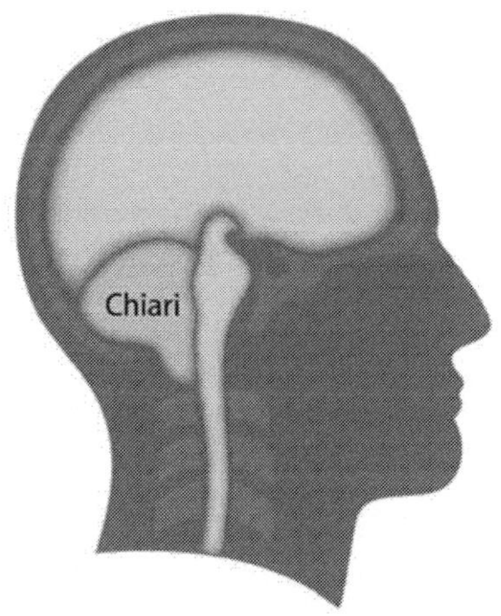

Figure 2-8: Chiari Malformation

Although the definition of Chiari, especially Type I, (Figure 2-8) appears simple at first, confusion arises from several sources. First is confusion over the many names used to refer to Chiari Malformations. Unfortunately, this confusion arose early in the 1900's when students of another German physician, Arnold, managed to attach their mentor's name to the Chiari Malformations. By publishing a paper describing a couple of cases – which many in the medical community feel added nothing to the knowledge of Chiari – these students were successful in associating Arnold's name with Chiari's. This trend has continued over the years with different doctors and researchers using different terms in research publications to refer to the Chiari Malformation.

Listed on the next page are different names and acronyms that are, or have been, used in reference to Chiari:

- **Chiari Type I/II** - The original definition of Chiari.
- **Arnold-Chiari** - Some people use this term to refer to all types of Chiari, whereas others reserve Arnold-Chiari to refer to Chiari II associated with Spina Bifida.
- **Tonsillar Herniation** - Refers to the cerebellar tonsils protruding through the opening of the foramen magnum.
- **Tonsillar Ectopia** - Ectopia means a body part which is out of position, so this term refers to the cerebellar tonsils being out of position.
- **Cerebellar Herniation** - Similar to tonsillar herniation, refers to the cerebellum, or part of it, protruding out of the skull.
- **Cerebellar Ectopia** -Part of the cerebellum being located out of position.
- **Hindbrain Herniation** - Hindbrain refers to the cerebellum and brainstem, so this term is used as a general term which can encompass different types of Chiari.
- **CM** - Chiari Malformation
- **CM I** - Chiari Malformation Type I
- **CM II** - Chiari Malformation Type II
- **ACM** - Arnold-Chiari Malformation
- **ACM I** - Arnold-Chiari Malformation Type I
- **ACM II** - Arnold-Chiari Malformation Type II

Although first identified more than a century ago, Chiari was extremely difficult to diagnose until the introduction of Magnetic Resonance Imaging (MRI) technology about 20 years ago. With MRIs, doctors could obtain detailed pictures of the anatomy in question and begin to study the structures involved in more detail. While the widespread adoption of MRIs has been a definite boon for Chiari patients, it has also muddled the picture when it comes to defining Chiari in a number of ways.

First, as more and more people underwent MRIs, it became clear that a certain number of people – actually quite a few – have cerebellar tonsils that are located below the foramen magnum. While these people fit the classical definition of Chiari, they have no symptoms associated with it, and it is not clear that they will ever develop symptoms.

This type of finding is often referred to as incidental or asymptomatic Chiari.

Once this discovery was made, further research showed that across the general population there is actually a range of what could be considered a normal position of the cerebellar tonsils, both above and below the foramen magnum. Not only did this finding call into question the original, static definition of Chiari, but it has also caused many problems for Chiari patients in terms of diagnoses.

Some doctors and specialists have interpreted this finding to mean that a Chiari Malformation is normal and nothing to worry about. Unfortunately, this has led to patients – sometimes with severe symptoms – not getting the proper treatment and medical attention they need. Instead they are told that their symptoms are likely due to something else, or all in their head.

A second revelation, and an extension of the first, that came from the new imaging technology is that the size of the Chiari malformation is not related to the severity of symptoms or outcomes after treatment. While intuitively it would seem that the more the cerebellar tonsils are positioned out of the skull the worse the condition would be, research studies, involving many patients, have looked at symptoms both before and after treatment, and failed to find any connection with the size of the herniation (as measured below the foramen magnum). In other words, some people can have large malformations, well above 5mm, and have few or no symptoms. Similarly, people can have malformations below 3mm (the original definition) and have severe symptoms.

In a study of 364 patients by Milhorat, nearly half of the patients with herniations less than 5mm actually had developed syrinxes (syringomyelia) as well.

This finding has since led to a third problem with the traditional Chiari classifications. Namely, that some people with essentially no signs of herniation on MRI exhibit Chiari symptoms (and even may develop syringomyelia). People with Chiari-like symptoms, but no MRI indication of a cerebellar herniation, are often referred to as Chiari 0. However, Chiari 0 is quite controversial, made more so by some physicians who have tried to expand the use of Chiari surgery to treat things like Chronic Fatigue Syndrome.

Still, while controversial, recent research has provided evidence that Chiari 0 may be for real. In 2005, Sekula examined 22 Chiari 0 patients and found that while they did not show Chiari malformations in the traditional sense, he identified four distinct anatomical measurements in the posterior fossa region (the back of the skull where the cerebellum is situated) which were significantly different between the Chiari 0 patients and a group of healthy volunteers.

Further straining the traditional Chiari classification by types (I/II) was the identification by Tubbs; of 22 children with features of both Chiari I and Chiari II. The authors of this study labeled the group Chiari 1.5 because the children seemed to fall in between the standard definitions of Chiari I and Chiari II. Specifically, none of the children had spina bifida, yet like with Chiari II, more than just their cerebellar tonsils – their brainstems as well - were descended into the spinal area.

In summary, research has identified three problems with the traditional definition and classification of Chiari:

1. People may have significant tonsillar herniation without any symptoms or neurological problems.
2. People can have herniations less than 3mm-5mm and have severe symptoms.
3. There are patients labeled Chiari 0 and Chiari 1.5, who do not fit in the classification scheme.

The confusion surrounding what Chiari is has caused a great deal of problems for patients. As will be discussed further in Chapter 3, the lack of a simple, objective definition of Chiari is one reason that people often go years before being properly diagnosed, are frequently misdiagnosed as suffering from something else, or told outright there is nothing wrong with them.

New ideas take time to spread through the medical community, and some doctors still rely on the old definition of Chiari (at least 3mm-5mm descent), while others believe that since some people with herniations don't have symptoms, that in general Chiari is no big deal. Fortunately, there are also some very smart people, both doctors and engineers, at the forefront of research who are actively seeking a new, objective, and testable definition of Chiari.

The Search for A New Chiari Definition

The findings discussed previously mean that diagnosing Chiari is not as simple as looking at an MRI and measuring the location of the cerebellar tonsils, but as will be discussed further in the next chapter, an accurate diagnosis is subjective and a matter of judgment.

As the Chiari pioneers realized that the size of the malformation could be misleading, they began to look at other factors, such as whether the normal flow of CSF was disrupted. As MRI technology advanced, it became possible to look not only at a static picture of the body structures in question, but through cine-MRI, to examine the flow of spinal fluid as well. While not exact, this advanced type of MRI did – and still does - provide neurosurgeons another source of information upon which to base their opinions.

As cine-MRI (also known as phase-contrast MRI) began to take hold, researchers started looking for ways to use the advanced imaging techniques to measure CSF flow quantitatively. Studies have shown that Chiari patients do have abnormal CSF flow characteristics, but the results are sometimes mixed and CSF flow has yet to produce a new standard for defining Chiari; and despite its popularity, some neurosurgeons – off the record – question the usefulness of cine MRI.

What Causes Chiari?

In the end, a new definition of Chiari may arise from an understanding of what causes it. Although the way Chiari is currently defined makes it sound like a brain malformation, there is actually significant evidence that Chiari results not from too big of a brain, but rather from a skull that is too small. Over the past 15 years or so there has been growing evidence that Chiari is really due to lack of bony development in the posterior fossa region (where the cerebellum is situated), which results in a space which is too small to accommodate a normal brain. Specifically, several researchers, using slightly different techniques, have shown that Chiari patients on average have smaller posterior fossas than healthy people.

For example, in 1993, Stovner compared the skull dimensions of 33 Chiari patients to 40 healthy controls, and found that, "the posterior cranial fossa was significantly smaller and shallower in patients than controls." Similarly, in 1997, Nishikawa devised a volume ratio to study whether the brain was crowded in the posterior fossa region of 30 Chiari patients versus 50 healthy controls. He found that despite the actual brain volume being about the same between the two groups, there was significantly more crowding in the Chiari patients than the control subjects. Additionally, in 1999, Milhorat found in his landmark study that the posterior fossa volume of 50 Chiari patients, as measured by MRI, was smaller than that of 50 matched control subjects. In fact, there is now so much evidence that Chiari patients have unusual skull shapes and dimensions that most Chiari experts now refer to Chiari as characterized by the underdevelopment of the posterior fossa. However, while Chiari patients have been shown to have small posterior fossas on average, a true quantitative definition of Chiari based on skull dimensions has yet to be proposed.

Having said this, the Sekula study referenced above showed how such a definition, if and when it is developed, might be useful. Specifically, they looked at 22 patients who were suffering from Chiari like symptoms and compared their MRIs to 25 people with no evidence of Chiari or syringomyelia (they had been treated for trigeminal neuralgia). While the authors used the term Chiari-like in their publication, the term Chiari 0 is often used, controversially, to refer to people with Chiari type symptoms and no herniations.

The patients were given a complete exam, and filled out both a symptom check-list and a personality assessment. The personality assessment was designed to identify anyone with emotional problems or signs of depression. In addition, the group underwent MRIs which were then reviewed by a physician who did not know their diagnosis.

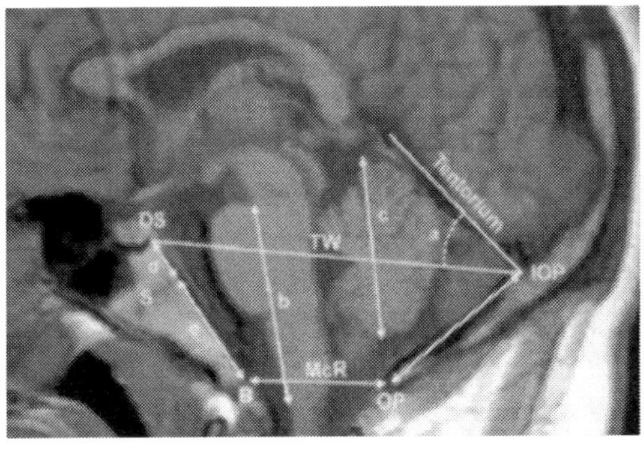

Figure 2-9: Skull Base Dimensions
Source: Sekula RF Jr, Jannetta PJ, Casey KF, Marchan EM, Sekula LK, McCrady CS. Dimensions of the posterior fossa in patients symptomatic for Chiari I malformation but without cerebellar tonsillar descent. Cerebrospinal Fluid Res. 2005 Dec 18;2:11.

Based upon the results from other studies, the team decided to look at nine different measurements in the posterior fossa region. (Figure 2-9) They found that in the Chiari-like group, 4 of the nine measurements were significantly different from the control group, namely the clivus, the basiocciput, and the basisphenoid were all smaller in the Chiari group, and the tentorial angle was steeper. So even though these patients did not meet the traditional definition of Chiari, it is possible (but not definite) that they would meet a new definition of Chiari.

Tight Filum Terminale

While the small posterior fossa theory is gaining acceptance in the medical community, it is not the only theory on what may cause Chiari. A Spanish neurosurgeon, Dr. Royo-Salvador, hypothesizes that a tight filum terminale leads to Chiari by pulling down on the spinal cord. The filum terminale is a fibrous, thread-like extension of the bottom of the spine. The filum is normally elastic, but sometimes it becomes fatty and can be abnormally tight. When this occurs, it essentially pulls down on the spinal cord.

A tight filum is a recognized cause of tethered cord syndrome and can cause bladder and bowel problems and leg weakness, but Royo-Salvador proposes that the spinal traction caused by a tight filum also can lead to Chiari, syringomyelia, and scoliosis. He published a report indicating that a simple surgery to cut the tight filum improved Chiari symptoms in a number of patients. Unfortunately, his report did not indicate how he selected patients for this procedure and the outcomes were not well defined.

Beyond Royo-Salvador's publication the evidence regarding a tight filum as a possible cause of Chiari is mixed. One research group did find that children with lipomeningoceles – fatty tissue that protrudes out of the spinal cord – had an unusually high rate of Chiari malformation. One possibility for this was that the defects were tethering the spinal cord and causing downward traction. However, this same group subsequently performed a study using cadavers where weights were attached to the bottom of the spinal cord to simulate a tight filum or tethering at the bottom of the cord. They found that the mechanical force induced by the weights was dispersed very quickly moving up the cord and that they did not effect the position of the cerebellar tonsils at all. However Ellenbogen published the case of a 3 year girl who developed Chiari as a result of a fatty, tight filum. The report included MRI images that were taken both before and after Chiari developed.

For now, there is some skepticism regarding the idea that a tight filum can cause Chiari, but there does seem to be some type of connection between Chiari and tethered cord syndrome which is worth exploring.

Acquired Chiari

Most cases of Chiari are considered to be congenital, meaning that people are born with the structural abnormalities which will eventually lead to symptoms. While this may be true, Chiari can also be an acquired problem. Basically, any mass inside the skull, such as a tumor or cyst in the posterior fossa region, can cause crowding and force (herniate) the cerebellar tonsils out of the skull. In addition, Chiari can also result from problems with the CSF system, such as hydrocephalus, which result in the tonsil being forced out due to pressure.

While there are documented cases of acquired Chiari due to tumors, etc., a more controversial cause of acquired Chiari is trauma. There are many anecdotal reports of people developing symptoms and being diagnosed with Chiari after traumas such as car accidents. In fact, Milhorat found that 24% of symptomatic patients reported some type of trauma as a precipitating event in developing symptoms. However, the question is whether trauma only plays a role in sparking symptoms, or whether it can actually lead to the cerebellar tonsils herniating. In other words, do some people already have a Chiari-like anatomy and an accident, for reasons that aren't clear, triggers their symptoms, or can trauma actually cause an anatomical change?

Several people have reported to Conquer Chiari that they have MRI evidence that the whiplash from car accidents actually caused their cerebellar tonsils to herniate. Unfortunately, such cases have not been published in the medical literature and subjected to the peer review process, so many doctors remain cautious in saying that trauma can actually cause acquired Chiari. Complicating the situation is the fact that many of these cases have legal ramifications due to lawsuits over car accidents and workers compensation claims.

Chiari II

The discussions above refer to Chiari I. Since Chiari II is almost always associated with spina bifida, it is believed to be a result of the spinal defect. In spina bifida, the spinal cord does not close properly during development.

One theory on Chiari II is that this opening alters the CSF pressure, which in turn can cause parts of the brain to descend out of the skull.

A second consideration is the idea that CSF pressure in the skull is necessary for normal skull growth. In other words, during development CSF pressure builds to a certain level in the skull, which essentially pushes out the skull plates and guides normal skull development. When the spinal cord does not close, the proper CSF pressure is not maintained resulting in lack of skull growth and herniation of the brain. Interestingly, while this theory of skull growth was very popular a number of years ago, some developmental biologists now feel the theory is outdated.

Given the amount of research attention focused on spina bifida, it is surprising that the link to Chiari has not been explored in more depth, but there are actually very few publications on this subject. Another subject which is not written about or discussed as much as it should be is whether Chiari I and Chiari II are related or are they distinct clinical entities. In other words, are Chiari I and Chiari II due to the same underlying cause; do they lie on the same spectrum with Chiari II being more severe?

The prevailing wisdom is probably that they are two separate conditions, however as mentioned earlier in this chapter there are people with features of both Chiari I and Chiari II. In addition, if proper CSF pressure is required for normal skull growth, and Chiari I patients tend to have small posterior fossas, one has to wonder if a temporary drop in CSF pressure – such as due to an opening which then heals on its own – may be the problem.

Common Questions About Chiari

How Many People Have Chiari?

Although this is a common question, there is not yet a precise answer to how many people have Chiari in the US. The best way to determine the prevalence of Chiari would be to randomly select a large number of people off the street, in the thousands, and examine them with MRIs and neurological tests. Unfortunately, this is prohibitively expensive and unlikely to be done anytime soon.

However, there are a number of data points which can be used to estimate the prevalence of Chiari. Based upon these Conquer Chiari, in consultation with our advisors, has decided to use a conservative estimate that 1 in 1,000 people have Chiari (0.1%). This translates to **300,000** people in the US alone with Chiari.

Conquer Chiari derived this estimate based upon the following:

1. **AANS Surgical Procedure Survey** – In 1999, the American Association of Neurological Surgeons conducted a survey to quantify what types of surgical procedures are performed each year. According to this survey there were over 3500 Chiari decompressions performed in 1999. From this, a prevalence estimate can be extrapolated:

Number of Decompressions Performed in 2006	5,000
Number of Reoperations (20%)	1,000
New Surgical Cases in 2006	4,000
Total New Cases per Year	8,000 (Assume 50% surgical)

Finally, published reports indicate an average age of diagnosis of around 30 years. With 8,000 new cases per year, this would translate roughly into a prevalence of 300,000 – 400,000. Note that the assumption that 50% of cases are surgical is based upon published interviews with leading Chiari surgeons.

2. **Syringomyelia Prevalence** – Dr. Marcy Speer (Duke) performed an analysis to determine the prevalence of syringomyelia (which is most commonly caused by Chiari). In this analysis, she estimated that the number of Chiari related syringomyelia cases in the US range from 141,000 – 209,000. Published reports of patient series have shown that the percent of Chiari patients who have syringomyelia ranges from 30%-70%. These two ranges can be combined to produce a Chiari prevalence estimate which ranges from 200,000 – 700,000.

3. **Meadows et al.** – In the June, 2000 issue of *"Journal of Neurosurgery"*, Meadows published a study which reviewed over 22,000 head and cervical MRIs from a hospital database. He found that 0.7% of the MRIs demonstrated herniation of the cerebellar tonsils of at least 5mm (the traditional definition of Chiari). Extrapolated to the general population, this would mean that more than 2 million people meet the classic definition of Chiari. However, this type of extrapolation is not statistically sound, but this study does show that an incidence rate of 0.1% is fairly conservative.

4. **Epidemiological Research at UCSF** – Dr. Stephen Hulley, a nationally recognized epidemiologist and retired Chair of Epidemiology at UC San Francisco, is performing a true epidemiological study of the incidence and prevalence of Chiari using a large HMO medical database. Although this work is not yet published, he presented initial findings at the UIC/Conquer Chiari Research Symposium 2007 which indicated that a prevalence estimate of 300,000 is reasonable.

Based upon these data points, Conquer Chiari believes that about 300,000 people in the US have Chiari; (Figure 2-10) shows how this compares with other neurological diseases.

Figure 2-10: Disease Prevalence

Disease	# of People Affected In US
ALS	30,000
Huntington's	200,000
Chiari	300,000
MS	400,000
Parkinson's	500,000

Note: Huntington's refers to total number at risk genetically
Sources: ALS Association, Huntington's DSA, National MS Society, NINDS

Who Gets Chiari?

It is generally believed that Chiari affects people of all races, however without rigorous epidemiological studies it is difficult to say if some races are more prone to Chiari than others. A study from New Zealand did indicate some racial differences, but more research is required in this area. Similarly, the existing published literature seems to indicate that females are affected at a slightly greater rate than males, but again definitive data is lacking. Because of this Chiari is described as affecting people of all races and both genders.

In terms of age, although most cases of Chiari are congenital, symptoms can develop at any age. Among adults, for reasons that are not clear, the average age of diagnosis appears to be around 30 years. However this can be misleading because many people go several years before an accurate diagnosis, and average age among adults does not take into account the significant number of children who are diagnosed at a young age. As the use of MRIs continues to expand, it is likely that people will be diagnosed more quickly.

Is Chiari Genetic?

Ongoing research at Duke University has identified more than 100 families with two or more members affected by Chiari. Given this, the Duke researchers feel confident that at least some percentage of Chiari cases is genetic in origin. Their work has continued and the team recently published a report identifying several genetic variations which were unusually common in tested Chiari patients.

While this progress is exciting, it is important to realize that the research is in its early stages, and:

- It is not yet clear what percentage of Chiari cases is genetic.
- What gene, or more likely genes, influence the development of Chiari is not yet known.
- There is no genetic test to say whether someone has a Chiari gene.
- There is no way to determine what the risk is of having children born with Chiari.

In addition to genetics, there may be a large environmental component to Chiari. Different researchers have been able to induce Chiari in rodents by exposing the developing embryo to different agents. In one such study (Marin-Padilla), a single dose of Vitamin A to pregnant hamsters resulted in both Chiari I and Chiari II in their offspring, along with abnormal skull shapes characteristic of what is found with Chiari.

There is a good chance that it will turn out that both genes and environmental factors play a role in the development of Chiari.

Is Chiari Fatal?

Although severe cases of Chiari II in young children, especially when accompanied by multiple birth defects, can be fatal; in general Chiari I is NOT considered to be a fatal condition. However, there are several reports in the medical literature regarding sudden death associated with Chiari, including:

- Three people, one child and two adults, who died suddenly after a minor trauma to the head; Chiari was found during autopsy.
- Several cases of sudden respiratory arrest, including two children.
- An adult with a history of headaches and fainting. The headaches were diagnosed as migraines, but the person died suddenly and Chiari was found after they died.
- Two 25 year old men

Sudden death due to Chiari, like those listed above, is thought to be related to brain stem malfunction, likely due to the pressure placed on it by the herniation. While sudden death associated with Chiari can be frightening, it is important to put these events into perspective.

A medical literature search revealed about 10 reports of sudden death related to Chiari since 1984 (the earliest report). During that time there have been thousands and thousands of people with Chiari who have lived with their symptoms, or no symptoms, and did not require emergency care. Assuming conservatively that about 10,000 people per year are found to have Chiari on

MRI (in the US alone), that would translate to 230,000 people since 1983 with Chiari. Thus, 10 cases out of more than 200,000 is a miniscule number.

Of course, the one unknown in an analysis like this is that we don't know how many deaths might be due to Chiari which are not discovered and we don't know how many deaths, even if they are attributed to Chiari, are not reported in the medical literature. In fact, Conquer Chiari has received a couple of emails from family members whose relatives were found to have Chiari after their unexpected death. But even accounting for these unknowns, it is likely that sudden death is a rare event compared to the total number of Chiari cases. It is also important to note that in the cases listed above, the people did not know they had Chiari and had not been treated surgically.

A related question is whether Chiari can affect a person's natural lifespan. This is a much more difficult question to answer, because even if Chiari is not a direct cause of death, one has to consider whether living with a chronic condition like Chiari, can lead to other health problems which in turn can impact a person's lifespan. This may be especially true for people with syringomyelia with limited mobility, which can lead to weight gain and other problems. In addition, given the high rates of depression among Chiari patients, there is some indication that Chiari patients may be at an increased risk for suicide as compared to the general population.

As will be discussed later in the book, research has shown that people with one chronic health problem often end up with additional chronic problems and that living in chronic pain can have very serious negative health affects. Thus, although it has not been studied directly, it is not out of the question that Chiari/syringomyelia may have an impact in this area. However, it is also important not to jump to any conclusions and to wait for research which examines this subject to be carried out.

Symptoms

Causes

One of the more complicated, and confusing, aspects of Chiari is that it can cause many different symptoms. With eye problems, ear problems, headaches, and weakness in the arms and legs, for many patients it seems like Chiari can impact every part of the body. This is not far from the truth; in fact, the diversity of Chiari symptoms, and the way it can look like so many other diseases led Dr. Ray D'Alonzo, a patient advocate, to dub Chiari the duck-billed platypus of diseases.

One reason that Chiari can involve so many different bodily symptoms is because it can affect the brain and nervous system several different ways, including:

- Direct compression of the brainstem;
- Direct compression of the cerebellum;
- Direct compression of the cranial nerves;
- Damage to nerves in the spine;
- Disruption of the natural flow of CSF;
- Elevated CSF pressure in the skull/brain;

Each of these affected areas can lead to multiple symptoms, so it easy to see how the list of Chiari related symptoms can grow to be quite long.

A second reason that Chiari patients tend to endure many symptoms is because as mentioned above Chiari is often accompanied by several anatomical abnormalities. For example, some Chiari patients also have a kink in the brainstem, or natural instability in the top part of their spine, which of course can lead to problems.

Finally, anytime someone is dealing with a major health issue, secondary symptoms tend to come into play. In other words, chronic neck pain and muscle atrophy caused by Chiari/SM can lead to a general imbalance in how muscles are used which can cause pain in additional areas. Between primary and secondary symptoms, trying to understand what is related to Chiari and what isn't can be very difficult and usually isn't worth the time or energy.

Many & Varied

A 2004 study (Mueller, Oro) documented, in dramatic fashion, the wide range of symptoms that can accompany Chiari. The research involved the self-reported symptoms of 265 Chiari patients who ranged in age from 12-78. In all, 13 symptoms were reported by more than half of the patients, and a whopping 49 symptoms were reported by at least 2 patients. In addition, 95% of the patients reported suffering from 5 or more symptoms. Not surprisingly, headache was the most commonly reported symptom (Figure 2-11) with 98% of the group saying they suffered from them. Dizziness, neck pain, blurred vision, fatigue, nausea and problems in the arms and hands were also very common.

The sections on the next few pages discuss some of the most common problems Chiari patients face in terms of symptoms and the research, or lack thereof, which accompanies each. Obviously, these represent just a subset of the wide spectrum of possible Chiari symptoms.

Figure 2-11: Common Symptoms

Symptom	%
Headache	98
Dizziness	84
Difficulty sleeping	72
Weakness in arms/hands	69
Neck pain	67
Numbness/tingling in arm, hand	62
Fatigue	59
Nausea	58
Shortness of breath	57
Blurred Vision	57
Tinnitus	56
Difficulty swallowing	54
Leg weakness	52

- (20%-50%) – depression, body weakness, balance problem, memory problems, leg/foot numbness, hoarse voice, chest pain, facial numbness, anxiety, slurred speech, arm pain, abdominal pain, photophobia
- (<20%) – tachycardia, trouble hearing, vomiting, double vision, word-finding problems, vision loss, blackouts, apnea, vertigo, loss of peripheral vision, nystagmus, earache, nosebleeds, snoring, thoracic pain, hypotension, wake up choking, leg pain, palpitations, hypertension, abnormal gag reflex, face pain/tingling

Source: Mueller DM, Oro' JJ. Prospective analysis of presenting symptoms among 265 patients with radiographic evidence of Chiari malformation type I with or without syringomyelia. J Am Acad Nurse Pract. 2004 Mar;16(3):134-

---

Personal Experience: I had ignored some serious symptoms for years, so by the time I was on the path to a diagnosis I had a laundry list of issues. Here are the ones I can remember: *Extreme headache especially with coughing, climbing stairs, etc; extreme neck pain; shoulder pain; weakness in right hand (hand started to curl up); leg weakness; balance problems aka walking into doorways; fullness and ringing in ears; hoarseness; trouble finding the right words (brain knew what to say, but voice didn't listen); trouble swallowing which caused me to gag on many types of foods; light sensitivity; frequent urination...You get the idea.*

The Chiari Headache

No other symptom defines Chiari like the *Chiari headache*. Chiari headaches are usually described as starting in the back of the head and sometimes radiating forward to behind the eyes. The pain is described as a feeling of intense pressure, or even explosive in nature, and is brought on or aggravated by straining (known as a Valsalva maneuver), coughing, sneezing, posture, singing, laughing, etc. The pain can be so intense that many people end up avoiding activities, such as laughing or bending over, which bring on these terrible headaches.

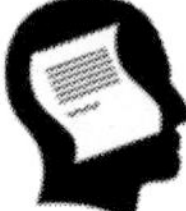

Personal Experience: Before I was diagnosed, and even for a period of time after surgery, I used to get several Chiari headaches a day and found that lying down flat on the floor would usually help get rid of them. Interestingly, even when I didn't know what was going on, I described the feeling as if there were a fist in the back of my skull squeezing my brain.

Over the years, researchers have speculated on what actually causes the Chiari headache. One theory posited the notion that headaches are aggravated during a cough by tonsillar movement compressing nerve roots in the spine.

Another headache theory speculated that the pain arose because of a difference in pressure between inside the skull and inside the spinal area. Neither of these theories had substantial data to back them and were not well accepted by the research community.

However, a theory published by Heiss, a neurosurgeon at the National Institutes of Health, provided data which showed that there is a CSF pressure spike in Chiari patients when they cough. Specifically, Heiss showed that the peak CSF pressure during coughing was higher in Chiari patients who suffered from cough headaches than in Chiari patients who didn't get cough headaches and healthy people.

Unfortunately, knowing what causes a Chiari headache doesn't help people get through them. Some people have found that over the counter medicines, such as ibuprofen and naproxen, can help to some degree, and some prescription medications are available, but others have struggled to find any relief from crippling headaches.

Complicating the headache situation is an apparent link with migraines. Although the published research is limited in this area, some Chiari experts believe there is some type of link between Chiari and migraines, for example Chiari patients may be more prone to developing migraines.

Unfortunately, some people with Chiari, especially women, are told that their headaches are "just migraines" and thus their access to effective treatment can be delayed for years.

Neck & Shoulder Pain

Pain in the neck, shoulder, and upper back is another very common problem with Chiari and can be due to several causes. First, the nerves which serve these areas originate in the top part of the spine and so can become compressed by the herniated tonsils. Second, syrinxes (which will be discussed in more detail later in this chapter) are common in the upper cervical region and thus can also damage the nerves in this area. Third, recall that Chiari patients often have unusual anatomy in the upper spine which can translate to problems with the muscles in the neck, shoulders, and back. Finally, once one muscle is affected by nerve damage in the neck and shoulders, it can affect how the rest of the muscles work. Instead of working together to perform a task, muscles can start to work against each other which in turn leads to pain and loss of function.

Interestingly, for reasons that are not entirely clear, it appears that the right side of patients, meaning the right side of their neck and their right shoulder, is affected more often than the left side.

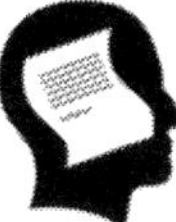

Personal Experience: The atrophy on the right side of my upper body was so bad that my right shoulder actually drooped down very significantly. In looking back at picture from that time it is easy to see how with the shoulder pulling down like that it put extra tension on my neck and caused considerable pain.

Balance Problems (Ear)

The human balance system – also known as the vestibular system – is a delicate system which involves a number of parts. In order to maintain balance, the body integrates input from three sources: the eyes, muscles and joints, and the inner ear. The inner ear has fluid-filled structures which send balance information to – of all places – the cerebellum. Obviously, if the cerebellum is compressed, like with Chiari, the system may not work properly.

Beyond being a common symptom, there is also evidence that vestibular problems may be an accurate indicator of symptomatic Chiari. Specifically, a 2002 study (Kumar) looked at the vestibular test results of 77 confirmed Chiari patients. The vestibular testing – a series of 6 tests – revealed abnormalities in more than half of the patient group. In fact, 75% of the group showed abnormal results to a test which involved irrigating the ears.

The researchers further divided the patients into groups based on symptom severity. In the group with the most severe symptoms, a remarkable 18 of the 19 patients had abnormal vestibular testing results. In addition, the test results were strongly suggestive of posterior fossa related problems. In a group with milder symptoms, the vestibular results were abnormal in 82% of the patients. Interestingly, two patients in this group who did not have surgery later became asymptomatic, and once they were symptom free, their follow-up vestibular testing became normal. Although it is not routinely used in assessing patients, based on these results, vestibular testing appears to be a strong predictor of symptomatic Chiari malformation.

Eyes

Chiari can affect the eyes in several ways. One of the most common is a rapid, involuntary movement of the eyes known as nystagmus. Similarly, Chiari can cause blurred vision, double vision, and sensitivity to light. It is likely that Chiari actually causes these symptoms, but there are additional eye problems which may or may not be related to Chiari.

Specifically, there appears to be a connection between Chiari and strabismus, which is when the eyes don't align properly (think cross-eyed). In fact, one study found that strabismus related to Chiari can be treated effectively with Chiari decompression surgery, rather than the standard strabismus eye surgery. It may be that in these cases Chiari affects the muscles which position the eyes properly, or it may be that Chiari patients are just more prone to developing strabismus.

Apnea/Respiration

One of the most serious Chiari symptoms, and one that is only recently being recognized, is sleep apnea. In the human respiratory system, the act of breathing is constantly monitored and adjusted in order to maintain the proper levels of oxygen, carbon dioxide, and pressure. To accomplish this, the central respiratory center (the part of the brain that controls breathing) receives signals from throughout the body which travel on afferent nerves. The respiratory center then processes this information and makes adjustments by sending commands to different parts of the body, such as the diaphragm.

An example of this system in action is when a person starts to exercise. Muscles work harder and send signals for more oxygen. The body responds, automatically, by increasing the breathing rate and adjusting whether the breaths are shallow or deep. All of this occurs in the part of the central respiratory system that controls involuntary breathing - the brainstem - just above the spine.

There is, however, a second part of the breathing control center which allows for voluntary control over breathing. Located in the cerebral cortex (which is responsible for higher order processes) this part of the brain takes over when a person consciously changes their breathing, for example to sing, or to take slow deep breaths in an effort to calm down.

This complex interaction between nerves carrying signals from the body, two parts of the brain deciding what to do, and nerves carrying commands back to the body, changes when a person goes to sleep. The voluntary breathing control center essentially shuts down. In addition, the involuntary center's response to stimulus (both inside and outside the body) is reduced. Finally, the muscles of the airway relax which results in an increase in resistance to the natural flow of air.

The changes in breathing during sleep are particularly evident during the REM (rapid eye movement) stage of sleep, which is considered to be when a person dreams. During REM, breathing becomes very irregular and will switch quickly from rapid breaths to slow breaths and from shallow ones to deep ones.

During the altered breathing states of sleep, problems, which can be quite serious, sometimes develop. The term apnea refers to a temporary stop in breathing. Sleep apnea is a disorder characterized by repeated incidents where a person stops breathing, partially wakes up, then starts breathing again. The frequent episodes of apnea and arousal often lead to daytime exhaustion.

In general, there are three types of sleep apnea: obstructive, central, and mixed. Obstructive sleep apnea occurs because something physically blocks, or obstructs, the airway (muscles for example). In central sleep apnea, the problem lies with the respiratory control center itself, which for some reason fails to signal the body to breathe. Mixed refers to someone who suffers from episodes of both types of apnea.

While millions of people in the US who don't have Chiari suffer from sleep apnea, there is significant evidence that the rate of apnea in Chiari and syringomyelia patients is much higher than in the general population. Several studies which have looked at the night time breathing of Chiari patients using formal sleep testing has found apnea rates ranging from 60%-75%, which is much, much higher than the rate in the general population. In addition, rates of central sleep apnea – which is considered to be more serious – have also been found to very high among Chiari patients. Finally, decompression surgery for Chiari has been shown to be effective in treating sleep apnea.

The precise mechanism by which Chiari is linked to sleep apnea is not known, however there are a number of possibilities. First, the Chiari malformation itself may compress the brainstem, which is where the breathing center is located. Second, Chiari is also known to compress and interfere with the function of the cranial nerves which are also important for breathing at night. Finally, Chiari is also known to cause problems in the throat area, such as swallowing, raspy voice, etc. It may be that in some cases of Chiari, the muscles of the lower throat become weakened, and this weakness leads to an obstruction of the airway during sleep.

Unfortunately, Chiari can also affect regular daytime breathing as well. Although uncommon, there are case reports in the literature of respiratory arrest associated with Chiari.

Arms/Legs

From a high-level point of view, body parts such as the extremities (arms, legs, hands, and feet) are served by both sensory and motor nerves. Therefore, when problems develop, they can come in the form of sensory disturbances and/or muscle weakness. When sensory nerves are affected, problems can include both loss of feeling in certain areas, and feeling unusual sensations such as tingling. When motor neurons are affected, muscle weakness and atrophy can ensue. In either case, pain is always a distinct possibility.

Although problems with the arms, legs, hand, and feet are fairly common with Chiari, as a class they have not been studied very much. There has been some research on the specific types of damage that syringomyelia can do, which is discussed further in later chapters.

Neuropsychological – Cognitive

Since Chiari involves the brain, it is natural to assume that the compression of brain tissue would cause some cognitive problems. While there is abundant anecdotal evidence that this is the case – with many Chiari patients referring to a brain fog and many parents reporting learning difficulties with their Chiari children – there has been virtually no research in this area, so it remains an open question.

Skeptics might point out that the part of the brain affected by Chiari, namely the cerebellum, is believed to control only motor functioning, not higher order thought processes. While this was true at one time, more recent research has shown that the cerebellum is likely involved in a wide variety of cognitive functions and activities.

In fact, there is significant indirect evidence that Chiari may in fact be responsible for cognitive impairments. Research involving damage to the cerebellum – not related to Chiari – has shown significant deficits in intelligence tests due to problems such as tumors.

Beyond the cerebellum, Chiari has the potential to affect more than just one part of the brain. The effects of blocking the natural flow of spinal fluid on other parts of the brain are not known. What has been shown, however, is that a long-term increase in intracranial pressure, which is common with Chiari, can have far-reaching cognitive effects.

In addition, one study involving children with Chiari II and spina bifida (Vinck) tried to isolate and assess the cognitive effects of Chiari. The researchers administered standard intelligence tests to a group of children with spina bifida, some of whom had Chiari II and some of whom didn't. The results showed that the children with Chiari II scored significantly lower on tests of Verbal IQ, Performance IQ, and Total IQ. For example, the average Total IQ score for the group without Chiari II was 94.5 – close to the general population average score of 100 – however, the average score of the group with Chiari II was much lower at 72.6.

While this is suggestive that at a minimum Chiari II can have cognitive effects, it is not conclusive. It is well known that some children with spina bifida have cognitive deficits, which are largely attributed to accompanying hydrocephalus (excessive CSF in the brain). While these researchers tried to control for the effects of hydrocephalus, it is difficult to separate what impact hydrocephalus may have versus the actual Chiari.

One of the most intriguing pieces of evidence that Chiari may indeed have a cognitive impact comes from an Italian study (Buoni) which found that a number of children with Chiari were found to have abnormal EEG results. An EEG is a device which measures and records the brain's electrical activity through sensors placed on a patient's scalp. Specifically, the tests showed what is called intermittent rhythmic delta activity (IRDA), which is considered a non-specific abnormal result.

However, before reaching the conclusion that Chiari causes cognitive problems, it is important to keep in mind that Chiari patients can suffer from cognitive deficits which are not directly caused by Chiari. For example chronic pain, medications, depression, and unrelated conditions all must be considered as possible contributors to any cognitive problems, so while there is some evidence that Chiari can impact cognition, it is too early to say for sure that it does.

Neuropsychological – Depression/Anxiety

According to the Mueller study cited above, both depression and anxiety are major problems for a significant number of Chiari patients. However just like with cognitive issues, it is difficult to say whether Chiari directly causes depression or if depression is a result of the chronic pain and disability that can accompany Chiari. Beyond Chiari, research has shown that high rates of depression, and anxiety, are linked to both chronic pain and disability. In fact, one study (Dersh) found that more than half of people with a disabling spine problem suffer from major depression and are much more likely to have a personality disorder than the general public.

Whether caused directly by Chiari – which is entirely possible – or indirectly, depression, anxiety and related symptoms are a major problem for Chiari patients.

Pediatric Symptoms

Young Children

Although children and adults share many Chiari symptoms, there is some evidence that the most common symptoms among children may be different than among adults. Specifically, a 2002 study (Greenlee, Menezes) found that oropharyngeal problems – having to do with the throat – were the most common presenting symptom among very young children.

The study reviewed the medical, radiological, and treatment records of 31 pediatric Chiari patients. Surprisingly, 11 out of the 16 children under the age of 3 (69%) presented with oropharyngeal problems, including:

- Aspiration
- Reflux
- Choking
- Dysphagia
- Stridor
- Chronic cough
- Hoarseness
- Poor weight gain

Many of these children were on antacids or other drugs and some had undergone multiple gastrointestinal procedures. It should be pointed out that while other researchers have noted oropharyngeal problems in pediatric Chiari patients, no other studies have reported this level of oropharyngeal problems.

However, since very young children are often unable to effectively communicate what they're feeling and experiencing, the idea that oropharyngeal problems can be associated with Chiari is worth keeping in mind.

Scoliosis

Among older children; scoliosis, an abnormal curvature of the spine, is a common problem among Chiari and syringomyelia patients. However, since the exact link between the two is not known, it is difficult to say whether scoliosis is a symptom of Chiari, whether they are both due to some other underlying problem, or whether they are just coincidentally associated.

Also, given the large number of children who develop scoliosis at some point, scoliosis as a "symptom" by itself is not very useful in identifying Chiari. There are over 500,000 people in the US with scoliosis and over half of them are idiopathic (meaning the scoliosis is due to an unknown cause).

Realistically, only a small fraction of those cases are likely associated with Chiari. To order an MRI to check for Chiari for every one of these cases would be cost prohibitive. In addition, an MRI for children often involves sedation and can be a traumatic event for both the child and their family.

Since ordering blanket MRIs for every scoliosis patient is not reasonable, doctors must rely on their judgment and experience to determine when an MRI is necessary. The good news is that there is general agreement in many cases. Research has shown that MRIs rarely reveal anything in what are considered typical scoliosis cases, so most doctors will not order an MRI if there is nothing unusual about the patient's scoliosis. At the other end of the spectrum, patients with severe neurological deficits in combination with scoliosis, are very likely to have Chiari or syringomyelia, so MRIs are routinely ordered.

Going even further, research out of the University of Iowa (Morcuende) found that pediatric patients with both a severe curve (greater than 45 degrees) and abnormal neurological findings had an 86% chance of finding CM and/or SM on MRI, suggesting criteria for when an MRI should be ordered.

Practical Tip: *What's In a Name?* Sometimes symptoms can be confusing because of their strange names. The following chart translates a few of them.

Figure 2-12: Symptom Definitions

Name	What It Is
Allodynia	Pain in response to something that should not cause pain
Aphasia	Trouble finding the right words to use when speaking
Ataxia	Difficulty walking due to loss of muscle coordination
Atrophy	Wasting away of muscle
Cephalgia	Headache
Diplopia	Double vision
Dysesthesia	Unusual, unpleasant sensations
Dysphagia	Trouble swallowing
Kyphosis	Hunchback
Nystagmus	Rapid involuntarily eye movements
Photophobia	Sensitivity to bright lights
Scoliosis	Abnormal right-left curvature of the spine
Strabismus	Cross-eyed
Tachycardia	Rapid heart beat
Tinnitus	Ringing in the ears
Vertigo	Dizziness

Syringomyelia

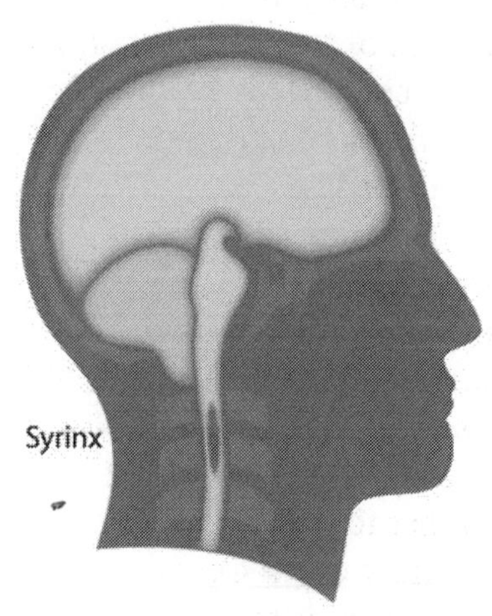

Figure 2-13: Syringomyelia

One of the most serious symptoms associated with Chiari is actually another medical condition known as syringomyelia. Syringomyelia refers to the development of a fluid-filled cyst, or syrinx, inside the tissue of the spinal cord. (Figure 2-13) Over time, a syrinx can expand and put tremendous pressure on, and damage, the sensitive nerves in the cord.

Although it is considered a medical condition unto itself, it is believed that syringomyelia is always the result of something else, like Chiari. Research has shown that anywhere from 30%-70% of Chiari patients also have syringomyelia, however there is currently no way to predict who will develop a syrinx and who won't. Symptoms specific to syringomyelia include loss of sensation and weakness in the arms, legs, hands, and feet, inability to regulate body temperature, and bladder and bowel problems. Pain in the neck, shoulders, and upper back is very common and is referred to as the cape effect of syringomyelia. As a syrinx expands it can cause permanent nerve damage and even lead to paralysis. As will be discussed later in the book, the nerve damage caused by a syrinx can also lead to unrelenting neuropathic pain that is difficult to treat.

Did You Know: While Chiari is the leading cause of syringomyelia, it can also be caused by spinal injuries (post-traumatic), tumors, and arachnoiditis. In some cases, known as idiopathic syringomyelia, the underlying cause is not clear.

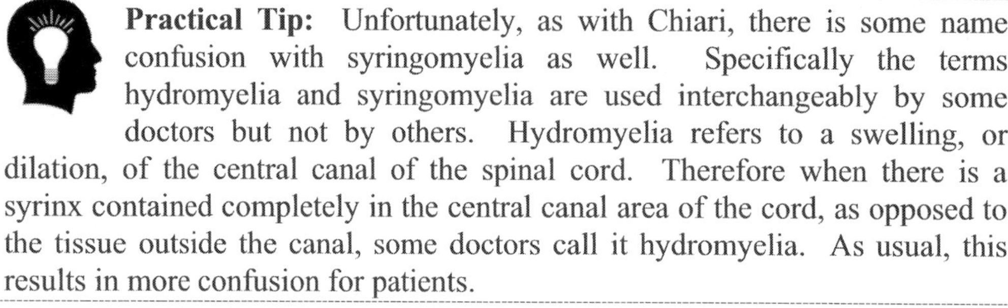

Practical Tip: Unfortunately, as with Chiari, there is some name confusion with syringomyelia as well. Specifically the terms hydromyelia and syringomyelia are used interchangeably by some doctors but not by others. Hydromyelia refers to a swelling, or dilation, of the central canal of the spinal cord. Therefore when there is a syrinx contained completely in the central canal area of the cord, as opposed to the tissue outside the canal, some doctors call it hydromyelia. As usual, this results in more confusion for patients.

Over the years there have been many theories as to how a Chiari malformation leads to the development of a syrinx. Gardner kicked it all off with a theory that stated if a Chiari malformation blocks the natural flow of CSF out of the brain, it will be redirected and flow down the central canal of the spinal cord instead, which in turn will create a syrinx. However, it has since been shown that in most adults the central canal closes off and would not allow this type of CSF flow, so this theory has largely been abandoned.

Today, one of the most popular theories is called the piston theory. Developed by surgeons at the National Institutes of Health (Oldfield, Heiss), this theory holds that with Chiari the cerebellar tonsils act like a piston, and with every heartbeat, they drive down into the spinal area and create a pressure wave of CSF. This pressure wave crashes into the spinal cord and forces CSF inside. There is some evidence to support this theory, including the fact that tonsils have been shown to move on MRI, some type of pressure wave does flow down during the cardiac cycle, and dye studies have shown that CSF can flow into the spinal cord along the outside of veins and arteries through what are known as the perivascular spaces. However, the theory is also somewhat counterintuitive.

Engineers have pointed out that for a syrinx to form - and bulge out - the pressure inside the cord itself should be higher than in the subarachnoid space outside the cord (where the CSF is). In other words, a balloon is blown up by creating higher pressure inside the balloon, not by forcing air into the balloon from the outside. Recently however, computer simulations and models of the spinal system have shown that at certain points during the cardiac/CSF cycle the pressure environment in the spinal cord may allow for both the flow of CSF into the cord and the expansion of the syrinx itself.

The piston theory is by no means the end of the story and researchers continue to propose new ideas for how syrinxes form. In 2004 Levine proposed a completely different theory, including a different source for the syrinx fluid itself. Specifically, Levine proposed that with Chiari, activities such as coughing, straining, standing up, etc., create a pressure imbalance between the skull and spine. This in turn leads to abnormal expansion and contraction of blood vessels in the spine and cause stress and damage to the spine. This damage leads to a breakdown of the blood-spine barrier and allows fluid to leak from blood vessels and create a syrinx.

In 2006, an established syringomyelia researcher, Greitz, introduced the Intramedullary Pulse Pressure Theory. This theory states that normally pressure waves are in unison between the spinal cord tissue and the CSF space. However, when there is a small narrowing of the CSF spaces, the pressure waves are no longer synchronized and the cord tissue starts to distend and fills with extracellular fluid, basically filling from the inside rather than the outside.

Finally, the immune system may actually play a role in syrinx formation as well. A study which involved creating syrinxes in rats by injecting them with kaolin (Lee) found a significant immune response in the central canal of the spinal cords near the injection site.

No matter what the underlying mechanism of syrinx formation turns out to be, syringomyelia is a very serious by-product of Chiari. For some people, the pain and disability associated with syringomyelia will dominate their experience with Chiari.

Related Conditions

Hydrocephalus

Hydrocephalus involves an abnormal accumulation of cerebrospinal fluid in the brain. It is commonly seen with Chiari II, and usually requires a shunt to be put in surgically to drain the extra CSF. It can also be found sometimes in children with Chiari I and again may require shunting. When hydrocephalus is found with Chiari, in general the hydrocephalus is treated first surgically, then the Chiari is evaluated and treated if necessary. Hydrocephalus is a major disorder onto itself and details of its theories, symptoms, treatments, and impact are beyond the scope of this book.

For more information about hydrocephalus, visit the Hydrocephalus Association, a non-profit dedicated to providing support, education and advocacy for individuals, families and professionals.

Hydrocephalus Association: **www.hydroassoc.org**

Complex Anatomy

As mentioned previously, beyond the herniated cerebellum itself, Chiari patients often have complex anatomy in the head and neck region. This can include, but is not limited to:

- Small posterior fossa
- Congenitally fused vertebrae
- Kinked brainstem
- Flattening of the skull base
- Misaligned odontoid process

While several surgeons have noted these abnormalities in published cases, to date there has not been a systematic analysis of the anatomy of Chiari patients (beyond posterior fossa volumetrics). Thus, while it is logical to assume that patients with complex anatomical issues may be more difficult to treat and have poorer outcomes, this has not been established scientifically.

Genetic Conditions/EDS

Chiari has been noted to co-exist with many genetic disorders. In fact, a 2006 paper (Germain) which reviewed the medical literature for such references, found reports of 17 distinct genetic disorders co-existing with Chiari. This does not mean that every one of these conditions is linked to Chiari in the sense that they are related – it could just be that one patient happened to have both – but it is likely that some of them are.

One such condition which has received a great deal of attention lately is Ehlers-Danlos Syndrome (EDS). EDS is actually a group of connective tissue disorders characterized by problems such as hyperelastic skin, extremely mobile joints, fragile blood vessels. These problems all stem from deficiencies in collagen, which is the core of connective tissue and provides strength and structure.

At the 2005 American Syringomyelia Alliance Project Conference, Dr. Thomas Milhorat of the Chiari Institute gave a presentation on their group's observations regarding Chiari and EDS. Basically, The Chiari Institute had identified a subset of Chiari patients who appeared to have some variant of EDS. This in turn led to surgical complications for these patients, such as cranial settling. Because of this, the TCI doctors began to take certain precautions with patients they believed had EDS and used specific surgical techniques to treat them.

According to Milhorat, TCI has identified enough patients in this group that the association between Chiari and EDS is not likely to be due to chance. However, how many Chiari patients may fall into this category is difficult to specify because the patient group at TCI is biased towards these types of patients; it could be less than 1% or as high as 5%.

For those who would like more information on this subject, there is a video of Milhorat's presentation available at:

www.northshorelij.com/body.cfm?id=6456

Tethered Cord

In recent years, several Chiari experts have begun to examine the relationship between Tethered Cord Syndrome (TCS) and Chiari. Clinically, some Chiari patients are being treated for tethered cord before undergoing Chiari surgery. On the research front, scientists are beginning to look at whether a tethered cord can play a role in the development of Chiari. The work on Chiari and TCS is very preliminary and there have not yet been many publications on the subject. To make matters worse, TCS has generated quite a bit of controversy on its own, without Chiari even being in the picture.

Tethered Cord Syndrome is a condition where the spinal cord tissue attaches abnormally to the bones of the spine. The resulting tension causes symptoms such as bladder and bowel incontinence and weakness of the legs. Sometimes skin abnormalities develop over the attachment point, and can be a clue to the underlying problem. TCS is usually treated surgically by "freeing" the cord. Success of the surgery is mixed with many patients experiencing relief from some symptoms but not others.

TCS can be due to a number of different factors, such as spina bifida or fatty deposits, but recently much attention has been paid to the role that the filum terminale plays in tethered cord. The filum terminale is a fibrous thread which connects the very bottom of the spinal cord to the coccyx bone. If the filum terminale is unusually thick, or tight, it can essentially place the spinal cord in traction and pull it down. For children, as their spinal cords grow, they will be pulling up on an anchor that is too strong.

Because the cord is mechanically pulled down, TCS can often be seen on an MRI, which shows that the conus - a lower section of the spinal cord - is abnormally low relative to the bony vertebra. Specifically, the conus is usually located at the L1/L2 level, and MRI evidence that it is lower than this is a strong indication of tethered cord. If a cord is tethered due to the filum terminale, the surgery to correct it is fairly simple; the filum terminale is cut, or sectioned, and the tension on the cord is released.

While the traditional diagnosis of TCS relies on imaging evidence, beginning in 1990, some physicians began to speculate that a subset of patients might be suffering from tethered cords which do not show up on MRIs. Referred to as occult tethered cord, the theory is that even though the conus is at the normal level, the filum terminale is abnormally fatty, thick, or tight, and thus puts the cord under tension. These physicians began to section the filum terminale based on symptoms - such as intractable urinary incontinence - rather than MRI results.

Naturally, since the surgeons were basing their decisions mostly on their own judgment, controversy began to grow over this practice. Conservative surgeons pointed out that there was no clear evidence that these patients had tethered cords and that the risks of surgery were not warranted. More aggressive surgeons pointed to their own track record of success in improving patients' symptoms with the relatively simple surgery.

The controversy surrounding surgery for occult tethered cord was highlighted recently in the May, 2006 issue of the *"Journal of Neurosurgery: Pediatrics"*, which published several papers on the subject. The papers were based upon a professional society meeting of neurosurgeons in December, 2004 which discussed and debated the subject, and included the results of a survey (Steinbok et al.) done at the meeting.

The survey was taken based upon 4 hypothetical case studies. In each case, the patient was the same clinically, but the MRI results were different. Specifically, the case involved a 6-year old girl suffering from incontinence with only minor neurological signs. The MRI results varied as follows:

- Case 1: Low-lying conus; thick, fatty filum
- Case 2: Normal conus; normal filum
- Case 3: Normal conus; some fat in filum
- Case 4: Normal conus, thoracic syrinx, no Chiari

For each case, the surgeons were asked whether they thought TCS was present and whether it should be operated on. Not surprisingly, there was near unanimous agreement for surgery with Case 1, due to the presence of both symptoms and radiological evidence.

The controversy, however, came to the forefront with the responses to Case 2. The surgeons were nearly evenly split with 29% recommending surgery, 35% against surgery, and 35% saying they were unsure.

Highlighting the reliance many surgeons have on objective tests, the addition of a small MRI finding of some fat in the filum tipped the scales towards surgery for Case 3, with 76% agreeing that surgery should be recommended.

The surgeons were split again for Case 4 with a syrinx but not Chiari, with 43% for surgery, 39% against, and 14% unsure.

Beyond highlighting the deep controversy over surgery for occult TCS, it is interesting to note that these results are reminiscent of a similar survey on decompression surgery which also revealed a wide range of opinions in the surgical community. Based upon the survey results, the authors naturally call for rigorous controlled trials to examine this issue further, and as we will see below, the lack of such trials is one of the major problems with this surgery.

The meeting also included surgeons arguing for and against surgery for occult TCS. Arguing in favor of surgery was Dr. Nathan Selden, a pediatric neurosurgeon from Oregon Health & Science University, who presented the results from a medical literature review on surgical outcomes. Using search terms such as tethered cord, filum terminale, and voiding dysfunction, Selden searched the literature from 1964 - 2004 for studies which reported surgical outcomes on children with no MRI evidence for, but symptoms of, tethered cord due to a tight filum terminale.

In all, Selden found 7 such studies (including his own experience with 6 patients) representing a total of 161 patients. In support of the pro-surgery position, overall 87% of patients improved after surgery, with improvement referring to bladder problems and based primarily on informal patient reports. For those studies which involved formal urodynamic testing, a significantly lower 63% of patients demonstrated objective improvement.

It should also be pointed out that there were no serious complications and only 3 minor complications were reported for the entire group of patients.

While these results seem impressive, it is important to keep in mind - as Selden readily admits - that the referenced publications are considered weak scientifically due to methodological problems. In addition to the fact that only 161 patients are represented overall, all the studies were retrospective (meaning the cases were examined after the fact), there was no standard, objective measure of outcome, and perhaps most importantly there were no control groups.

A control group is a scientific device which helps validate the treatment being assessed. A control group would generally receive a standard treatment which the new treatment can then be compared to; or in some cases a sham treatment. There can be a powerful placebo effect with surgery, and well respected studies (published in the *"New England Journal of Medicine"*) have shown that patients with arthritic knees experience an improvement of symptoms even after a mock surgery. A more rigorous study of the filum terminale surgery might randomly assign patients to one of three groups: medication, filum surgery, and fake surgery. That way the results from the groups could be compared directly.

The lack of strong evidence that the surgery is effective was just one of the arguments made by Dr. James Drake, of the University of Toronto, in his paper against surgery for occult tethered cord. Drake also points out that there is an unclear definition of the syndrome, the pathogenesis and natural history are not known, and there are no objective clinical tests.

In terms of definition, Drake highlights that different clinicians use different definitions to determine when occult tethered cord is present. In other words, even setting aside the imaging, there is not one set of symptoms that doctors agree constitute occult TCS, and without such a definition it is difficult to even begin to evaluate the syndrome objectively. One doctor may be very accurate in using his judgment to identify good surgical candidates, but another might not.

In terms of the natural history of occult TCS, Drake argues that some assume, mistakenly, that all cases will progressively get worse, thus necessitating surgery. Yet, according to Drake, there is no evidence that this is the case, and there are even some indications the opposite may be true.

Similarly, no evidence has been published on how a tight filum terminale is supposed to translate into symptoms. While there are theories that the tension disrupts blood flow, the theoretical basis for the occult tethered cord has not yet been developed.

In terms of diagnosing based on symptoms, Drake stresses that the symptoms associated with occult tethered cord are actually very common. Specifically, urinary continence among school aged children is very prevalent, with some reports showing that more than 16% of children suffer from some level of incontinence (and this may continue into adulthood). In addition the neurological signs and symptoms that sometimes accompany the tethered cord can actually have many different causes. Thus, absent an objective clinical test, or at least a more rigorous symptomatic definition, it is very difficult to diagnose occult TCS.

Finally, Drake brings to his argument the underwhelming evidence (as discussed above) to support the effectiveness of the surgery. Thus, he concludes, absent clear scientific evidence, there is no basis for subjecting patients to even limited surgical risk.

While there have been several publications since this debate, they continue to lack the scientific methodology necessary to say conclusively that surgery should be used for occult TCS. A report by Metcalfe et al. in the October 2006 issue of *"Journal of Urology"* is one such study.

The authors report on their experience with 36 children who were referred for sectioning of the filum due to severe bladder and bowel problems. While their results are impressive, with 92% of patients reporting an improvement in constipation and 72% an improvement in urinary problems, the study was retrospective in nature with no clear inclusion criteria, and no control group was used. In addition, it is interesting to note that when objective urodynamic testing was used as the outcome measure, the success rate dropped to 57%. In addition, even the authors point out that they were only referred children with severe problems, and those children represented a tiny fraction (.04%) of the total cases they evaluated.

At this point, much like with Chiari, the diagnosis of TCS can be as much art as science and a patient is likely to get different opinions from different doctors. Perhaps stronger magnets will allow MRIs to show a subtle difference in the filum, or even somehow measure its tension, but until then the controversy surrounding TCS, and its potential link to Chiari, is likely to persist.

Pseudo-Tumor Cerebri

Idiopathic intracranial hypertension (IIH), also known as pseudotumor cerebri (PTC) and benign intracranial hypertension, is a condition characterized by an increase in intracranial pressure (the pressure of spinal fluid in the head) with no apparent cause. Like Chiari, its main symptom is a pressure headache, made worse by straining, coughing, etc. Since both IIH and Chiari are fundamentally tied to the CSF system, perhaps it should not be surprising that there appears to be some type of connection between the two.

Recently, there have been a couple of studies published which indicate that a percentage of Chiari surgeries fail due to the presence of IIH in addition to Chiari. However, this research is early-stage, and the exact link between Chiari and IIH is not understood. It could be that the sustained increase in pressure associated with IIH eventually leads the cerebellum to herniate out of the skull and creates a Chiari malformation. If this were the case, then decompression surgery would help symptoms associated with direct compression of the malformation, but would not relieve the symptoms associated with the elevated pressure of IIH.

It may also be the case that the blockage caused by a Chiari malformation, which we know can elevate the intracranial pressure, may lead to a fundamental change in the CSF system and eventually IIH. In this case, even though the region around the Chiari malformation is decompressed surgically, for unknown reasons, the intracranial pressure remains high.

A third possibility is that both Chiari and IIH are manifestations of a more fundamental problem, such as a too small posterior fossa (the skull region where the cerebellum sits). Perhaps some people with a small or abnormally shaped skull develop IIH, while others develop Chiari, and still others develop both.

Finally, it may be that Chiari surgery itself plays a role in the development of IIH. There appear to be some cases where symptoms associated with IIH don't appear until after Chiari surgery. How, and even if, decompression surgery could lead to IIH is not at all clear.

Despite the unknowns, from a clinical point of view identifying IIH in Chiari patients is important so that proper treatments can be pursued.

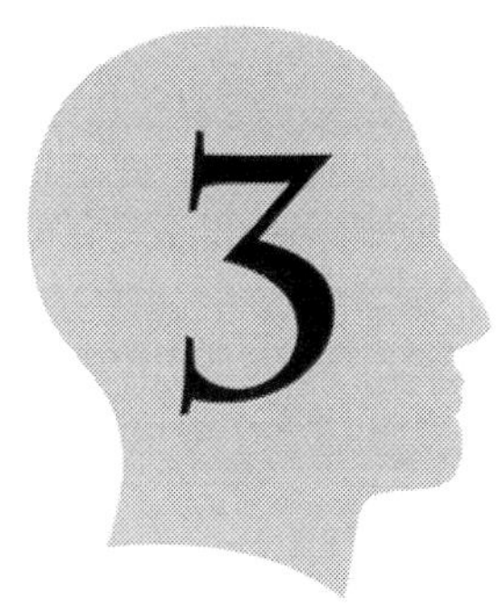

Diagnosis

"Since I was a kid I had all these different symptoms that couldn't be explained"

~Chiari Patient~

Judgment Call

It is important to understand that there is no single, objective test to say whether someone has Chiari, or how severe it is. While some might say that the MRI is used to diagnose Chiari, this is only partially true. As will be discussed shortly, the MRI is a necessary test, but by itself is not sufficient to say definitively that someone has symptomatic Chiari. Rather, the diagnostic process involves several factors which a doctor, often a neurosurgeon, will take into account in making an informed, intelligent decision. In the end whether the specific symptoms someone is experiencing are due to a Chiari malformation is a judgment call.

Specifically, diagnostic factors include:

1. MRI evidence of abnormal anatomy, such as cerebellum tonsils out of position, narrow or blocked CSF spaces, crowding or compression of brain tissue, bony abnormalities, and/or the presence of a syrinx.
2. Patient reported symptoms and whether they are consistent with and likely to be caused by Chiari or syringomyelia. For example, if someone's only symptom is a non-descript headache, and the MRI shows tonsillar herniation but no crowding, it may be difficult to say definitively that the headaches are due to Chiari. If, however, the headaches are described as crushing pressure in the back of the head brought on by going up the stairs, laughing, or singing, and the MRI shows significant herniation with crowding of other brain structures and blocked CSF flow, it is much more likely the headaches are due to Chiari.
3. Neurological signs and whether they are consistent with and likely caused by Chiari or syringomyelia. A neurological sign is an objective result from a neurological exam, for example; abnormal leg reflexes. Similar to symptoms, the mere presence of neurological signs does not necessarily indicate Chiari, but rather the physician must evaluate whether the findings are likely caused by Chiari or a syrinx.
4. The individual physician's own experience and judgment in treating Chiari. While many cases are cut and dry, others are not so clear and will rely more on an individual physician's judgment. With the current state of testing, diagnosing symptomatic Chiari remains subjective and dependent on an individual to make the call.

Because diagnosing Chiari is not straightforward and involves a rather expensive imaging test (the MRI), patients follow many different paths to being diagnosed, and will often hear different opinions from different doctors.

Many Paths to Diagnosis

The paths people take to being diagnosed with Chiari are as numerous and varied as its many symptoms. In fact, the first hints of an accurate diagnosis are sometimes based on the major symptoms that are present. For example, someone with extreme balance problems may end up seeing a specialist in balance disorders, who identifies a problem with the cerebellum and orders an MRI. Or, someone with pain in their arms and legs may end up seeing an arthritis specialist, who notices something unusual and does a thorough neurological exam, which finally places the patient on the track to an accurate diagnosis. No matter how they get there, and what doctors they see along the way, in the end the vast majority of Chiari patients will end up seeing a neurologist or a neurosurgeon for a final diagnosis.

While Chiari can become symptomatic at any age, many people are diagnosed as young adults in their late 20's and early 30's. The reason for this is not exactly clear. It could be that symptoms naturally get worse as people age and begin to become significant around this time. However, since many people are also diagnosed as children, and in turn many people diagnosed as adults can recall symptoms from their childhood, one has to wonder if the average age of diagnosis will drop as awareness of Chiari spreads through the medical community and diagnostic technology improves. It could be that the early adulthood average diagnosis is an artificial artifact of the rather recent introduction of critical MRI technology, and the lack of knowledge about Chiari, even among physicians.

No matter their age, for some people, the path they follow is short and an accurate diagnosis comes quickly, for far too many however, the path is long, torturous, and littered with missed diagnoses, misdiagnoses, self-doubt, and bitterness.

Missed Diagnoses

"When I was about 26 years old I started going numb on the right side. If I bent over it felt like my head would explode and heaven forbid if I sneezed or coughed, I thought I would pass out and the pain in back of my head and shoulders was unbelievable." ~Louise~

Louise (above) represents a typical Chiari story (if there is such a thing). Suffering from a variety of progressively worsening symptoms for years, in her mid-twenties, the symptoms became so severe and disabling that Louise was essentially in a crisis. Doctor after doctor had brushed off her complaints and ascribed them to stress, or other factors. Only when her symptoms were crippling, was an accurate diagnosis finally made.

Research involving hundreds of patients has shown that the average Chiari patient may suffer from symptoms for more than 5 years before being accurately diagnosed. During that time, they will likely see numerous doctors, often from different specialties, to no avail. Time and again, they are told not to worry, there is nothing really wrong with them, or ironically, that it is all in their head. This is in fact a major problem, namely that many Chiari patients are told their symptoms are psychological in nature.

Milhorat's landmark study of over 300 Chiari patients found that over half of the patients had been told by a doctor that they suffered from a mental problem.

The effects of being told over and over again that nothing is wrong can be devastating. Not being believed leads people to doubt themselves, and this in turn can lead to depression and social isolation. Often, since there are no visible symptoms, and without validation from the medical community, friends and family will question whether there really is something wrong, or if a person is just being overly dramatic and trying to get attention. The irony is that eventually, living with the symptoms and pain, and being rejected by the medical community can in fact lead to problems with depression and anxiety, further complicating the diagnostic situation.

Inside, a person may know that something is wrong, but going years suffering from progressively worsening symptoms without knowing the cause is a terrible burden, as reflected by this Chiari patient:

"It started Friday morning. By Friday night I could not lift my head off the pillow. If I turned my head either way my finger tips felt numb. I was scared but I did not know what to do. The headache continued all weekend until Sunday night when I started getting slowly better... It was then that I decided that either my headaches would get better and I did have a mental problem, or they would get worse and, maybe then, someone would believe me or maybe I would just die from a brain tumor or something. I had been having headaches since I was 16. I had been seeing doctors about them since I was 18." ~Carol~

Once a person has been told by several doctors that there is nothing wrong, the inherent trust that is critical for an effective doctor-patient relationship is severely compromised. Patients become extremely bitter towards the medical community and their ineffectiveness in identifying what is wrong with them.

This bitterness can manifest in several ways. Some people essentially give up and resign themselves to a life of pain and misery. Those who continue to search for answers naturally carry the burden of their past experiences into the exam room when they meet with new doctors. Expecting the worst in these situations often leads to the worst, as the patient anticipates another letdown and the physician can not help to sense the strong emotion in the patient and react to it, distracting the always too short session from the core problem. Thus, the cycle continues and the patient sinks further into hopelessness and despair.

There is also a physical price to be paid for delayed diagnoses. Besides the obvious of having to deal with numerous disabling symptoms, research has indicated that the time between the onset of symptoms and surgical treatment may influence the final outcome after treatment. In other words, the longer someone goes between symptoms and an accurate diagnosis and treatment, the worse their eventual outcome is likely to be.

It is important to note that not all studies have shown this, but it makes a certain amount of sense, especially with syringomyelia. As one neurosurgeon noted in a private conversation; as a syrinx expands and puts pressure on nerves it is impossible to say when it will cause permanent nerve damage.

The question then becomes, why are so many Chiari diagnoses missed and why are so many patients told that nothing is wrong with them? The answer is both simple and complex. The simple answer is that most first-line physicians – and even many specialists - are not familiar with Chiari and don't know what to look for. In addition they will likely only encounter a few cases over the course of their career. In diagnosing, doctors will, out of necessity, start by thinking about the most likely possible causes, in effect playing the odds. Pam, a nurse practitioner, describes it this way:

> *"[A] provider is not going to jump to a "worst case scenario" but will rule out the most common disease processes first thereby requiring multiple office visits. This can be very frustrating for a patient who not only has to pay for an office visit, trial different medications, and also expect the provider to have a crystal ball."*

If Chiari is not in their diagnostic thought process, then it is unlikely they will ever diagnose it, especially when presented with common symptoms such as headaches and dizziness for which there are many possible explanations. If, however, the doctor is good, or the patient gets lucky, an MRI will be ordered based on the symptoms or a neurological finding.

Unfortunately, often even this is not enough. Unless a radiologist is specifically looking for Chiari, it can be missed completely. In a study which reviewed MRIs of patients with pseudo-tumor cerebri (elevated intracranial pressure) for evidence of tonsillar herniation, the researchers found that the original reading of the MRIs completely missed 50% of the cases with some degree of herniation. In fact, a number of the patients had significant Chiari malformations of 5mm or more, but there was no mention of this on the MRI reports.

So, if a front-line doctor (such as a family doctor or pediatrician), is not looking for Chiari, and can find nothing wrong, why do they so often throw it back on the patient as making it up or having psychological problems? This is where the answer gets more complex.

The first factor to consider is that doctors, above all, are human beings with human emotions and frailties. When presented with a patient who keeps coming back, time and again, with the same complaints, and they can find nothing wrong, different doctors will react differently. Some doctors will admit they don't know what is wrong; some will refer the patient to someone else so they don't have to worry about it anymore; and some, because they are human, will react inappropriately.

For some doctors, to say to a patient that they don't know what is wrong, is like admitting they failed. And because of a combination of training which makes them feel knowledgeable and supremely capable, and certain personality types, this is difficult for certain doctors to do. They in effect say to themselves, *since I can't find anything, and the tests we currently have don't show anything, the problem must not be physical. If there were a physical problem, I would be able to find it and fix it. The problem in diagnosis does not lay with me, the doctor, so it must be because of the patient.*

This is an ugly truth to confront, and it should be stressed that many doctors are not like this, but research and the experience of thousands of Chiari patients demonstrate that some undoubtedly are. When confronted with a problem they can't solve, they simply don't know what to do, or how to exit gracefully, so they push back on the patient, often with disastrous results.

A second factor to consider is whether there is an inherent bias in the medical community in the type of care that women receive and how doctors treat them. Many people strongly believe that there is, namely that women are less likely to be believed then men. This may be especially true when the problem is not readily visible and involves vague or common symptoms, such as headaches.

This bias, if it in fact exists, can come into play in two ways. First, for women who have Chiari, such a bias would translate into dismissal of symptoms, not receiving further testing or referrals to specialists, and perhaps most damaging, sourcing of the problem as emotional in nature, rather than physical. Second, for mothers who believe there is a problem with their child (who actually has Chiari), such a bias results in statements such as, *you're overreacting, your child is just trying to get attention,* or *it's just growing pains.*

Interestingly, the research on whether there is a systemic bias against women in the medical system is mixed. Some studies have shown such a bias, but other, large, national studies have not. Still other studies have actually shown that women tend to receive more doctor visits, tests, and prescriptions than men for general complaints such as headache and dizziness.

Practical Tip: While it is very difficult not to take it personally when a doctor tells you there is nothing wrong with you, or it is all in your head, or that you are overreacting and your child is fine, that is one of the best things you can do. Stay calm, say thank you for your time, leave quietly, and as a modern health care consumer find another doctor.

Misdiagnoses

In addition to the problem of diagnoses that are missed completely, Chiari is often misdiagnosed as something else as well. Again, because of the many possible symptom manifestations associated with Chiari, and the general lack of awareness regarding it, many physicians will ascribe the neurological signs and symptoms to something else. Chiari (and syringomyelia) have been misdiagnosed as MS, Chronic Fatigue, migraines, cluster headaches, ALS (Lou Gehrig's), and carpal tunnel syndrome; to name just a few. Chiari is just not in the front of many physicians' minds as a possible cause to watch for.

Obviously, a misdiagnosis just adds more confusion to an already muddled medical situation and results in critical delays in getting proper treatment. In addition, a patient may end up taking medication, or even undergoing procedures that are ineffective and unnecessary.

It would be interesting to see what percent of Chiari patients are outright misdiagnosed during their journey. Given that the average time to diagnosis is several years, the number is probably staggeringly high.

Fortunately, there are some indications that awareness may be growing among front-line providers. In the past year, more and more parents have reported that their pediatricians were able to either identify Chiari outright, or at least recognize that something was wrong and refer them to a specialist for a diagnosis. In addition, one neurosurgeon who has published articles on Chiari stated in a private communication that; primary care doctors have begun to ask him for more information because they think they may be missing the diagnosis.

Sudden Onset

"Get up, you're fine," said my husband. "It wasn't that bad of a fall. Get back up on your snowboard and let's go."

"But I'm not fine. I'm tingly all over. Something's wrong." Thus began my journey into the realm of Chiari malformation and syringomyelia. One airlift and two MRIs later I knew that I had experienced neurological symptoms after a relatively minor fall because a large syrinx left my spinal cord distended and ill-protected." ~Nancy~

Nancy's experience is at the other end of the diagnostic spectrum. A triggering event, often a minor trauma, leads to the rapid onset and progression of symptoms which are obviously neurological in nature. Because of their sudden onset, and especially if they are getting worse quickly, an MRI is ordered and the underlying Chiari and/or syringomyelia is discovered. The time from symptoms to surgery for patients like this is measured in weeks not years.

Patients like Nancy do not have to confront years of doubt and frustration, but rather they are quickly dropped into the world of Chiari, usually the last place they expected to be. To them, the diagnosis of Chiari is not a validation, but an outright shocking event.

Surprisingly, people who experience a rapid onset of symptoms and a quick diagnosis are sometimes found to have not only very large Chiari malformations, but enormous syrinxes as well. More than one patient that falls into this group has reported being told by their doctor they can not understand how they didn't have symptoms before or are even surprised they are able to walk.

Some researchers have speculated that the development of a syrinx in the spinal cord is actually the body's coping mechanism to help alleviate the problems of a Chiari malformation at the cranio-vertebral junction. Perhaps in people with large syrinxes and no symptoms, their bodies did just that; compensated for the disruption of a Chiari malformation with the formation of a syrinx, and this in turn postponed the onset of symptoms. It should be stressed again that this is just speculation and that as discussed in the previous chapter, why people become symptomatic, and the exact role that trauma plays in this, are currently not well understood.

Precipitating Factors

The most revealing research in the onset of symptoms – and thus diagnosis – comes from Milhorat's landmark study of 364 patients. In this group of patients, about half (47%) clearly identified a precipitating event which, in their own opinion, sparked their symptoms. The most common factor cited was trauma, including whiplash type injuries and direct blows to the head and neck. Other precipitating events cited included coughing, infection, pregnancy, and even air travel. See (Figure 3-1) on the next page.

The link between physical trauma and Chiari is not well understood

Figure 3-1: Precipitating Factors

Factor	# of Patients	% of Patients
None	193	53%
Trauma*	89	24%
Infection	27	7%
Coughing, Sneezing	24	7%
Pregnancy	16	4%
Other**	15	4%

* Trauma includes whiplash and direct blows to head/neck
** Other includes sexual intercourse, epidural anesthesia, lumbar puncture, and air travel

What is not clear from this data is whether there was a precipitating event for the other half of the group, which for whatever reason they could not recall. If trauma does play a role in the onset of symptoms, then it seems likely that some people might have experienced a minor trauma, perhaps in their childhood, which they simply can't remember or didn't seem significant at the time.

The entire subject of trauma as it relates to Chiari is a difficult one, made more so by the legal ramifications associated with it. Conquer Chiari is often contacted by both patients and lawyers trying to determine if a car crash or work related injury can "cause" Chiari. The legal context of this question is beyond the scope of this book, but scientifically it is an interesting question which deserves more research attention than it gets. Specifically what role does trauma, in any form, play in either sparking symptoms or making them worse?

It is worth pointing out again, as stated in Chapter 2, that even if trauma is found to trigger symptoms, that doesn't necessarily mean that a specific traumatic event, like a car accident, can cause Chiari per se, meaning that the trauma didn't cause the cerebellar tonsils to herniate out of the skull. While this may be possible, the prevailing scientific thought is that Chiari is most often congenital (meaning people are born with an abnormal anatomy) and what causes an individual person to start experiencing symptoms, and start looking for a diagnosis, is not exactly known.

Having said this, one way for the average person to think about this aspect of Chiari – and this is speculation by the author and not supported by scientific research – is that developing symptoms is like a point system. Picture a point scale from 0-100, and assume each person with Chiari is born with a certain anatomy, and based on this anatomy, has a trigger point, at which symptoms will become noticeable. For one person this may be at 30 points, for another, it may be at 75 points.

Now, as we go through life, we accumulate points on this scale. (Figure 3-2) As we age, we accumulate points from activities such as coughing, sneezing, and especially traumas. Even getting older adds points because the dura thickens as we age. All these activities add different numbers of points to an individual's Chiari scale; say 15 points for going through labor, 5 points for a bad case of bronchitis, and 30 points or more for a trauma such as a fall or car accident. People accumulate points differently based on their daily life as well. Those with physical labor jobs accumulate points faster than those with desk jobs; people involved in contact sports accumulate points quicker as well.

When a person gets near their trigger point, they may start to experience some minor symptoms, like an occasional headache or some tingling. However, once the threshold is crossed, the symptoms become very noticeable and prominent, and people begin to recognize that something is wrong and look for a diagnosis.

While markedly unscientific, this model does show how some people can experience a rapid onset of symptoms with a recognized precipitating event, while others do not. An individual could be well below their symptom trigger level when they are involved in a fall or car accident which instantly propels them into the symptom range of the point scale. In contrast, someone else may sneak up on their trigger level over many years and begin to cross the boundary only due to natural aging and their daily activities.

Whether this model at all represents reality is anyone's guess, but it will be a critical breakthrough in understanding Chiari once it is understood how and why people become symptomatic.

Figure 3-2: Chiari Symptom Scale

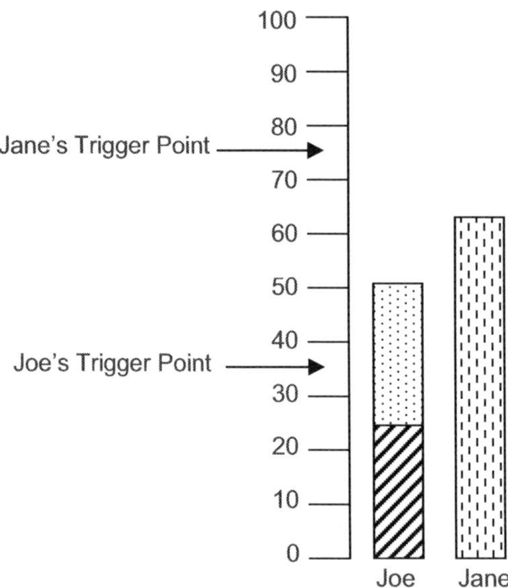

In this example (refer to the "*Chiari Symptom Scale*") both Joe and Jane are 30 years old and have anatomy associated with Chiari; small posterior fossa and herniated cerebellar tonsils. Joe's anatomy is a little more severe however, so he has a symptom trigger point around 50, whereas Jane's is closer to 75.

Joe's daily activities (the diagonal lines) don't have much effect on his Chiari; he works in an office and does not participate in sports much. However, recently he was in a car accident (dotted region) which put him clearly over the trigger point and sparked Chiari symptoms

Jane on the other hand has not experienced any major trauma but leads a very active life. She is on her feet all day at work and participates in numerous activities, including some extreme sports. If she had Joe's trigger point, she would have already been symptomatic for some time, and a bad fall or other trauma will likely spark symptoms as well. Even without any added trauma, Jane will eventually become symptomatic as she gets older.

Personal Experience: Like so many others, I went years before being diagnosed with Chiari and syringomyelia. However, in my case, the delay was mostly my own fault. I had written off symptoms for years. Every day when I'd come home from work, I would have a terrible headache in the back of my head, which would require me to lie down for a period of time. In addition, there was constant pain in my neck, and my right shoulder drooped down noticeably. At night, my legs hurt terribly and were starting to get weak. I had developed significant balance problems and would often stumble when standing up or bump into doorways as I went through.

Unfortunately, none of this sunk in as meaning that something was wrong. I thought the headaches were related to sinuses and the neck and shoulder pain were from athletic wear and tear. The balance problems were again due to sinuses and my legs had hurt my entire life, so that was nothing new. I didn't go from doctor to doctor, I just stayed away from them until I finally brought up the neck pain, which led to an x-ray, which led to an MRI and my shocking diagnosis.

What's interesting is that a few years before this a physical therapist almost put me on the path to a diagnosis. I went to my family doctor because the pain in my shoulder, neck, and upper back were getting so severe that it was becoming very limiting. My doctor sent me to a physical therapist who took one look at me and said that the muscles on my right side were atrophied and that he thought there was a nerve problem.

Unfortunately, when I brought this up with my family doctor, he disagreed, and the idea that there might be something significantly wrong was dismissed. Eventually, the pain subsided a bit and I learned to live with it for a while longer.

Now, I can't help but wonder what my outcome would have been if, at that point in time, my doctor had agreed with the physical therapist and started investigating. Would an earlier diagnosis and surgery have led to no deficits and residual problems?

Pediatric Diagnosis

The diagnostic process can be more complicated in children for a couple of reasons. First and foremost, the main diagnostic tool, the MRI, requires the patient to remain very still for an extended period of time. Obviously, this is not easy for a young child, especially when the machine is making loud noises. Because of this, children often have to be sedated to get an accurate MRI. This extra hurdle, plus the high cost of the test leads some physicians to be very conservative when it comes to ordering an MRI.

A second complication is that children can not always verbalize what they are feeling. Instead, their symptoms may result in changes in behavior, attitude, and affect, which may be written off as developmental phases. Even as a parent, it can be difficult to distinguish when something is truly wrong. However, many parents have reported knowing deep down that something was not right.

Sometimes with young children, the first clue is lack of proper development, either physically or cognitively. Very young children with Chiari can have trouble swallowing (an abnormal gag reflex) which can lead to failure to thrive issues. In addition, Tubbs, a researcher at the University of Alabama, has noted a connection between Chiari and growth hormone deficiency in some children. In older children, as noted in the discussion on symptoms, unusual presentations of scoliosis are a strong indication that an MRI should be done.

The evidence that Chiari can affect cognitive development in children is more anecdotal in nature, but many neurosurgeons also take it as a given. If a child seems to have developmental issues – especially if they come on suddenly – in today's quick to label environment, it can be difficult to get professionals to even consider a physical cause such as Chiari.

Concerned parents should ensure that their child is evaluated neurologically for any objective signs of a problem. If a neurological exam shows something, physicians will begin to include conditions such as Chiari in their diagnostic thought process. Perhaps the most important thing for parents to remember, is to believe in yourself and be an effective advocate for your child.

Believe In Yourself

Until technology advances to the point where there is a simple, inexpensive Chiari test, or awareness of Chiari and its many symptoms spreads throughout the medical community, it is likely that diagnosis will remain a struggle for a significant amount of patients. As such, it is important for patients, or the parents of affected children, to be their own advocates in pursuing quality medical care.

"Listen to your body! You know better than anyone if something is wrong, and follow through." ~Sabrina~

People often know, without being able to articulate why, there is something wrong with their body. Similarly parents (usually the mom) just know, deep down, that there is something wrong with their child. The key, as Sabrina says above, is to trust yourself, believe in yourself, and follow through.

There are two keys to getting an accurate diagnosis of Chiari if that is what is suspected. First is to get an MRI to see if there is any evidence of tonsillar herniation or crowding. This alone can be difficult for some people. While some doctors will freely order an MRI, others – for various reasons – are often reluctant to order such a test.

If you find yourself in this situation, the best approach is to just ask, in a calm, straight-forward manner, for an MRI to see what is going on. An explicit request is harder to refuse than just a vague plea to do something.

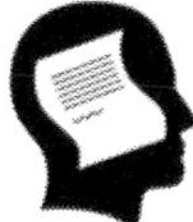

Personal Experience: While I have heard from countless people who have struggled with getting doctors to order tests and with their relationship with the medical community in general, not once have I ever had a doctor refuse something I requested outright.

Second is to find a doctor who can accurately interpret both the MRI results and the symptoms that are being experienced. Usually this means a neurosurgeon. Some people, when it is found there is a neurological problem are referred to a neurologist; however, since the primary treatment is surgical, this can add an unnecessary step and critical delay in getting proper treatment. It should be noted, however, that some neurosurgeons work with a neurologist when evaluating Chiari patients. In this case, it is best to follow whatever procedure the practice has established.

The medical system has changed drastically in the US over the past couple of decades. Gone are the days of the all-knowing family doctor who is familiar with all his patient's problems and will spend the time necessary to solve any problem. Lawyers, insurance reimbursement, the two minute office visit, and endless specialists are the realities of 21st century medical care, and patients must adapt to this new paradigm accordingly. It is critical that patients (or parents) be strong advocates for themselves and their children.

Believe in yourself and follow through.

Diagnostic Tests

While there is no single Chiari test, there are several tests which are commonly used to help diagnose Chiari, the most common of which are the MRI, the neurological exam, and the cine-MRI.

MRI

MRIs (Magnetic Resonance Imaging) have become tremendously popular over the past few years, with imaging centers literally popping up everywhere. Their popularity is fueled by their usefulness in diagnosing a range of diseases and injuries, from neurological disorders like Chiari to torn ligaments in the knee. Combined with their safety and the rapidly advancing technology, MRI has become the diagnostic tool of choice in many medical situations.

This is especially true for Chiari. Before MRI Chiari was very difficult to diagnose and study. MRI technology, with the ability to directly visualize the brain, skull, and spinal tissue revolutionized the diagnosis, treatment, and understanding of Chiari. With the widespread adoption of MRI, also came the realization that Chiari is much more common than once thought. In essence, the MRI heralded a new era for both Chiari patients and the medical professionals who treat them.

What It Is

Magnetic resonance imaging is aptly named because the process involves magnets (as everyone knows), resonance (think vibration), and imaging (creating pictures). The MRI machine is essentially a big magnet - most are powerful enough to pick up a car - along with sensing devices known as coils and a sophisticated computer.

MRI works because the human body is composed largely of water and fat, which both contain large amounts of the element Hydrogen. Individual Hydrogen atoms have a magnetic property with a certain direction, (think of the way a compass needle points). In general, the magnetic properties of all the Hydrogen atoms are pointing all over the place in a random fashion. However, when a body is placed inside a strong magnet, the magnetic properties of the Hydrogen atoms will tend to line up in the same direction, much like a compass needle points to the North Pole. This is where the Magnetic in MRI comes in. The MRI magnet lines up the Hydrogen atoms in an orderly way.

What happens next is, an energy wave (like radio waves) is directed at the Hydrogen atoms. This moves the alignment of the Hydrogen atoms to a different direction.

When the energy wave is turned off, the Hydrogen atoms will return to their alignment from the magnet. As they return to this state, they resonate - or vibrate - and give off electromagnetic energy that they absorbed from the energy wave. This is the Resonance in MRI.

Finally, a device known as a coil detects the energy given off by the Hydrogen atoms and sends the information to a computer. The computer uses that information, combined with what it knows about the magnets, and creates the detailed images we are used to seeing. This is the imaging part of MRI.

MRI machines are rated according to the strength of their magnets in units called Tesla (named after the physicist and inventor Nikola Tesla): the stronger the magnet, the better the image quality. High strength machines are considered to be .9 Tesla or higher, with the latest generation of products at 3.0 Tesla and even stronger ones in the pipeline.

One reason MRI has become so popular is the detailed images it can generate of soft tissue in the body. While an X-ray is useful for identifying bone fractures, the MRI can be used to examine the structure of the brain, spine, organs, veins and arteries, and joint ligaments and tendons.

A second advantage of MRI technology is its safety. MRI uses much less energy than an X-ray and there are no known safety issues with being exposed to the magnetic fields generated by an MRI machine. One very important safety precaution however is that people with metal in their bodies - such as aneurysm clips, orthopedic implants, etc. - may not be able to use MRI. The strong magnet can move metal which is in the body causing damage to the tissue around the metal. This is why MRI technicians ask a patient a laundry list of questions before every scan.

Because of its versatility, researchers (radiologists and medical physicists) are constantly developing new applications and finding new uses for MRI technology. Recent applications include using MRI to visualize blood flow and diagnose cardiac problems, and functional MRI which identifies brain activity based on how much blood is flowing to a particular part of the brain.

What It Means

The MRI is considered the gold standard in diagnosing Chiari. Although by itself it is not sufficient to say that someone has Chiari, at this point in time the vast majority of physicians consider it necessary for a diagnosis.

In other words, the MRI is the first step in the diagnostic process. If an MRI establishes that the cerbellar tonsils are herniated and misshapen, that there is insufficient space for the natural flow of CSF, and/or there is crowding of tissue or an abnormal anatomy then a physician will try to determine if the symptoms that are present are likely due to what is seen on the MRI.

The Experience

Unfortunately from a patient's point of view, the MRI, while safe, is not the most comfortable of tests. MRI units are very cramped and some people feel claustrophobic while inside. Procedure times are long and patients must be very still while being scanned. Injected contrast agents and coils that look like Hannibal Lechter's mask in *Silence of the Lambs* add to the discomfort. In general, the rooms are cold and the magnets in the machines are very loud as they turn on and off, so ear protection must be worn. However, MRI manufacturers are constantly working to improve the patient experience by creating more room, reducing the noise level, and reducing the amount of time required in the machines.

Different people react differently to the MRI experience. Some people are able to relax themselves and go into a kind of meditative state while inside. For others, the MRI will always involve anxiety and stress. No matter what type of person you are, the fact is that MRIs are a way of life for Chiari patients. During the first year alone, a patient can expect to undergo several scans, with repeated follow-up in the years to come. The quote below succinctly summarizes how most people feel about the MRI experience.

"Like many people, I've never gotten completely comfortable being in an MRI machine." ~Kathleen~

If you've never had an MRI before, the actual experience is a fairly lengthy process. You will likely be asked to arrive early to fill out the necessary paperwork and medical history. After waiting in a reception area, an MRI technician will ask you why you are there, explain what they are going to do, and ask you a series of questions to make sure it is safe for you to have an MRI (basically, do you have any type of metal in your body). Depending on the facility and the type of clothes you have on, you may be asked to change into surgical scrubs.

The actual MRI room can be cold. Once inside, you lie down on what is essentially a hard bed. If you need a contrast agent, which is an injection of a dye, a technician will insert a needle into your arm so it doesn't have to be done in the middle of the scan.

Depending on the equipment, what is called a coil may be attached over your face like a mask. You will either be given ear plugs for protection, or headphones, through which you can listen to music and hear the technicians. Once you are settled, the "bed" will slide into the actual MRI, and you will be in a small tube. There are lights in the tube, but there isn't really anything to look at, so you might as well close your eyes. The technicians can hear you and speak to you, and you will have a panic button to push if you need to come out.

Over the next 20 minutes to an hour, the MRI will make a series of bizarre and loud noises as it does its work. Every now and then the bed will move to a different position. During that time, it is critical to stay as still as possible so that the machine can get an accurate picture.

If you require a contrast agent, the bed will slide out of the machine in the middle of the procedure so that the dye can be injected for the rest of the scans. When the scans are done, the technicians will come into the room and the bed will slide out of the machine.

It can be disorienting coming out of the closed space like that, so it is important to be careful getting up off the bed and you may want to take a moment to reorient yourself.

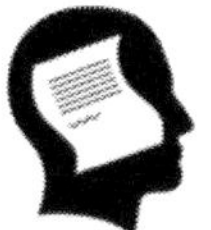

Personal Experience: While I do not get claustrophobic, going for an MRI is not something I look forward to. During the scans, I tend to fall asleep, but then I twitch in my sleep and the techs wake me up to tell me not to move. After that, I try to stay awake and just think about pleasant things until it's over. Sometimes, I wonder if I could get out of the machine by myself if I had to (for example, if there was only one technician and they had a heart attack). The longest I've been in a machine in one setting is 2 hours as part of a research study. While I survived, it is not an experience I would like to repeat. For me, the hardest part of getting MRIs is that being in the machine tends to hurt my neck and my neck muscles will be sore for hours or days after the test.

Practical Tips: MRI

Don't take any valuables in case you have to change - While lockers are provided, it is best to leave jewelry and money either at home or in the car.

- Wear clothes without any metal - If you wear cotton clothes with no studs or metal buttons, you may be able to wear your own clothes for the test.
- Take music - Many facilities allow you to bring a CD to listen to during the scan. Having your own music can help make the experience less stressful.
- Go to the same facility/machine for scans - As doctors monitor your progress, they will compare MRIs from the present to previous ones. So if possible, go to the same imaging facility for all your MRI scans.
- Keep MRI/medical records - Before you leave, ask the MRI technician for a copy of your MRIs and keep them in a safe place. Keep all your MRIs, x-rays, and medical records together so that if you go to a different doctor, you have everything you need.

- Don't try to read MRIs yourself – While it may look like Chiari malformations are obvious on an MRI, the images are very difficult to interpret. Do not try to read the scans yourself and make a diagnosis or determination if you're getting better/worse. It is difficult to wait for a doctor's appointment, but it is better than needlessly scaring yourself over a trivial imaging artifact which you thought was something important.
- FONAR stand-up, multi-position MRI – If you are extremely claustrophobic, or have some other difficulty with a standard MRI, or are trying to avoid sedating a child, consider what is known as an upright MRI. FONAR is an MRI manufacturer which has a machine which allows people to sit upright for the test, with nothing in front of them. For more information about this type of MRI, including where they can be found, visit: www.fonar.com. Note, you should check with your doctors to see if they are comfortable with using an image from this type of machine.

Neurological Exam

The neurological exam has been around for hundreds of years and is the most basic tool in the neurologist/neurosurgeon's diagnostic arsenal. While decidedly low-tech - the exam involves very simple devices for poking and prodding - the neurological exam can reveal a tremendous amount of information for a well trained, experienced physician and remains a mainstay in the diagnostic process for many neurological problems, including Chiari and syringomyelia.

The neurological exam provides a physician a way to explore what is happening inside the body, more specifically to the nervous system, by examining how different parts of the body respond to different forms of stimulus and various functional tasks. The stimuli can range from temperature probes to needle pricks to reflex hammers, and the tasks can be as simple as walking across a room to more complex tests of manual dexterity.

What It Is

The neurological exam works because the human nervous system is highly organized. When you touch something, cells in your skin send electrical signals along nerve fibers to the brain. Similarly, in order to move, the brain sends electrical signals to your muscles, which in turn send signals back to the brain so you have an internal sense of where your body parts are and how they are moving.

The nerve fibers that carry all this electrical messaging are laid out like a system of roads.

Major bundles of nerve fibers, like highways, run down the spinal cord. At each spinal level, or segment, groups of nerve fibers branch out into the body like primary roads (more on spinal segments in a bit). As the nerves get closer to their final destination - like your shoulder or thumb - the nerve fibers branch out even more to serve specialized cells.

Like with any set of roads, a map can be used to help navigate the nervous system. Scientists have been investigating how people respond to stimuli for hundreds of years, but the neurological exam itself began to evolve in the late 1800's. The medical researchers of the time began to realize that different types of sensation - temperature, touch, pain - were affected differently by injury and disease, and traveled different pathways to the brain. Normal responses to stimulus were characterized, as were normal joint movements. As knowledge of the nervous system advanced, testing for sensation became more prevalent. By the 1950's, the neurological exam contained many of the features present in today's exam.

The guideposts along the human nervous system roadmap are the spinal segments from which nerve bundles branch out. As discussed in the brief introduction to anatomy, the spine is composed of 7 cervical, 12 thoracic, 5 lumbar, and 5 sacral segments with the cervical segments at the top and the sacral segments at the bottom. Each spine segment is denoted by its region and number. C4, for example, is the fourth segment down the cervical region. L3 is the third segment down the lumbar region. The nerves that branch out from the spine at each segment serve - or map to - a specific location in the body, called a dermatome. The cervical segments generally serve the neck and shoulders, the thoracic region maps to the chest, the lumbar region maps to the hips and the front of the legs, and the sacral segments map to the back of the legs and part of the feet.

What makes this mapping useful is the fact that damage to the nerve root will cause a loss of sensation in the area served by that nerve. So if doctors detect a loss of sensation, or muscle strength, in the shoulders, there is likely a problem at the C4 level.

In addition to mapping dermatomes, different types of stimulus can be used by doctors to aid diagnosis. Your skin and organs contain different types of receptors which specialize in responding to touch, pressure, pain, vibration, and temperature. Different types of receptors, known as proprioceptive cells, provide information on movement and position. The different types of receptor cells send their information along different sized nerve fibers – which mean the signals travel at different speeds – and along different routes. So by combining responses to different stimulus, along with motor functions such as strength and gait, doctors can begin to get a picture of the location and extent of damage to the nervous system.

A complete neurological exam is an extensive procedure which involves many tests. In addition to evaluating a patient's medical history and mental status, in general the tests can be grouped into the following categories:

- Cranial Nerves
- Motor Function
- Coordination and Gait
- Reflexes
- Sensation

Because specific diseases present different neurological symptoms, a neurologist or neurosurgeon will usually tailor an exam to the specific patient and situation and focus on a few key areas.

"The thoroughness [of the exam] depends on whether a syrinx is present, whether it is a follow-up or an initial visit, and how important the findings will be in the surgical decision making." ~Dr. Ghassan Bejjani, Neurosurgeon~

Sometimes this can be disconcerting to a patient who may feel that the doctor in question is not being thorough. This is generally not the case however, as neurologists and neurosurgeons do not need to perform every test and identify every neurological deficit to form an intelligent opinion.

Below is a brief description of some of the tests that comprise a neurological exam and what they mean.

Cranial Nerves

The cranial nerves are 12 pairs of nerves that originate in the brain as opposed to the spinal cord. They are responsible for sensation and function in the cranial area, including but not limited to, facial movement, eye movement, pupil dilation, smell, taste, swallowing, and sticking your tongue out.

Tests to assess cranial nerve function might include whether strong odors can be detected, whether someone can smile or frown, and whether there are problems swallowing. Because of their location, cranial nerves are commonly compressed by a Chiari malformation, so these tests can be particularly useful in determining if a Chiari malformation is actually pressing on, and compromising, other brain structures.

Spontaneous Venous Pulsations (SVP's)

In the vast majority of people, the veins in the retina in the back of the eye can be seen to pulsate when a doctor looks through the pupil. For people with elevated intracranial pressure – the pressure inside their head – these pulsations tend to not occur. Elevated intracranial pressure (ICP) can be associated with a Chiari malformation. So if a doctor observes the lack of SVP's, it is a good indication of high intracranial pressure and might indicate a Chiari malformation.

Motor Function

When a doctor evaluates motor function, he is essentially checking whether the nerves that supply your muscles are working. A doctor will evaluate muscle size, tone (flaccid vs. rigid), and strength and look for weakness, imbalance between right and left sides, and muscles that are either too rigid or too soft.

Muscle strength is rated on a scale from 0-5, (Figure 3-3) and is measured by a patients ability to resist force. Basically, the patient tries to hold his arms (or legs) in a specific position while the doctor applies force. Evaluations might include tests for the biceps, triceps, wrist, hand, hip muscles, quadriceps, hamstrings, and ankles.

Figure 3-3: Motor Strength Assessment Scale

Score	Description
0	No muscle movement
1	Some visible movement
2	Full range of motion, not against gravity
3	Movement against gravity, but not resistance
4	Movement against resistance, less than normal
5	Normal strength

The effects of syringomyelia, more so than Chiari, are usually evident in evaluating motor function as a syrinx will directly damage motor nerves, thus affecting the corresponding muscles.

Syringomyelia can often be identified by its effects on the neck, shoulder, and upper back area, where it can cause weakness and outright muscle atrophy. In fact, syringomyelia traditionally has been described as affecting the "cape" muscles, meaning the area of the shoulders, back, and neck where an old-fashioned cape would hang on someone. The effects of a syrinx can be seen by reduced size and strength in muscles in this area, even to the point where a person's shoulder will droop down considerably due to muscle atrophy.

The hands are another critical area in looking for signs of a syrinx. People with syringomyelia tend to lose strength in one or both of their hands, and in many cases the hand will noticeably shrink in size over time and possibly curl up. Finally, abnormal muscle stiffness in the legs is common with syringomyelia.

Coordination and Gait

These are the tests that make you feel like you've been pulled over by the state police for DUI. The coordination and gait tests can reveal problems with the nerves that provide feedback on muscle movement and position, balance, and cerebellar function. Tests for coordination include:

- Rapid alternating movements such as touching your thumb to the tips of your fingers in succession.
- Point to point movements - the old touch something with your finger, then touch your nose (may be done with eyes closed)
- Romberg test - Named after the 19th century German neurologist who developed it, the Romberg test involves standing with your feet together and eyes closed for about 10 seconds. If you lose your balance, it indicates a problem along one of the highways in the spinal cord.

Gait, or walking, requires many nerve functions to work together and is a good indication of problems in the nervous system. In addition to walking normally, a doctor may observe how a patient walks on their toes, walks on their heels, or walk heel-to-toe along a line.

Reflexes

The neurological exam tests what are called deep tendon reflexes. Basically, a doctor uses a small hammer to strike a tendon and watches the response. In many CM/SM cases, there will be an exaggerated response movement, indicating a problem - or lesion - of the muscle nerves in a specific location. As discussed earlier, the location of the problem can be deduced by identifying which reflexes are abnormal. The exam might include testing the following reflexes:

- Biceps - Correlates to C5, C6
- Triceps - Correlates to C6, C7
- Forearm - Correlates to C5 ,C6
- Abdomen - Correlates to T8-T12
- Knees - Correlates to L2-L4
- Ankles - Correlates to S1,S2

Reflexes are graded on scale from 0-4, (Figure 3-4) with 0 being no reflex, and 4 being an abnormally strong reflex with clonus - a series of muscle contractions.

Figure 3-4: Reflex Grading Scale

Score	Description
0	No reflex
1+	Hypoactive (less than normal)
2+	Normal
3+	Hyperactive (more than normal)
4+	Hyperactive with clonus (like a muscle spasm)

Abnormal reflexes indicate a problem with the associated nerves, which in the case of Chiari and syringomyelia, means the nerves are being compressed or stretched.

Sensation

As mentioned earlier, the sensations of touch, pain, temperature, vibration, and pressure are carried along different nerves and pathways. By testing with different stimulus at different locations, a doctor can locate potential problems. A sensation exam might include using a Q-tip to test for light touch, a tuning fork to test for vibration, and pin pricks. The exam will test sensation on the arms, legs, and other areas depending on the findings and patient history.

Abnormal sensations in a given area, such as the shoulder, can be used to pinpoint both the type and location of a neurological problem.

What It Means

Before the development of advanced imaging technique like the MRI, which can clearly identify Chiari malformations and syrinxes, the neurological exam was the main diagnostic tool for neurological diseases. Despite rapid and impressive advances in imaging, the exam is still critical for CM/SM patients as it can identify the type and extent of any neurological deficits, important factors when evaluating treatment options.

"[The neurological exam] is a way to assess whether the disease is causing any deficits warranting surgical intervention...[I look for] evidence of sensory deficits, weakness, ataxia, dys-coordination, lower cranial dysfunction, and lack - or presence of - spontaneous venous pulsations." ~Dr. Ghassan Bejjani~

As discussed previously, an MRI alone is not sufficient to determine whether any anatomical abnormalities (meaning a Chiari malformation) are actually causing symptoms or problems. The neurological exam offers a means to objectively assess the impact that Chiari, and/or syringomyelia is having on the nervous system and provides both the physician and patient critical information in deciding what to do next.

The Experience

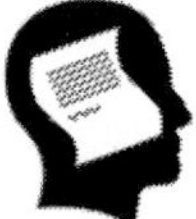

Personal Experience: For me, the neurological exam was an eye-opening event. Even though I had been told by one neurosurgeon that I had Chiari, when I went to another neurosurgeon for a second opinion, I was still in denial about the seriousness of my problems. The exam itself was fairly brief. The surgeon tested the strength in my hands and arms and checked some of my reflexes with a small hammer. Next, he asked me to walk across the room (it was a small room), which I did easily.

This is when the exam got interesting. Over the next couple of minutes, I was asked to do a series of things which before the exam I would have bet a million dollars I could do easily: walk across the room on my tip-toes, walk on my heels, unbutton my shirt with one hand, and stand with my feet together and my eyes closed. It turns out I would have been deep in debt, because I could not walk on my tip-toes without losing my balance, I could barely walk on my heels at all, and to my astonishment I could not, no matter how hard I tried, work the button on my shirt with only one hand. Reality really began to sink in however when I stood with my eyes closed. After a few seconds, even though my eyes were closed, it felt like the room was spinning away from me and the doctor had to support me as I started to fall over.

Even though the exam was brief and far from comprehensive, the surgeon had seen enough to form an opinion based on the results and the MRI he already had. He told me that while my gait seemed ok, as soon as my system was stressed at all (for example by walking on my toes), it was clear that my nervous system was being compromised by the Chiari and the syrinx. Knowing this, we quickly turned to a discussion of what to do about it (which will be addressed further in the next chapter).

Cine-MRI (Phase-Contrast MRI)

MRI technology has revolutionized medicine in general, not just the diagnosis of Chiari. Because of its wide-ranging uses, vast amounts of time and money are spent each year in trying to improve both its accuracy and capabilities. One by-product of all this work, which applies directly to Chiari, was the development of phase-contrast, or cine-MRI, which allows for the visualization of the flow of cerebrospinal fluid. Thus, cine-MRI can be used to determine if a Chiari malformation is blocking the natural, back and forth flow of CSF between the brain and spine and by how much.

What It Is

Cine-MRI uses the same hardware as a regular MRI, meaning the actual machine is no different. However, the operator will program the MRI a little differently and the computer that generates the image(s) will interpret the data it receives differently in order to show the movement. The technical details of how this works are beyond the scope of this book.

The Experience

From a patient's point of view, the experience is the same as undergoing a regular MRI.

Do You Need It?

Cine-MRI is quickly becoming a standard test for Chiari diagnosis, especially among University based surgeons, but there is still a question as to its value. As mentioned in the discussion on what Chiari is, once it was determined that the traditional definition of Chiari (greater than 3mm-5mm of tonsillar descent) may not be valid, doctors looked for additional information to aid in the decision making progress.

At first, cine-MRI looked to fit the bill perfectly as it could clearly show whether CSF flow was disrupted. However, research has not really shown, from a clinical point of view, what benefit it brings to patient outcomes, and some surgeons – at least privately – question its value.

One way to think about the value of cine-MRI is to consider in what situations this information may change a doctor's opinion or course of action. Along these lines, one private practice neurosurgeon (neurosurgeons not associated with a university generally do not conduct a lot of research and tend to be more conservative in both their approach and their use of new technology) told Conquer Chiari that he sees value in this type of MRI only for borderline cases. In other words, in many cases even a regular MRI clearly shows that there is not adequate room for CSF flow, and conversely many cases may clearly show normal space around the cerebellum. For cases which aren't so clear using regular MRI however, cine-MRI can show whether CSF flow is being affected.

Another situation in which cine-MRI adds value beyond an anatomical MRI is in looking at syrinxes to see if they are active. If the fluid in a syrinx is under pressure, research has shown that it vibrates with every heartbeat, which is clearly visible using cine-MRI. In contrast, often after decompression surgery the fluid in a syrinx will no longer move or vibrate with the cardiac cycle. Although this has not been studied extensively, presumably a syrinx in which the fluid is pulsing with every heartbeat is more likely to expand and become worse than one that is not reacting in this fashion.

While the clinical value of cine-MRI may still be open to debate, it has proven to be a valuable tool in the research arena. Although quantitatively measuring CSF flow can be tricky, there is active research in this area to determine if there are specific CSF flow characteristics unique to Chiari patients, which in turn could be used to make clinical decisions.

Other Tests

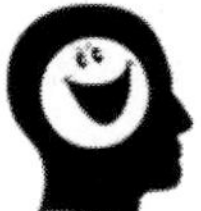

You Gotta Laugh! While traveling to St. Petersburg to get yet another consult from a neurologist, my 13 year old daughter, (who is diagnosed with a syrinx on the T 7-11), and I were talking about a wide variety of subjects. She suddenly inquired of me, did I know that cat skins emit radiation? I immediately thought of her Manx cat Peachy, who we adopted as a stray.

I replied, "How can that be? I have never heard of such a thing, and how would she have ever been in contact with radiation as she is always inside? And if that is the case, she needs to stop sleeping with you."

She looked at me funny and asked "Mom, what are you talking about?"

I said, "Peachy [the cat], it doesn't make sense about this radiation, where did you hear that?"

She started to laugh hysterically and said "CT scans mom."

Beyond the basic MRI and neurological exam, there is no precise list of medical tests which every Chiari patient should have. Some doctors will order X-rays and/or CT scans, others won't. Largely, the types of tests depends on the path a specific person takes to a final diagnosis; and often, the specific tests are a result of the type of doctor being seen and the primary symptoms that started the ball rolling.

For example, a person with fullness in their ears and balance problems may see a specialist who does a variety of hearing and vestibular testing prior to an

MRI. Similarly, for a person suffering from neck pain and tingling in their arms and hands, a physiatrist (a doctor of physical medicine) may order what is known as an EMG to check the function of the nerves in that area.

Basically, the way the US medical system is set up, each type of medical specialist tends to rely on certain types of tests and will look for the most common problems in their field of expertise. This is an important point for patients to understand, especially as it relates to a poorly understood condition like Chiari. Namely, that a physician's view of what Chiari is is often based largely on the type of doctor they are, and whatever limited direct experience they have with it.

In other words, an orthopedic surgeon may be familiar with Chiari related scoliosis, but may not be aware that Chiari can cause problems with swallowing, breathing and even sleep apnea. Similarly, an eye doctor may have seen eye related symptoms associated with Chiari during their career, but is likely not aware of current treatment options.

Recognizing that the way the medical system is structured, with narrowly defined specialists, means that it is virtually impossible for every doctor to be knowledgeable and current on conditions such as Chiari, can save a lot of frustration. While it is understandable that patients want whatever doctor they are seeing to have all the answers, this is simply not realistic.

Even with specialists that one would expect to be familiar with Chiari, such as neurologists and neurosurgeons, patients need to be cognizant of how each doctor's background may influence how they view Chiari and how they deliver a diagnosis. For example, many patients have reported being told by neurologists that while the MRI showed a Chiari malformation, that Chiari doesn't really cause any problems and is benign. Others have reported that neurologists have told them that yes they have a Chiari malformation, but there is nothing that can be done about it, so they should just learn to live with it.

This is not to pick on or denigrate neurologists. There are many neurologists who are very current in their understanding of Chiari, however because Chiari is (at this time at least) fundamentally a surgical problem, neurologists – who treat problems medically – have a different view of it than neurosurgeons. By their very nature, doctors will tend to focus on things they can effectively treat, which is why for Chiari most people end up seeing a neurosurgeon.

Neuropsychological Evaluations

One area of testing which would really benefit Chiari patients if it were used more often is neuropsychological evaluations. NPEs, as they are known, encompass a wide variety of tests to determine if there are any cognitive or emotional problems due to a neurological cause. In general, an NPE is administered by a high-level professional, can take several hours, and can be very expensive, which is likely one reason they are not routinely used.

However, when administered properly, NPEs are sophisticated tests based on a large amount of scientific evidence and can be used to pinpoint specific functional problems.

As discussed in the previous chapter, there is growing evidence that Chiari can have a negative effect on the cognitive functioning of patients, and there is even stronger evidence that many Chiari patients suffer from mood and anxiety problems. Unless these issues are clearly identified and diagnosed, they will be left untreated and can potentially limit patient outcomes.

Identifying cognitive and emotional problems is especially important for young and school-aged children with Chiari. While school teachers and administrators are likely to be unfamiliar with Chiari, they will be more familiar with how to handle any developmental or learning problems that may be associated with Chiari. It is important for parents to recognize that there may be these types of issues and to address them in terms that a school is familiar with.

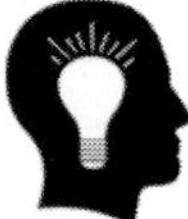

Practical Tip: If you have a child with Chiari, you should research and understand your rights when it comes to their education. Find out what the process is to have your child evaluated through the public school system and negotiate a plan of action with the school. Numerous resources can be found on the web to help parents with this.

Genetic Tests

Chiari is often diagnosed in early adulthood when people are either starting or beginning to plan families. As such, one of the primary concerns of any parent, or future parent, is will my children get Chiari? Will they have to go through what I have gone through?

Similarly, parents who are not affected often have the same question when their child is diagnosed with Chiari. Will they have to worry about their children getting Chiari?

As discussed in the previous chapter, there is some evidence that there may be a genetic component to Chiari. This means that evidence from families with multiple members who have Chiari indicates that some percent of the cases (how big or small a percent is not known) may be hereditary in nature. Based on this, most people want to know if there is a Chiari gene and if there is a genetic test to see if someone will develop Chiari.

While there is active research in this area, the gene, or more likely genes, involved in any proposed Chiari hereditary transmission have not been identified, and as such today there is no genetic test. It is also important to keep in mind that even if a genetic test were developed, environmental factors during a person's life may turn out to play a large role in whether symptoms develop and how severe they may become, which would limit the usefulness of such a test.

Reacting to the Diagnosis

In general, people react in one of two ways to being diagnosed with Chiari. For people whose symptoms came on suddenly, the diagnosis can come as quite a shock, and the thought that there is something seriously wrong is difficult to comprehend. Someone who was healthy and active may have trouble accepting that they face a serious medical issue.

In contrast, for people who have struggled for years to find out what is wrong with them, and have been told over and over it's all in their head; a final diagnosis can become a watershed moment with strong feelings of relief and vindication. Their long-held belief that something was wrong is validated and there can be a sense of victory over those who doubted them.

Interestingly, there is anecdotal evidence that some people experience a rapid worsening of symptoms after they are diagnosed. There are a couple of reasons that this could occur. First, it could be that they only began to seek medical attention when the symptoms were entering a more severe stage and the deterioration would have occurred independent of a diagnosis.

But, it is also possible that there are psychological factors that are brought into play by the diagnosis itself. Once someone is made aware they have a disease, it is possible they become more in tune with what is going on with their body. This can mean that symptoms that were in the background prior to a diagnosis are brought to the forefront and even amplified by a sense of hyper vigilance. It is also possible that the mind-body connection is such that there is a mental letdown as the significance of the diagnosis sinks in and with this comes a corresponding physical letdown.

Another common response people have to being diagnosed is to try to connect every single symptom they have (or sometimes have ever experienced) to Chiari. In other words, people will wonder whether this pain or that peculiarity is due to Chiari. While this may be one way in which the mind tries to get a handle on the Chiari diagnosis, or perhaps a need for validation that the symptoms are real, it can also become a distraction and interfere with patient-doctor communication.

Patients often get frustrated because they expect their doctor to listen to every symptom they have and discuss how it relates to Chiari. Unfortunately, this is an unrealistic expectation, and from a clinical point of view the doctor only needs to understand the most troublesome symptoms (much like the neurological exam does not need to include every possible test). This is one case where the patient can help themselves by realizing that they don't need external validation of all their symptoms. Symptoms are inherently subjective, so if you are experiencing a symptom it is real.

Given the broad array of symptoms that Chiari can cause, it is also difficult to say whether a given symptom is "due" to Chiari, and it is even harder to say if it will get better with treatment. As was discussed in the previous chapter, the situation is further complicated by the fact that if someone has been suffering from Chiari symptoms for years, second-order symptoms can develop, which aren't normally attributed to Chiari, but can be a result of life-style changes due to Chiari. Teasing out what is due to Chiari, what may be a second-order symptom, and what may be a normal ache and pain can prove to be an exercise in frustration, and often not worth the effort.

Parents of young Chiari patients may be especially hard hit by the actual diagnosis. The resulting emotional turmoil comprised of fear, anger, and even guilt that they might have done something to cause this, can bring overwhelming stress into the family dynamic. The thought of surgery on a young child, and not knowing what the future will bring becomes a living nightmare for parents.

"I felt like I had been hit by a truck. I was totally unprepared for it. I thought the whole thing was handled poorly and for a whole month I was in a daze...I'm trying to wade through all the information. I could think about nothing else, I was completely consumed. I kept thinking, how I am going to let them open up his skull? How could I get through it...[he] was going around saying, 'I have to have surgery and I could die.' Every time I heard that I cried. It was really hard because he's only 7 years old... I was a wreck." ~Nancy~

For both adult and pediatric patients, the Chiari diagnosis is an extreme event, and while it was discussed in the Introduction, it is worth repeating. The time immediately following diagnosis is a whirlwind of confusion, emotion, and medical jargon. While people are trying to come to grips with what has occurred they are also faced with the stark reality of having to make major decisions either for themselves or their children.

Adding to the confusion is the general lack of awareness regarding Chiari. When most people are diagnosed, they have never heard of it and have no idea what it is or what to expect. So in addition to having to deal with the emotional shock of an illness, they immediately must try to educate themselves.

This lack of awareness extends to family, friends, business associates, and schools as well, which makes the step after being diagnosed all the more difficult. That step, of course, is telling others.

Telling Others & Talking About Chiari

"My Chiari story differs according to my audience. It isn't as though any version is incorrect, but where my narrative starts, what it focuses on, and how much emotional content I let it convey depends on many factors." ~Sue~

Sue, like many Chiari patients, has developed her own strategy for telling other people about Chiari, and her strategy is a good one. One thing every Chiari patient must face is how and when to tell other people. The first time a newly diagnosed patient tells someone they have Chiari is likely to be filled with emotion driven by shock and fear of the unknown. However, once the reality begins to sink in, people realize that this situation, namely deciding who to tell and how much to reveal, is one which will be faced over and over for many years to come. Each person must decide who to tell at work, in social circles, etc. Parents much decide who in their children's lives needs to know: principals, teachers, coaches, dentists...the list goes on.

Obviously, there's no right or wrong answer to how to tell someone about Chiari, especially a loved one, but based on the experiences of other patients, there are some steps which can be taken to make the job easier.

The first thing to remember is that 99% of the general public (this is not a scientific number) don't know what Chiari is, so the job of telling someone about a diagnosis by default includes educating them, to varying degrees, about Chiari. Each person must be their own Chiari ambassador, and they should not resent this fact. Some patients get angry at people for not knowing about Chiari, but this is likely misplaced anger. There is no reason for most people to have heard of Chiari, and it is only through positive action that awareness will spread.

This is where Sue's approach comes into play, because there are many different audiences for the Chiari story, and they don't all need, or want, to hear the same thing. A close friend may be willing to listen to symptom details or the emotional turmoil of facing surgery, but this may be inappropriate for a work colleague who is just curious why someone has been absent. Either way, each is an opportunity for a patient to spread the word about not only himself, but Chiari in general.

Each person has their own story, so in turn must develop their own method and style of telling others. However, listed below are some tips to consider when dealing with this inevitable task.

Practice a short explanation

In the business world, entrepreneurs (those starting their own business) are told to develop what is known as an elevator pitch about their company and product idea. The concept is that they should be able to convey the general idea in the time it takes to ride an elevator in an office building. To get comfortable telling people about Chiari, develop a short, elevator explanation and **practice it**. Try different phrases on people to see what works and what doesn't, and don't be shy about practicing it in front of a mirror over and over. There may be times when explaining Chiari in a clear, concise manner is very important (such as an employment situation or to a teacher, dentist, etc.). A sample elevator explanation may be, *"Chiari is a serious neurological problem where part of the brain (point to the back of your head) ends up crowding the top of spinal cord causing all kinds of problems."* This short explanation actually conveys a good deal of information and allows people to begin to frame a mental picture of Chiari. It tells people that Chiari is neurological in nature, that it can be a serious life event, and if you remember to point it even tells people where the problem area is.

The explanation can of course be extended to create different, longer versions which can be used when there is more time. The key, just like any public speaking, is to be prepared and practice. The more you practice, the easier it will become, the more natural it will sound, and the more effective you will be in getting your message across.

Don't use medical jargon

Once you have the basics down, it's easy to slip into med-speak and throw out words like foramen magnum and CSF flow. However, this is not a good idea. Try to remember what it was like when you first started learning about Chiari and how confusing all the new words were (or still are). Don't try to sound like a neurosurgeon, using plain English when telling others about Chiari is much more effective.

Be prepared for common questions

As you gain more experience telling other people, you will realize that there are common questions people will ask. It is best to be prepared for these questions with short, factual answers. Being prepared will make you sound very knowledgeable, will keep people engaged, and will help spread awareness of Chiari, making life easier for both yourself and future patients.

Here are some common questions with short answers:

Q: How many people have it (most people, when first hearing about Chiari, will struggle to remember/pronounce the name and will instead use the pronoun it)?
A: We don't know for sure, but we think about 1 in 1,000 which means about 300,000 people in the US. It affects people of all ages.

Q: What are the symptoms, what does it do?
A: The most common symptom is a severe, disabling headache in the back of the skull which is made worse by exertion, coughing, sneezing, etc. However, it also causes a ton of symptoms like balance problems, leg weakness, trouble swallowing, etc., and eventually it can lead to paralysis (this lets people know that it's serious).

Q: How were you diagnosed or how did you find out you have it?
A: *Supply your own story here, but keep it short!!*

Q: How do they treat it?
A: The only real treatment is a very traumatic surgery where they create more room around the brain and spine. The surgery doesn't always take away all the symptoms and fails outright about 20% of the time.

Q: Wow, I've never heard of it…
A: I know, most people haven't, even a lot of doctors. Before MRIs it was difficult to diagnose. The lack of awareness is a real problem. People can go years before being properly diagnosed. But now that we've talked about it, you'll likely hear about another case in the next few months.

Obviously, these are just a few of the most common questions people are likely to ask. To effectively talk about Chiari with other people requires a commitment to understand the fundamentals yourself, so you can explain them to others.

Use comparisons that people are familiar with

One way to help talk about Chiari is to provide a frame of reference that people are familiar with. Interestingly MS, or Multiple Sclerosis, is a neurological disease which affects about the same number of people (estimates for MS range from 250,000 – 500,000 in the US) as Chiari, and the similarities don't end there. Many of the symptoms of MS are similar to Chiari, even to the point of Chiari being misdiagnosed as MS as mentioned previously. In addition, MS often strikes young adults just like Chiari and outcomes are widely variable, meaning that some people are mildly affected and some are completely disabled.

Obviously MS and Chiari, while similar, are different diseases and the comparisons should not be taken too far. One major difference is that MS is treated with drugs and Chiari with surgery, but perhaps the biggest difference is that virtually everyone has heard of MS and very few have heard of Chiari. But that's why it can be useful to compare Chiari to MS, because it provides a benchmark for people to begin to think about and understand Chiari.

If you're curious why MS is well known and Chiari isn't, one of the main reasons is that the advocacy groups for MS are extremely vocal, well organized, and have been active for decades. In fact, MS research gets a significant portion of the National Institute of Neurological Diseases and Stroke annual research budget, and MS advocacy groups were in no small part responsible for much of the overall increases in the National Institutes of Health (NIH) annual budget.

Say Chiari over and over

Chiari is a person's name, and many people are not good at remembering names. When talking about Chiari, try to work in the actual name several times so that it is likely to stick in people's minds.

Let the other person guide the discussion

Many people are uncomfortable talking about medical issues, especially of a personal nature. One way to alleviate this is by starting with the elevator explanation, and then letting the other person lead the discussion. So rather than dumping years of frustration and anger on one person in a 20 minute session, try to read what the other person is interested in. For example, one person may focus on the medical and scientific aspect and ask detailed questions about treatment and outcomes, while someone else may focus on the impact it can have on people's lives and families. Letting the other person be the guide in the type and amount of information that is given will greatly increase what they learn, and retain, about Chiari.

Don't be negative, be matter of fact

It's a fact of life that negativity, and especially anger, turn people off. Many people will tune out someone who is ranting, or venting a lot of emotion and anger. Unfortunately, it is also very natural for people with Chiari, especially if it took them years to be diagnosed or if they are severely affected, to have a lot of negative emotions associated with it. So while it may be difficult, it is also very important to not be negative when talking about Chiari. It is often best to just be matter of fact, or even understated. This way more information will be conveyed in a clear manner.

It's also a fact of life that people like, and respond to, fighters. They want to see people persevere through adversity and show resolve and a determination to win. People most of all want to hear that someone will be ok; that it's a tough break but they'll get through.

In general, people don't want to hear how difficult it can be to get out of bed, or get through a day of work or parenting, or how the pain is so all consuming.

This can be true even among close friends and family. It doesn't mean they're callous and don't care, it just means they don't know how to handle something like that. It is difficult to hear about someone's pain and suffering, especially a loved one, and not be able to do anything to help.

Obviously, people need to be able to vent their emotions and express their anger and frustration. It is just important to carefully consider who to do this with. Before unloading emotionally on someone, be sure they are ready, and willing, to take the load.

Be prepared for, "My sister's cousin had..."

It is human nature to try to relate to what someone is saying; in fact in one sense that is the basis of communication. Because of this, people often respond to being told about Chiari with some medical story of their own. It may be a bad back, or it may be some surgery that some friend or relative had. It really doesn't matter, it's just a natural response. While the story may seem completely irrelevant and nothing like Chiari, it is best to ignore this fact when talking about Chiari. If it provides a way for people to relate, and if it keeps them engaged, all the better.

Don't judge how other people react

This may be the single most important piece of advice when it comes to talking about Chiari with others. Don't judge how other people react to what you are saying. While some people may seem very empathetic and immediately show insight into the Chiari struggle, many won't and will end up saying strange and inappropriate things.

This does not mean that they are saying these things to be malicious, it is often more likely the case that they just don't know how to handle what they are hearing. Disease is an uncomfortable subject for many people, and their stress response to it may come across in a negative way. If, as a patient, you take it as a personal insult, you are letting Chiari interfere with relationships just when you need them the most. Give people time to digest what they are hearing and don't place any expectations on what they may or may not say when initially told about Chiari.

Many patients report that they feel alone because no one seems to understand what they are going through. This is true at the most fundamental level; it is impossible to really understand how much pain someone is in or how hard it is to do certain activities, but this does not mean people don't care. If someone is empathetic and can offer emotional support all the better; but if they say the wrong thing, is it really worth getting upset over? Save your strength and redirect it in a positive direction. When the time is right, take the time to educate and make people aware. Until then, sometimes it is best to look inside for validation, no one knows what you're going through like you do.

Awareness sheets

Conquer Chiari has developed single page Awareness Sheets to help people tell others about Chiari. These pdf files are great for emailing to friends and family, or for taking to meetings with teachers and even doctor appointments. They provide a simple description of Chiari (or syringomyelia) along with some key facts and have been used by thousands of people in the Chiari community. The sheets can be found on the Conquer Chiari website at:

http://www.conquerchiari.org/awareness/awareness%20education%20sheets.htm

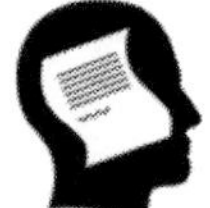

Personal Experience: I remember (sort of) the first time I told someone I had Chiari. I had just been given the results of the MRI and I had no idea what Chiari was or what it would mean, but I remember wondering how I was going to tell my wife. Our first child was only a couple of months old and thinking about the future was like standing on the edge of the abyss and looking down.

Since that time, and over the ensuing years, I've lost track of how many times I've told people about Chiari. Now, there is no anxiety when I talk about it, no embarrassment or discomfort, just an attempt to pass on some bit of information which will stick in a person's mind; an opportunity to educate one more.

It wasn't always like that. Beyond my family, I didn't really like to talk about it with anyone else. I literally hated the thought that people might feel sorry for me or take pity. I also didn't like the thought of people thinking of me in any way different than their original impression. I was used to being strong and capable and I was not adjusting well to not being able to do things.

Some of my reluctance came from the incredibly inappropriate things people would say in response. When I told my boss I was putting in for short-term medical leave and why, he stammered for a second, then mumbled, "Well, they're doing wonderful things in medicine these days." When I told a co-worker I was going in for brain surgery, they just nodded and asked if I was still going to some party that Friday.

Despite this, I eventually made the decision that not talking about it was unproductive. I was in the restroom at a restaurant when a guy came stumbling in, apparently from the bar. As he stood next to me, he blurted out, "Hey, what's that scar?"

At first I cringed. It was late in the day, I was tired and my head hurt. The last thing I wanted to do was try to explain to some drunken buffoon the nuances of Chiari. But then it hit me, why not? Why not take the opportunity? He was interested and in one sense a captive audience.

So, I started with a simple explanation (thus began the elevator explanation) and let him ask a few questions, which to my surprise were reasonably intelligent.

For that moment on, I decided if people asked I would answer. Now, of course, it goes further than that; I often talk about it whether people ask or not. When people ask me what I do for a living, I have an opportunity to talk about Conquer Chiari and how Chiari affects so many people.

I can understand why some people don't like to talk about it, I was in that place; but I would also encourage them to try. It's a simple choice really, talk about it or try to avoid it. If you choose to talk, the tips above worked for me, I hope they work for you as well.

The Incidental or Asymptomatic Diagnosis

While the widespread use of MRIs has revolutionized the diagnosis and treatment of Chiari, it has also created a new type of Chiari patient, if that's what you can call it, and muddled the diagnostic picture somewhat. MRIs can be ordered for many reasons, and the sheer number of scans performed each year has led to a new phenomenon, the incidental, or asymptomatic, Chiari diagnosis.

Some people, who don't really have what could be considered classic Chiari symptoms, are found to have significant tonsillar herniation on MRI. And it turns out this is not a rare event. Research has shown that what can be considered the normal position of the cerebellar tonsils is actually more like a range from above the foramen magnum to a couple millimeters below. The most striking example of the potential for confusion in this regard comes from a study of over 10,000 MRIs which found that fully 30% of people with tonsillar herniations of 5mm or more (the classic definition of Chiari) exhibited **no** Chiari-like symptoms; they were symptom free. As a side note, findings such as from this study has also led some physicians to inaccurately generalize that Chiari is benign and nothing to worry about.

An incidental Chiari diagnosis can mean one of two things. It can mean that the person in question is not yet symptomatic, but may develop symptomatic Chiari at a later time…or it can be a reflection of how tonsillar descent is not a good definition of Chiari (as discussed in Chapter 2) and the person will never become symptomatic.

Unfortunately for patients, it is not easy to tell which is the case. There is very little research on whether people with an incidental diagnosis ever become symptomatic.

An experienced physician can provide a judgment to the patient on whether their anatomy, such as the size of their posterior fossa and the space for CSF to flow is consistent with Chiari or not, but this does not always provide a sufficient level of comfort for patients.

"The neurosurgeon's words were clear enough, "Your daughter has Asymptomatic Chiari."...we didn't know how to react! We had prepared ourselves for getting details about decompression surgery... Now, we were hearing news we weren't quite sure was good news or bad news". ~ Bruce~

An incidental diagnosis can be very unsettling for patients. With a definitive diagnosis, something can be done, however unpleasant the experience. With this type of diagnosis, the pain comes from not knowing what the next day will bring. The anticipation of future problems may always lurk in the back of the mind.

This can be especially troubling for someone who has some symptoms, but who is told that they are not likely due to Chiari. They then must decide whether to consult more doctors to get more opinions and are still facing the prospect of not knowing what is wrong.

Because of the lack of knowledge regarding a clear definition of Chiari, an incidental diagnosis is a mixed bag for patients. On the one hand they likely will not undergo a traumatic surgery; on the other hand, the seed is planted in their mind that they may have a health time-bomb ticking away inside their head.

Slit-like Syrinx

The problems associated with an incidental diagnosis can extend to syringomyelia as well. It turns out that if you put enough people into an MRI, you will find that some will actually have evidence of a syrinx, even though they don't have any symptoms. Just as with Chiari, the problem arises, are they just pre-symptomatic, or will they never have a problem.

In 2002, Dr. Ulrich Batzdorf - a somewhat legendary neurosurgeon in the Chiari world - examined this phenomenon and proposed that there are a set of people which have what he calls slit-like syrinx cavities. He defined the slit-like syrinx cavity as being narrow in width, not accompanied by factors that disrupt CSF flow, like Chiari, and generally asymptomatic in nature.

To support his claim, Batzdorf looked at the medical and imaging records of 32 patients, with slit-like syrinxes, who had been seen between 1992 - 2000. On average the syrinxes were less than 2mm wide, and in no case was the spinal cord enlarged due to the syrinx.

Neurological exams were completely normal for 12 patients, while 20 had minor sensation or motor related findings. There were no indications of many of the signs that are normally present in syringomyelia.

The patients were tracked for an average of 38 months and were evaluated with follow-up MRIs and neurological exams. Follow-up MRIs showed that not a single cavity changed in size during the 3 years. Similarly, follow-up neurological exams were uneventful.

Batzdorf believes that the slit-like syrinx cavity is not actually a syrinx, but is a remnant of the central canal which is visible on MRI in some people. The central canal is the very center of the spinal cord. When we are children, it is like an open tube, but as we age, it collapses and becomes closed off. Early theories on syrinx formation held that CSF flow was blocked by a Chiari and flowed back into the central canal from the brain. However, this has since been shown not to be true since the central canal is closed in most adults.

However, Batzdorf believes that in some people, the canal doesn't collapse completely, and thus can look like a thin syrinx on an MRI. Supporting this concept is a study by Petit-Lacour of 794 MRIs, which found that 1.5% of the images showed a visible central canal, with cavities ranging in diameter from 2mm - 4mm.

Whether it involves Chiari or syringomyelia, without a clear theory of how and why people become symptomatic, the incidental diagnosis will remain a confusing problem for patients.

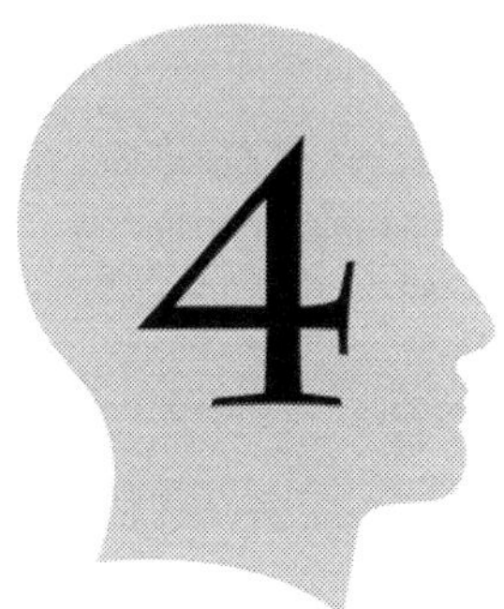

4 Treatment

Surgery, from the Greek, meaning "hand work"

~Wikipedia~

Little Agreement on Standard of Care

The first thing to understand about Chiari treatments is that there are very few options available to patients. The only real treatment is surgery (posterior fossa decompression), performed by a neurosurgeon, to relieve the pressure caused by the herniated cerebellar tonsils. By default then, absent surgery, the only other option is to wait and see what happens, monitor the situation with regular MRIs, and try to manage the symptoms. Although it seems like it should be a simple situation given there is really only one decision to make – whether to have surgery or not – the reality is it is not always an easy decision.

The difficulty in making the decision arises partly from the emotion that comes with facing brain surgery. While some people will do anything to relieve their symptoms, others have difficulty imagining going through such a procedure and will do just about anything to avoid it. However, overshadowing the emotional part of the equation is the second important thing to understand about Chiari treatments. Namely, that there is a lot of disagreement among doctors about when surgery should be performed and how to perform it. The disagreement ranges from profound fundamentals, such as some neurologists who don't believe Chiari is a problem at all, to when surgery should be recommended, to questions such as whether the dura should be opened as part of the procedure.

The upshot of all this is that patients are likely to hear different things from different doctors. Depending on your point of view, this may be good or bad, but either way it underscores the importance of an educated patient who can ask intelligent questions, understand what is being recommended and why, and select a doctor they are comfortable with.

A 2004 survey of neurosurgeons (Schijman & Steinbok) highlighted the wide range of thinking among practicing neurosurgeons when it comes to treating Chiari. For their survey, the researchers designed 25 multiple choice questions and also included hypothetical case studies. They distributed the survey to 246 neurosurgeons world-wide and received 76 responses. The responses represented a variety of countries including - but not limited to - the United States, Great Britain, Japan, Argentina, Mexico, the Netherlands, Australia, France, India, and Turkey.

The survey involved four hypothetical case studies, which were used to solicit opinions on when surgery is recommended, plus additional questions on the details of each surgeon's preferred surgical technique. The first two cases presented a range from an asymptomatic patient with a significant malformation, but no syrinx, to a patient with headaches, Chiari, and a syrinx.

Opinions on when to operate vary greatly among neurosurgeons.

As Figure 4-1 demonstrates, there is general agreement at the extremes (Case 1 and 2B) - namely don't operate if there are NO symptoms and NO syrinx, operate if there ARE symptoms AND a syrinx - but not much agreement in the middle grey areas (Cases 1A, 1B, 2, 2A).

In fact, for Case 2 (headaches, Chiari, no syrinx), the surgeons were almost divided down the middle with 46% saying they would operate, while the rest would either monitor or order further tests.

Interestingly, for the case with an asymptomatic patient with a syrinx (Case 1B), 75% of the surgeons surveyed would operate. The authors point out that this is in contrast with an earlier North American based survey which showed that many surgeons would choose to monitor a situation like this

The third hypothetical case (3, 3A, 3B) was designed to see when surgery would be recommended in the case of progressive scoliosis. More than half the surgeons would try to stop the progression using decompression surgery even if no syrinx were present, and if a syrinx were present, 97% of the respondents would operate.

Figure 4-1: Surgery Decision For Hypothetical Cases

Case #	Symptoms/Diagnosis	% Would Operate
1	7 yr old with no symptoms 12 mm tonsils- no syrinx	8
1A	w/ 2mm wide syrinx	28
1B	w/ 8mm wide syrinx	75
2	9 yr old with headaches 10 mm tonsils- no syrinx	46
2A	w/ 2mm wide syrinx	64
2B	w/ 8mm wide syrinx	90
3	11 yr old w/progressive scoliosis 12 mm tonsils- no syrinx	58
3A	w/ small syrinx	85
3B	w/ 6mm wide syrinx	97

A fourth case described an asymptomatic, 12 year old child with Chiari and a long but narrow syrinx. The family does not want surgery, and the surgeons were asked if they would recommend any activity restrictions. Surprisingly, almost half said they would not restrict activities at all, and only 19% said they would recommend avoiding contact sports. More than half the surgeons did say they would explain to the family the risks of not operating.

While the situation can be confusing to patients, the good news is that the neurosurgical community is aware that there is disagreement. The surgeons know what the specific areas of contention are and are working to develop a consensus on how to treat Chiari. However, until such a consensus emerges, it is important for patients to understand the areas of controversy so that they can help craft a treatment plan they are comfortable with and that suits their individual needs.

Finding A Neurosurgeon

"I asked physicians in the area who they would recommend if their patient had a weird neurological condition and the same person was mentioned several times so I went to him."~Susan~

The first step in getting proper treatment for Chiari is to find the right doctor. While many patients are referred first to a neurologist, given that the only real treatment for Chiari is surgical, Conquer Chiari recommends that patients see a neurosurgeon for evaluation.

Thus, the question becomes how do you find a good neurosurgeon? There are many ways to go about it, and below are some suggestions. Keep in mind these are just suggestions, you may decide to use all of them, use some of them, or not to use any of them at all. There is no right answer, but like anything else, the more work you put into it, the better the result is likely to be.

1. **Set emotion aside.** This can be extremely difficult to do, especially if the diagnosis has come as surprise, or if you have been told for years there is nothing wrong. However, this is an important decision, and a methodical approach to the matter can help. If necessary, recruit a family member to help you through the process.
2. **Establish your criteria.** Everyone is looking for something different. What is right for one person may not be right for someone else. Think through what YOU, as a patient, feel is important in a doctor. Some items to consider:
   a. *Location-* Are you willing to travel or would you rather stay local near your support system. Think about this carefully, traveling when you are going to have surgery can entail a lot of added effort.
   b. *University Based or Private Practice-* Oftentimes, people want to know where the research is going on. This is a perfectly fine approach, however, keep in mind there are many surgeons in private practice, who have not published research on Chiari, who are perfectly

capable of treating Chiari patients. Think through carefully what you want.

c. *Someone who does a lot of Chiari surgeries or a general surgeon?* Like (b.) above, some people are only comfortable with someone who does many Chiari surgeries a year, and that is fine. But if you don't want to travel, another measure of a surgeon's skill is how many surgeries they do a year of any kind. A very busy surgeon is likely a skilled one (because many people want to see him or her) and has also built up a wide base of surgical experience.
d. *Is bedside manner important?* Do you care more about the surgeon's skill, or his ability to be compassionate and listen to you, or a combination of both. There is no right answer, just individual opinions.
e. *With what you know about yourself, do you have a straightforward case, or a complicated one with multiple problems?* Someone with a "simple" Chiari and no other abnormalities may be comfortable with someone who does not focus their practice on Chiari. On the other hand, someone with a complex anatomy, or whose surgery failed the first time, might want to get an opinion from someone with a lot of Chiari experience.
f. *Insurance and cost-* The harsh reality is that most insurances won't pay (or will pay less) to go out of region/network. You have to weigh the costs of going outside of insurance (if you have insurance) against the benefits to you.

3. **Create a list of candidates.** This is the step where you create a pool of potential doctors to match against your list of criteria. You can build the list from a number of sources, including:
   a. The professional societies' websites often contain databases of doctors which can be used to find ones in certain areas. The AANS site, *www.neurosurgerytoday.org* can be searched by ZIP code to find board certified neurosurgeons in specific geographic areas.
   b. If you live near one or more Universities with medical schools, their websites will list neurosurgical faculty.
   c. Ask everyone you know, especially people in the medical community, who they would go see.
   d. Use the internet - refer to site in (3a.) - to identify surgeons and other doctors who do research on Chiari and SM.
   e. A lot of people use chat rooms and message boards to find doctors. I would offer a word of caution here. Be careful about getting doctor recommendations from message boards. People who have had good experiences with doctors may not necessarily participate in chat rooms, so while it may be good input, it should be considered in the context of all the information gathered.

4. **Create a short list based on your criteria.** Do what research you have to do to create a short-list of candidates. You can use the internet and phone to learn more and eliminate people from your list based on what is important to you. Or create multiple lists, for example doctors near by, or doctors you would see if you decide to travel.
5. **Do more thorough research on the doctors that made the short list.** Ask everyone again about these specific doctors. Have they published any research? Have they won any awards? Are they listed in America's Top Doctors?
6. **Compare your list (plus research) to your criteria list and make a prioritized list.** From this, you can set up appointments and see who you like.
7. **Trust Yourself.** When you meet with the doctor do you get a good feeling? Can you communicate with him/her easily? In the end you may have to trust yourself to this person. Can you see yourself doing that? If so, you probably have found a good doctor for you. If not, consider seeing someone else.

Don't let other people tell you who you should see. Do the work yourself; be smart and do your homework, only you can decide who's right for you.

"Though brain surgery can't help but be scary, much of my fear was obliterated by my doctor's expertise and bedside manner."~Nancy~

Tips on Communicating With Doctors

Once you have selected a doctor, it is important to get the most out of your healthcare. The best way to do this is to understand how to communicate with your doctor. The doctor-patient relationship is not always a good one and too many patients end up being angry and bitter towards their doctor and the medical community in general.

Since your number one goal is a positive health outcome, it is best not to get bogged down in poor communication and misunderstandings. If you end up complaining about your doctor visits and saying your doctor just doesn't understand there is a good chance you may not be happy with your outcome. In fact, some research has shown that the quality of the doctor-patient relationship can influence medical outcomes, or at least how patients perceive their outcomes.

With this in mind, following are some suggestions (based on a series of Editorials in Chiari & Syringomyelia News) for communicating with your doctor and maximizing your healthcare. While the relationship involves two people, you can only control yourself in this situation, so it is best to focus on what you can do to ensure smooth communication. After all, would you rather go the extra mile and have a positive experience (and hopefully outcome) or gripe about your doctor and the medical establishment?

There are 4 keys to getting the most out of your healthcare: know your doctor, establish goals before each visit, be a skilled patient, and do whatever you can to find care you are comfortable with.

1. **Know Your Doctor.** In order to maximize your benefit in any situation, you need to understand the people involved. Not just a superficial understanding either, but a deep understanding that comes from putting yourself in their shoes, understanding their background and experience, and understanding how they think. Above all, doctors are human, and like every other person bring a host of preconceptions and experiences to the table. Consider the following:
   a. The way doctors are trained today, it is their job to heal, not to be compassionate. They think deductively to identify a problem and fix it. At the same time, at the end of their extensive training, subconsciously - and necessarily - they are extremely confident in themselves and their abilities. This creates two problems in some doctors. First, many doctors aren't interested or even capable of dealing with their patients as a whole person. They focus on a narrowly defined, fixable problem. If a patient's family is falling apart because of an illness, the stress at home will likely aggravate his or her symptoms. Yet when the patient reports worsening symptoms to the doctor, the doctor doesn't see a 'medical' reason for the worsening symptoms and the patient's point of view is dismissed, thus souring the patient-doctor relationship. The second issue comes into play when a doctor encounters a problem he or she can't identify or fix. There are many doctors who do not handle this situation well; "I operated on you, the MRI looks good, you should feel better.", is the thought process. Consciously, or subconsciously, the doctor ends up blaming the patient for not getting better with the first treatment. This again, sours the relationship.
   b. Medicine is becoming more and more reliant on technology to make diagnoses. As this reliance grows, doctors are losing their skill at talking with patients. It is much easier to look at blood work or an image than it is to listen to a patient complain about every ache and pain.

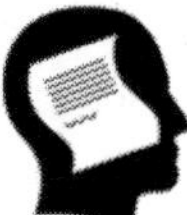

Personal Experience: I actually saw one doctor who sat with his back to me while he was asking why I was there. He didn't look me in the eye once during the entire visit!

c. A test is objective, whereas by definition a patient's report of symptoms is subjective. This is especially true with pain. Pain is purely subjective and can be very difficult to describe. Unless a doctor has personally experienced some type of severe, acute, or chronic pain, he probably doesn't have the context to really understand what a patient is reporting. At the same time, most patients have a strong need to connect with their doctor on a human level. After all, a patient has to place a great deal of trust in a doctor. This imbalance can leave patients feeling unvalidated and disappointed with their care.

d. Many doctors are under enormous financial, regulatory, and time pressure. Medicare reductions, soaring malpractice premiums, and insurance paperwork have put a large burden on doctors. Doctors are forced to spend more time and energy thinking about their business and have less time and energy to focus on their patients.

e. The internet has fundamentally changed the patient-doctor relationship. While the wealth of readily available information has been a boon to patients, doctors have had to adjust to patients who want to speak the medical jargon and discuss the latest research. To be fair, it is easy to jump to conclusions based on something off the internet and a patient may go into an appointment with their mind closed and unwilling to listen. Naturally, some doctors handle this better than others. Some are willing to have a real discussion with patients and some probably feel threatened by the amount of information available.

f. Doctors are individuals. Some went into medicine to save the world, some for the scientific challenge, and some for the prestige. Some will rely only on tests and some will listen to their patients. Some will be empathetic and some will end up saying very callous things. Some will be willing to engage in a discussion with their patients and some will have an 'I'm the doctor' attitude. This is a fact. It is up to us, as patients, to identify what type of person/doctor we are dealing with in order to develop a proper strategy for managing our own care.

2. **Establish Goals for Each Visit**. It is important to remember that you as a patient have much more time to think about your situation than your doctor does. Chances are he or she will begin to think about your case 30 seconds before knocking on the door as your file is being reviewed. You, on the other hand, have the luxury of thinking about the doctor's visit for

days in advance. As patients, we should use this time wisely and decide on one - or two at the most - goals for the upcoming visit. Do you want to try a different medicine? Adjust the dose? Bring up a new symptom? Ask a question about your MRI? Whatever the goal is, keep focused on it during the visit. This is not an easy thing to do. Doctor's visits can go off in many different directions, but no matter what path it takes, if you have one goal in mind, you can always return to it at the end of the visit.

3. **Be A Skilled Patient**. What is a skilled patient? Clearly the doctor is in control during a patient-doctor encounter, but there are ways to manage the visit to ensure a positive outcome. Like any skill, getting what you want from healthcare takes practice and patience. Luckily - or not - for Chiari patients, most of us will have a lot of opportunities to practice:
   a. Choose a strategy - Since you understand how your doctor thinks, now you can choose a strategy that will maximize your interactions with him. If he relies on tests, don't waste time talking about your symptoms and focus on the tests. If you think the tests aren't telling the whole story, ask about the limitations of the test or complementary tests. Play into what the doctor feels comfortable talking about. Some doctors respond well to direct patient requests. If that's not the case, try leading the doctor subtly into certain subjects. Is your doctor open to you bringing up recent research and asking scientific questions? If so, use the internet to your advantage, but keep in mind the training and experience your doctor has.
   b. Stay focused - Most doctors - particularly surgeons - have to see many, many patients a day. Don't clutter up the visit with irrelevant information. Think about what you want to say and how you are going to say it ahead of time, so the information comes out in a way that is easy to understand. If you want to talk about symptoms, remember not every little ache and pain is important.
   c. Don't look for validation where it isn't - If you have a compassionate doctor that validates your feelings, you are lucky. But if you don't, it doesn't mean the doctor can't help you. If your doctor doesn't provide the validation you need, look for it elsewhere - from family, friends, other people with the condition, or most importantly inside yourself.

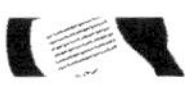

Personal Experience: I happen to have an excellent neurosurgeon and I am very confident in his abilities. But at the same time, I know he relies mostly on the MRI and his own observations and doesn't really want to hear about the lingering symptoms I may have. Why? Because they're not bad enough for surgery, so I just need to deal with them. It doesn't matter to me, he can still monitor my condition and take corrective action if necessary.

d. Stay in control - One of the key points in the hugely popular book, "The Seven Habits of Highly Effective People", is that you *can't* control how someone acts, but you *can* control how you react. Chances are high that when dealing with doctors over a period of time, a doctor will say or do something that will be very aggravating and frustrating. This doesn't have to ruin the situation. You can control how you respond to this. Think about your doctor's perspective, think about your emotional state, and remember they are people just like everyone else. It is a fact that you will get more out of your healthcare by checking your emotions at the door; that is simply the way it is. Obviously, this is not always easy to do.

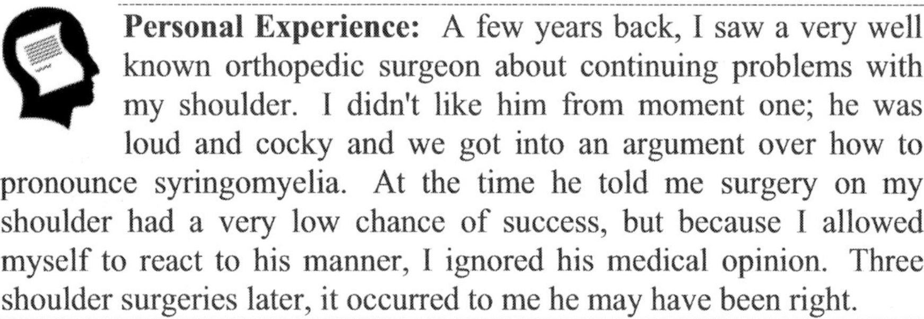

Personal Experience: A few years back, I saw a very well known orthopedic surgeon about continuing problems with my shoulder. I didn't like him from moment one; he was loud and cocky and we got into an argument over how to pronounce syringomyelia. At the time he told me surgery on my shoulder had a very low chance of success, but because I allowed myself to react to his manner, I ignored his medical opinion. Three shoulder surgeries later, it occurred to me he may have been right.

4. **Find Care You Are Comfortable With** - While in a sense medicine is a science, it is also still an art. Different doctors will approach the same situation differently. It is important to find a doctor that you are comfortable with. If one doctor is not working out, don't be afraid to look for someone else. It could make all the difference in the world.

A skilled patient has a strategy, is focused, and in control.

The Wait & See Approach

While most people associate surgery with Chiari, the reality is that the majority of patients who are evaluated for Chiari-like symptoms or tonsillar herniation do not have surgery right away. In fact, in casual correspondence several leading Chiari surgeons report that they only operate on between 25%-40% of the patients they see for Chiari. The rest fall into the wait and see category.

Sometimes the decision to pursue a wait and see approach is driven by the doctor. Reasons the doctor may advise against surgery include (but are not limited to): the patient's symptoms are not severe enough to warrant surgery, the symptoms aren't classic Chiari so it is not clear if the surgery will help, or the patient is not a good candidate for surgery due to other medical problems which should be addressed first.

Sometimes the decision to wait and see is driven by the patient. There are some people who have a difficult time with the idea of having surgery and choose instead to live with their symptoms. Whether they are afraid of complications or think they will be worse off, whatever their reasons, they would rather deal with the known, rather than the unknown.

In either case, the wait and see approach usually entails trying to manage symptoms and monitoring the situation with regular MRIs and doctor visits. Unfortunately, there is no standard for treating symptoms, and the treatments depend mostly on the specific symptoms that are most troubling. Certain medications can be used to try to relieve headaches, but in the end many patients end up adopting lifestyle changes to manage their symptoms. These modifications can range from restricting certain activities such as heavy lifting to major life changes such as a change in career or employment status.

There is also no standard for how often a person should be monitored with MRIs and doctor visits. Someone with few or no symptoms may be advised to just call if they experience anything unusual; whereas someone with significant symptoms who has chosen not to have surgery may be advised to have an MRI and check-up every six months to see if things are getting worse. There is not right or wrong answer as to how closely someone should be monitored, it is up to the individual and their doctor to strike a balance they are both comfortable with.

Alternative Treatments (Craniosacral Therapy)

Many people ask Conquer Chiari if there are any Alternative Medicine treatments for Chiari. The short answer is no. There is absolutely no scientific evidence that any type of complementary or alternative medicine is effective in treating the underlying problem of Chiari or syringomyelia.

This is not to say, however, that alternative treatments, such as acupuncture, can't be effectively used to treat symptoms. While it depends on the specific treatment, there is some evidence that certain alternative treatments can be useful in treating pain. However, even those treatments for which evidence exists of their effectiveness, do nothing to decompress the cerebellar tonsils or restore the normal flow of CSF.

It is also important to note that certain types of treatment, such as chiropractics, should not be pursued by people with Chiari. While this is controversial, and Conquer Chiari has heard from people with Chiari who claim it has helped, most physicians believe that chiropractics is not a good idea for people with Chiari and can in fact be dangerous. To this end, Conquer Chiari has also heard from patients whose symptoms became much worse after spinal manipulation. Because of this, patients are strongly urged to discuss this with their doctor before seeking chiropractic treatments.

Finally, one of the most commonly asked questions about alternative treatments is craniosacral therapy (CST). On the surface, craniosacral therapy seems like it would be a good fit for Chiari patients. Developed by an osteopath in the early 1900's, the foundation for CST is the rhythmic movement of the brain and spinal fluid. Therapists use an extremely gentle touch to manipulate the bones in the skull (cranium) and along the spine to the sacrum (tail) to supposedly release restrictions and improve the natural flow and rhythm of CSF.

However, CST is generally considered a sham by mainstream doctors and scientists, who believe its theories are groundless, there is no evidence of its effectiveness, and that practitioners are taking advantage of desperate people. Brid Hehir, a nurse/midwife, wrote in an opinion piece for the journal (*"RCM Midwives")*, "[CST] is disingenuous. Patients are being taken for a ride by people who, while being scornful of scientific medicine, seduce patients into believing they need to have sessions of worthless therapy...Parents can be vulnerable when it comes to their newborn babies, and will try any number of therapies [to help] an existing problem."

One reason CST is so controversial is that its underlying theories go against conventional medical knowledge. CST works under the assumption that the bones in the skull, which when we are born are not completely fused together, but joined by sutures, can be manipulated and that this manipulation will restore the natural rhythm of the brain and spinal fluid. The problem is that the skull bones fuse in childhood and most physicians believe can not be moved in adults.

A second problem with CST's theory is the notion of a natural rhythm of movement from the brain, down the spine to the sacrum. This is the heart of CST, because it is believed that restrictions of this rhythm lead to health problems and trained therapists can sense the rhythm and adjust it with gentle touch. As educated Chiari patients we do know that CSF moves rhythmically; however direct MRI imaging has shown that it moves in response to a person's heartbeat and breathing. This goes against CST's claim that there is a rhythm not attached to other bodily processes.

Although CST grew out of osteopathy, it has evolved and broadened to encompass a range of poorly defined techniques. As it has evolved, its claims have become somewhat outrageous. From the Craniosacral Therapy Association of UK's website, "Craniosacral therapy is a subtle and profound healing form which assists the body's natural capacity for self-repair.

In a typical craniosacral session, you will usually lie (or sometimes sit) fully-clothed on a treatment couch. The therapist will make contact by placing their hands lightly on your body and tuning in to what is happening by 'listening' with their hands. Contact is made carefully so that you will feel at ease with what is happening...*Treatment can aid almost any condition, raising vitality and improving the body's capacity for self-repair*."

Claims such as this, that CST can treat anything for everyone, attracted the attention of the Office of Technology Health Assessment at the University of British Columbia. In 1999, a team from this office, led by Dr. Green, undertook a review of the available published literature on CST in an effort to see if there was any merit to their claims. The researchers performed an exhaustive search of available databases using search terms such as craniosacral, cranial bones, cranial sutures, cerebrospinal pulse, and cerebrospinal fluid. What they found was very little evidence in support of CST and a pretty strong indictment against its theoretical basis. The research team identified 7 studies dealing with CST therapies and outcomes. Overall the studies were extremely poorly designed and presented little evidence of its success in treating patients. One study did find, however, that people with traumatic brain injuries were worse off after CST.

To summarize, there is no real evidence that CST works, and there are many warning signs that is a sham. Since this book is based on science, Chiari patients are advised to think carefully before pursuing CST.

Surgery

The technical name for Chiari surgery is *posterior fossa decompression*. The posterior fossa is the region of the skull where the cerebellum is situated and in this case, is the region of interest. Decompression refers to making more space and relieving the area which is compressed and under pressure.

The surgery is performed by a neurosurgeon, takes 3-4 hours depending on what all is done, and the patient is usually in the hospital for at least 2-3 days. Just as estimates for how many people suffer from Chiari vary, so do estimates of how many Chiari surgeries are performed each year. Estimates range from 3,000 to more than 5,000 just in the US each year, but these are just estimates and there is no official count.

There are two major goals of Chiari surgery. The first and foremost goal is to create more space around the herniated cerebellar tonsils and relieve the direct compression of the tonsils on the brainstem and/or spine. The second goal, which is really an extension of the first, is to restore the natural flow of CSF from the brain to the spine (and back).

After a successful decompression, it can be expected that the cerebellar tonsils will move up a certain amount and hopefully take on a healthier, rounded shape. In addition, if a syrinx is present, a successful surgery should hopefully result in a reduction in the size of the syrinx (not necessarily a total collapse) or at least prevent it from growing any larger.

Depending on a number of factors, Chiari surgery can be a big deal (to use a technical term). In an adult the trauma of the surgery itself, in that the muscles in the neck are cut, can be significant. Combined with the fact that patients have often been suffering from symptoms for years, and it's a procedure that should not be taken lightly. However, it should be noted that depending on what specific surgical techniques are used (see below) and if there are no complications, the surgery can be less traumatic today for certain patients.

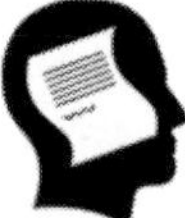

Personal Experience: As an active, fairly fit person I went into the surgery thinking it would be no big deal and I'd bounce back quickly. This was a mistake. It is major surgery and it is beneficial to be aware of that going in and plan accordingly.

Making the Decision

Before diving into the details of the actual surgery, it is worthwhile to spend some time on the decision to have surgery in the first place. After all, it could be one of the biggest decisions a person makes and it should be undertaken with careful thought and deliberation.

First and foremost it is important to realize that it is an individual decision and not one that someone else can make for you. Yes, many people will have opinions, some stated quite strongly, but in the end it is your body and your decision to make. The second thing to realize is that there is no objective measure or test to say when someone should have surgery. Rather, it is a complicated decision, with many factors, that is made in counsel with a, hopefully, trusted doctor.

Some of the major factors include:

- **Severity of Symptoms** – Obviously how severe a person's symptoms are is an important consideration. For someone with occasional, mild headaches the risk and trauma of surgery may not be worth it, but for someone with frequent, crippling headaches it probably is. Also, if symptoms are so severe that they endanger the patient by interfering with breathing or eating, they may necessitate surgery.
- **Symptom Progression** – Less obvious is whether symptoms are getting worse, or progressing. This can be difficult to evaluate, but if symptoms are progressing, especially rapidly, surgery may be required.
- **Neurological Signs** – Symptoms are inherently subjective and it can sometimes be difficult for a doctor to interpret what a patient is telling

them. However, neurological signs are objective. If there is evidence of cranial nerve compression or problems with the brainstem or spinal nerves which can be shown with a neurological exam then it is clear that the nervous system is compromised.

- **Syrinx** – For some doctors the presence of a syrinx along with symptoms is an automatic trigger to recommend surgery. One reason for this is because you can never tell when the damage a syrinx is causing will become permanent.
- **MRI, cine MRI** – Although not perfect, the MRI is the closest thing Chiari has to a gold standard test. The MRI can show whether the tonsils are compressed and abnormally pointy and also how much room there is for CSF to flow. However, an MRI is not usually the sole basis for the surgical decision.
- **Quality of Life** – It is also important to factor in how an individual's symptoms are affecting their overall quality of life. Are they interfering with their job, their daily activities and their personal relationships?
- **Patient's Desire to Relieve Symptoms** – In the end, for the patient it really boils down to whether Chiari is affecting them to the point where they are willing to undergo surgery in an attempt to get relief. This is an extremely personal decision, and people go about making it in different ways.
- **Surgeon's Experience and Judgment** – For the doctor, in the end their decision whether to recommend surgery (or agree to perform it) comes down to whether in based on their own experience and judgment, they think the potential benefits outweigh the risks.

Second, Third, and Fourth Opinions

Because the decision to have Chiari surgery is such a big one, many people seek second opinions (and third and fourth) before making their final decision. This is a reasonable approach, but before going down this road patients should realize that there is a good chance they will hear different things from the different doctors they see.

As discussed earlier in this chapter, research (and anecdotal evidence from patients) has shown that surgeons have a wide variety of opinions not only on when to recommend surgery but on the details of the surgery itself. If you are a person who wants to hear different opinions, weigh them against each other, and make an intelligent decision then you are likely to get this by seeking out opinions from different surgeons.

However, if you are a person who would feel overwhelmed by hearing different options and different views, then it may be better to stick with one surgeon, as long as you are comfortable dealing with that person.

In general, it is best to trust your instincts. If something you are hearing from one doctor doesn't sound quite right, or you can't picture yourself letting him/her operate, it is probably best to get a second opinion and see if you get a better feeling from a different doctor.

What is Done

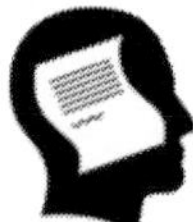

Personal Experience: The following is excerpted from the operative note in my medical records; the surgery was performed on 1/21/99. My personal memory of the OR is dominated by how cold it was when I was first rolled in, and how nice the heated blankets felt when I was finally situated on the table.

The patient was taken to the operating room where intravenous and inta-arterial lines were placed. General anesthesia was induced and the patient endotracheally intubated. Once the tube was secured, the Mayfield skull clamp was applied. The Foley catheter was placed. The patient was rolled into the left lateral decubitus position. The head position was fixed in the Mayfield head holder and the skin prepped and draped in usual fashion.

A linear skin incision was made and carried through the skin and subcutaneous tissue to the paracervical fascia. The paracervical fascia was incised with a cutting cautery. A midline subperiosteal dissection was performed. Self-retaining retractors were placed. The occiput was identified. Adhesions at the base of the foramen magnum were freed up. Craniotome was used to turn a small craniotomy flap in the suboccipital region. Measured that the patient would need 3.5cm to decompress. This was the distance that was taken.

The dura was opened. The CSF was under a good bit of pressure as were the cerebellar tonsils. The cisterna magna was drained. A dural graft was cut to length and sewed into place. Things were really quite nicely decompressed.

Meticulous hemostasis was achieved with bipolar cautery. Bone edges were waxed. The wound was thoroughly irrigated. Thrombin-soaked Gelfilm was placed over the dural defect. 2-0 Vicryl was used to close the paracervical musculature and paracervical fascia. The same was used for the subcutaneous tissue. Staples were placed on the skin. Evoked potentials were stable throughout.

This section will provide a brief, high-level overview of what Chiari surgery entails. Although it is not discussed until later in this chapter, it is important to understand that surgeons utilize a variety of different techniques to treat Chiari, so it is best to ask your surgeon specifically what he/she will do and why. For example, Chiari associated with hydrocephalus will almost always involve a shunt being placed to treat the hydrocephalus, and depending on someone's specific anatomy and how much bone needs to be removed, a cervical fusion may be required to provide spinal stability.

The following descriptions are not meant to be technical or all-inclusive. Rather they describe the most common techniques which are part of many Chiari decompressions. An individual surgeon may not utilize all of them depending on the situation and their personal preference. Additional surgical procedures are touched on briefly later in the chapter.

In addition, this chapter includes a series of sketches and pictures to help illustrate the Chiari surgery process.

As with most things, a picture is worth a thousand words, so perhaps the best way to get an idea of what Chiari surgery is about is to look at a video of an actual procedure:

http://www.or-live.com/memorialhermann/1327/ (surgery video)

The video clip is of Dr. Stephen Fletcher, a neurosurgeon at Hermann Memorial Hospital in Houston, performing a decompression on a child. Note, this site is not affiliated with Conquer Chiari and Conquer Chiari is not responsible for the content on this site.

In general Chiari surgery can be broken down into several steps:

Preparation– Perhaps the most noticeable part of patient preparation is shaving the hair to expose the back of the skull. How much is shaved will vary (see Tips for Women later in this Chapter). Unlike some brain surgeries, Chiari surgery requires general anesthesia, so patients are prepared accordingly. IV's are placed and presurgical medications are given. Once the anesthesia is administered patients are intubated – meaning a tube is placed down their throat to aid in breathing – and a catheter is placed. The patient is positioned for surgery (Figure 4-2) and the head is secured into place using clamps, (yes, they leave a mark).

Figure 4-2 Surgical Preparation

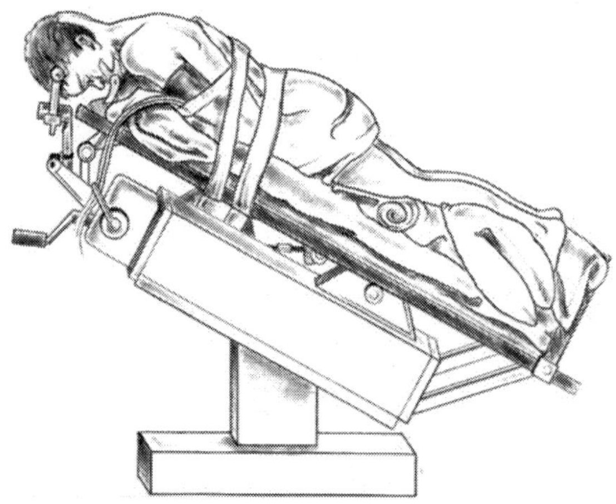

Incision– A straight line incision is made down the center of the back of the skull (Figure 4-3) from near the top down to the top area of the neck. The size of the incision may vary depending on how much bone the surgeon plans on removing. The muscle and tissue underneath are cut, pulled back and clamped to expose the skull.

Figure 4-3 Midline Incision

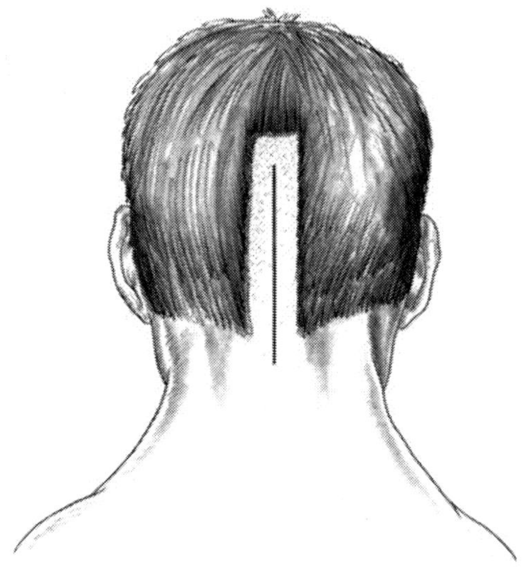

Craniectomy– Craniectomy is the technical term for removing part of the cranium, or skull. How much bone is removed will vary but 3cm-4cm vertically represents a typical amount. This is a major part of the decompression, the bone that is removed provides for more space around the herniated tonsils. A craniectomy combined with a laminectomy described below constitutes what is sometimes called a bony decompression (meaning that only bone is removed).

Laminectomy– With the cerebellar tonsils herniated into the spinal area, they are essentially compressed on one side by the bony vertebrae of the spine. For this reason, Chiari surgery usually entails a laminectomy, which refers to removing the back part of one or more vertebrae so that it is not compressing the tonsils. How many vertebrae are worked on depends on the size of the herniation. At this point, depending on the patient, some surgeons may choose to stop the decompression and close the incision.

Opening the dura– The dura is the outer covering of the brain and spinal cord and in many Chiari surgeries, the dura is opened over the cerebellar tonsils. The dura is cut and retracted in an upside down triangle shape (Figure 4-4). This allows access to the subarachnoid space and the cerebellar tonsils themselves.

Figure 4-4: After bone removal, the dura is opened

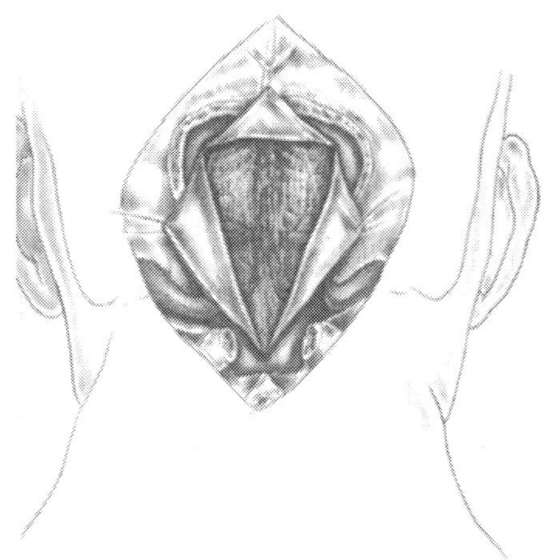

Intradural exploration– Once the dura is opened, surgeons may look for and remove adhesions and scar tissue which could be interfering with CSF flow. In addition, in some cases, surgeons choose to shrink the cerebellar tonsils using cauterization (heat) or remove them completely. This is known as tonsillectomy.

Duraplasty– After the surgeon is done working underneath the dura, a patch is sewn into the dural opening, which in effect expands the space underneath the dura and provides more room for the cerebellar tonsils and CSF (Figure 4-5). There are a number of different choices for the type of dural patch which can be used, including tissue taken from the patient's own body, dura taken from a cadaver, synthetic materials, and tissue taken from a cow.

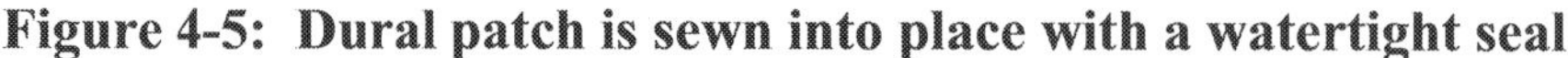

Figure 4-5: Dural patch is sewn into place with a watertight seal

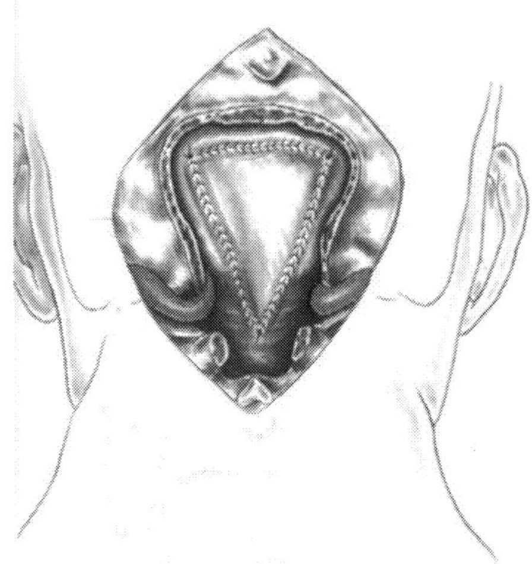

Chiari plate– Recently, some surgeons have begun inserting a plate (actually more like a metal grid) where the cranial bone was removed. Such a plate provides the muscles of the neck something to attach to. Without a plate, the muscles can attach directly to the dura. This can lead to headaches, because as the muscles are used they can pull on the dura underneath.

Dr. Bejjani, of the University of Pittsburgh, has put a video on the internet of a Chiari plate being put into place:

http://www.neurosurgery-web.com/Opening%20Page.htm

Closing– Finally, the surgical incision is closed in layers with the top of the incision usually being secured with staples. The staples run down the length of the incision giving the appearance of a zipper on the patient's skull and has led to the term "zipperhead" being used by some Chiari patients. (Figure 4-6)

Figure 4-6: Author's Surgical Incision Upon Discharge From Hospital

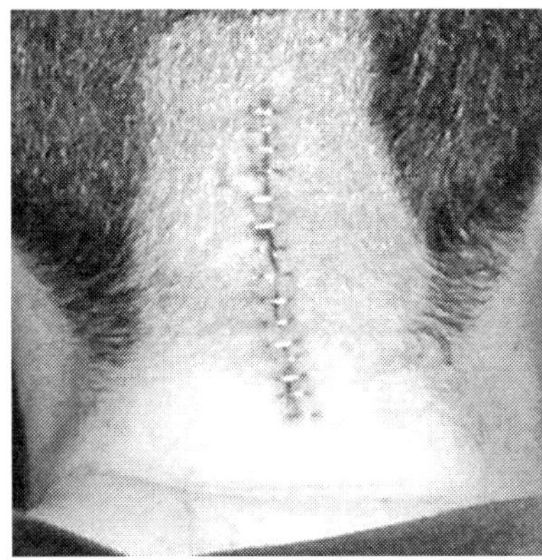

ICU– Immediately after surgery, most patients will spend some time in the Intensive Care Unit (ICU) of the hospital. The surgeon may instruct them to remain flat on their back for a specific period of time and the patient's breathing will be closely monitored. It is not usual for Chiari patients to require oxygen to help with breathing, especially the first night after surgery.

The ICU can be a quite a shock for family members as their loved one will likely be surrounded by machines and they may only have limited time for visitation (Figure 4-7).

Figure 4-7: Pediatric Patient In ICU Post-Surgery
Photo Courtesy of George Weir Photography

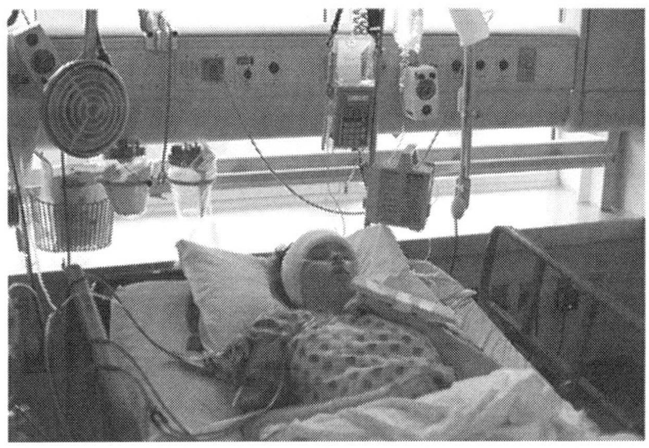

Leaving The Hospital– Depending on what was done during the surgery, for example whether the dura was opened, patients can expect to spend 2-3 days in the hospital after surgery before being discharged. If the dura was not opened, the hospital stay may be shorter. If there are post-surgical complications, obviously the stay may be longer.

Variations

As mentioned earlier in this chapter, there is no single standard for Chiari surgery. Rather, there are a range of techniques and options which neurosurgeons choose from based on how they were trained and their own experiences and preferences. Three major aspects of Chiari surgery where there is a real lack of consensus among the surgical community are:

1. Whether to open the dura
2. Whether to shrink or remove the cerebellar tonsils
3. What type of dural patch to use

The disagreement among surgeons was clearly illustrated by the same survey discussed earlier on when to recommend surgery. In addition to the hypothetical cases, the surgeons were also asked about how they perform Chiari surgery. As expected, these questions generated a wide range of responses. While 95% of the surgeons remove some of the skull as part of the decompression, the amount removed varied widely. When it comes to opening the dura, 76% of the respondents said they always open the dura, 20% said they sometimes open the dura, and 1% said they never open the dura. Detailed numbers on how many surgeons choose to shrink or resect the cerebellar tonsils were not provided, but preferences for dural grafts were. Specifically, thirty percent of the surgeons did report they prefer a graft from the patient, while 28% prefer to use a synthetic graft, 16% use a graft from a cadaver, and 6% still use material from a cow.

Opening the Dura

Whether to open the dura (the outer covering of the brain and spinal cord) during Chiari surgery is probably the most debated, and controversial, question. Those who advocate leaving the dura untouched - or not completely opening it - point out that cutting open the protective covering of the brain greatly increases the risk of complications, including CSF leaks, infections, and additional scarring of the dura itself. They believe that most of the benefits of decompression surgery come from removing the bone, both skull and vertebra, and that opening the dura is not worth the added risk. In fact, one study seemed to show just that; electrical tests during surgery showed that most of the decompressive effect on the brainstem occurred after the bone removal.

On the other hand, those who advocate opening the dura point out that one of the main goals of decompression surgery is to restore normal CSF flow and that there are often obstructions to this flow - from scarring and adhesions - underneath the dura. Their position is supported by several reviews which have showed that many failed surgeries are due to just such issues.

As if having two camps of surgeons weren't confusing enough, some surgeons have staked out a position in the middle by advocating approaches such as removing only the outer layer of the dura, or scoring the dura with small incisions that do not cut all the way through.

The topic was discussed in detail at the 2003 annual meeting of the Congress of Neurological Surgeons, where Drs. Ellenbogen, Muraszko and Mapstone reviewed the evidence both for and against opening the dura.

For the against side, they cited several studies which have shown fairly good surgical outcomes for either modified techniques, such as dural scoring or even no duraplasty at all. In two separate reports where just the outer layer of the dura was opened, a combined 8 of 10 patients were reported to have a successful outcome. Similarly, in one report of dural scoring, 7 of 8 patients with both Chiari and SM enjoyed symptom relief and a reduction in syrinx size.

In favor of opening the dura, the authors used Ellenbogen's own data, which showed that up to 40% of patients had extensive dural scarring which required opening of the dura to remove. In addition, up to 15% of patients had other types of obstructions to CSF flow under the dura. While the data is rather sparse, in studies which compared opening and not opening the dura directly, it appears that opening the dura results in a better success rate, especially in the long-term.

Opening the dura was also a hot topic of discussion at the 2007 UIC/Conquer Chiari Research Symposium, where it became clear that among pediatric neurosurgeons there is a trend towards not opening the dura. Several surgeons reported good results with leaving the dura intact for some patients, including shorter hospital stays and fewer complications. The emerging approach seems to be, to try a bony decompression first (at least for some patients) and if that doesn't work, to go back in and do a full duraplasty. With this approach, patient selection would seem to be the key, meaning that is likely that some patients can have a very successful outcome with the less invasive surgery. The trick, however, is to identify those patients.

It is also important to note that currently this trend is limited to pediatric patients. It is not at all clear if not opening the dura is viable option for most adult Chiari patients. As we age, the dura becomes thicker and scar tissue tends to build up, so it may be that leaving the dura intact will only be an option for children, but only time will tell.

Dural Scoring

Another emerging option is to manipulate the dura without completely opening it and sewing a patch in. One such technique involves scoring the dura with a number of shallow incisions. Another technique which has had preliminary success involves opening only the outer layer of the dura, but not cutting all the way through.

To examine whether this type of dura splitting technique is beneficial, Drs. Selden and Limonadi, at Doernbecher Children's Hospital in Oregon, designed a study which compared clinical outcomes, time in surgery, time in hospital, and costs incurred between a group of children with Chiari who underwent dura splitting as part of their surgery and a group of children with Chiari and syringomyelia who had a full duraplasty as part of their surgery. They published their findings in a November, 2004 supplement to the "*Journal of Neurosurgery*".

Over a period of approximately two years, the doctors operated on 24 children, 12 with Chiari only and 12 with Chiari and syringomyelia. The initial decompression was the same for both groups and involved removing a piece of the skull and part of the top vertebra. The group with syringomyelia also underwent a duraplasty, whereas the group with Chiari only did not. In the latter group, the top layer of the dura was split and the two sides were peeled back and sutured into place. This exposed the softer, underlayer of the dura, which was not punctured or opened in any way. Ultrasound was used during the procedure to ensure adequate decompression of the tonsils.

In order to track the clinical outcome of each group, the researchers carefully documented each child's neurological signs and symptoms before and after surgery. A score was assigned for each of the three primary signs and/or symptoms of each child: 2 = resolved; 1 = improved; 0 = unchanged; -1 = worse. The three numbers were then averaged to produce a single outcome score ranging from 2 (meaning all symptoms resolved) to -1 (meaning very poor outcome with every symptom worse).

After computing the outcome scores for each group, the scientists found virtually no difference between them. The syringomyelia/duraplasty group had an average outcome score of 1.53, while the Chiari/dura splitting group averaged 1.67.

The doctors did find, however, a significant difference between the groups in every other measure. The dura splitting group spent less time in surgery, in the operating room, and in the hospital overall. The costs incurred for the dura splitting group were also lower. On average, the duraplasty group spent a total of 249 minutes in the operating room and stayed in the hospital for 3.75 days. These numbers dropped to only 166 minutes in the OR and 3 days in the hospital for the dura splitting group.

Still Evolving

The techniques used during Chiari surgery are still evolving (which is a good thing), especially when it comes to the dura. In a paper published in February, 2007, surgeons from the University of Toronto described a simple modification to the standard duraplasty procedure.

In the traditional, and widely accepted, duraplasty, a Y shaped incision is made, the edges of the dura are pulled back and the patch is sewn over the opening. (Figure 4-8)

Figure 4-8: Standard Y Dura Incision

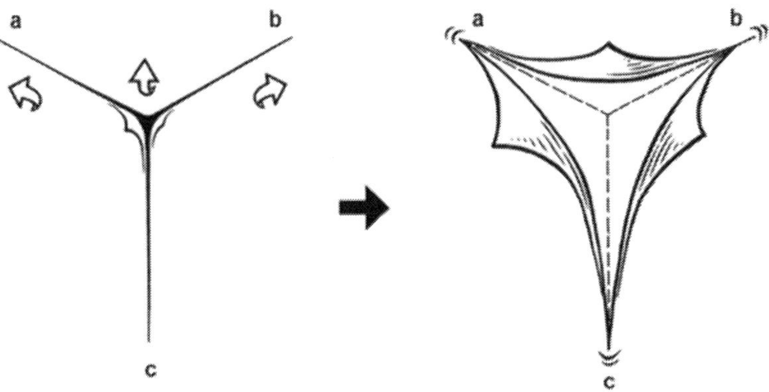

The variation described by the Canadian surgeons entails making two additional, angled cuts at the bottom of traditional Y incision (Figure 4-9).

Figure 4-9: Expanded Dura Incision

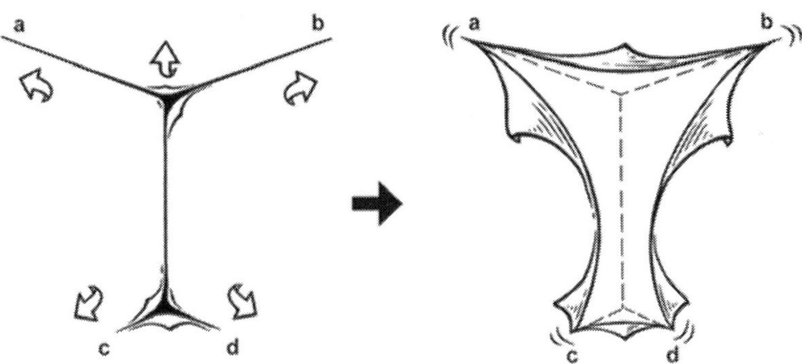

Source: Pirouzmand F, Tucker W. A Modification Of The Classic Technique For Expansion Duraplasty Of The Posterior Fossa. Neurosurgery. 2007 Feb; 60

Although the extra cuts are small, they allow the dura to be pulled open, or expanded, significantly more, especially at the bottom of the duraplastly. And as the surgeons point out, this area is right where the brain and spine meet and is where CSF flow is usually abnormal in Chiari patients. Thus, at least theoretically, creating more space there with an expanded duraplasty is a good thing.

Types of Dural Graft

The lack of consensus in Chiari surgery doesn't stop at the dura. The second major issue in which patients may confront a variety of opinions is what type of dural patch to use. Recall, that the goal of a duraplasty is to create more space for the tonsils underneath. This is accomplished by cutting open the dura and enlarging it by placing a patch into the opening.

Over the years, many different materials have been tried as dural substitutes, and today's surgeons have an array of choices, including:

- **From the Patient** – Many surgeons have begun to use tissue from the patient's own body for the dural graft. The tissue can be taken from a number of different places and has the advantage of eliminating any type of immune response to the graft. Some people also believe that this type of graft reduces the chance of infection. The downside, of course, is that there is another surgical site which needs to heal and may cause additional pain.
- **Cadaver** – Very popular a number of years ago, grafts from cadavers are being used less today because of safety concerns (see next section). Cadaver grafts can be made either from dural tissue directly or the pericardium, which is the membrane around the heart.
- **Cow** – Bovine grafts, such as DuraGuard (Synovis), are taken from the animal's pericardium.
- **Collagen** – Several manufacturers have recently come out with a new class of products known as collagen matrices. Collagen is a type of connective tissue which provides structure to body parts and has several advantages as the basis for a graft. Two of these grafts, Durasis (Cook Biotech) and DuraGen (Integra Lifesciences) both utilize animal collagen to form pliable, easy to work with grafts, which are actually absorbed by the body's tissue over a short period of time.
- **Synthetic** – Dural grafts can also be made from completely synthetic materials, such as Gore-Tex.

The basic question with dural patches is, does it really matter what is used? Surprisingly, there has been very little research published on this subject when it comes to Chiari surgery. However, at the 2007 UIC/Conquer Chiari Research Symposium Dr. Konstantin Slavin (UIC) presented the results of a randomized prospective study of 25 patients which compared two well-known graft products. One of the grafts required sutures to be put into place, while the other one did not.

Slavin evaluated the grafts on clinical outcome, complication rates, length of hospital stay and time in surgery.

Interestingly, there was no difference between the two grafts for outcome, complication rates, or length of hospital stay. Naturally, the graft which did not require sutures did result in shorter operating times. However, from this small study, and given the wide array of products on the market, it appears that choosing a graft really may just boil down to an individual surgeon's preference.

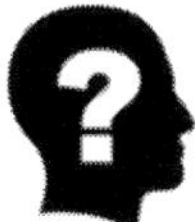

Did You Know? Dural grafts have been used for more than a century and have been based on a variety of materials. In the 1800's rubber and gold foil were tried (can you imagine?). These gave way to gelatin products in the first half of the 20th century and silicone later on.

Dural Patch Safety Issues

For all dural grafts, the spread of a virus or other type of infection from the graft to the patient is a serious concern. Human donors are screened for hepatitis B and C, HIV, and other diseases. Grafts that are derived from cow tissue (such as the collagen matrix DuraGen) are screened for evidence of Mad Cow disease and treated with powerful chemicals to kill viruses.

Unfortunately, the transmission of Creutzfeldt-Jakob disease (CJD), an always fatal neurodegenerative disease in humans similar to Mad Cow, has been documented in cases of human cadaver dural grafts. However, most of these cases occurred in Japan and were traced to a single brand produced before May, 1987.

The Centers For Disease Control in the US (CDC) has issued a number of reports on this topic. According to the CDC, between 1996 - 2003, the Japanese government identified 97 cases of CJD transmitted through a human cadaver dural graft. Of these 97… 93 of the affected patients received their grafts before 1987 and it is likely that the remaining four patients were given grafts produced before 1987. All but 11 of the grafts were traced to a single brand (LYODURA) - the brand could not be identified definitely in the other cases - and this manufacturer changed their procedures in 1987 to reduce the chances of CJD transmission.

While the effects of CJD are catastrophic, it is important to keep the relative risk in perspective. During the time period in question, there were over 100,000 LYODURA grafts used in Japan. Also, that specific brand was never intended to be distributed in the US, and very few have ever been used here. In 1997, a US Food and Drug Administration Advisory Committee recognized that using human cadaver dura carries an inherent risk for transmitting CJD, but went on to recommend that using such grafts be left to the discretion of the neurosurgeons, provided that the grafts are processed using acceptable safety measures. Interestingly, according to the CDC report an estimated 4,500 such dural grafts were distributed in the US in 1997, but after the FDA recommendation this number dropped sharply to only 900 in 2002.

Cerebellar Tonsils

The third major area of controversy in Chiari surgery centers around whether to manipulate the cerebellar tonsils. In this case, manipulation can range from reducing them in size through cauterization to cutting them out completely. A survey of pediatric neurosurgeons found that more than 30% favor some type of tonsillar manipulation. However, similar data for adults is not available.

Dr. Lazareff, a pediatric neurosurgeon at UCLA, is a proponent of tonsillar manipulation and has published research on a technique which relies predominantly on removing the tonsils as opposed to removing bone. According to Dr. Lazareff, most Chiari symptoms can be directly attributed to the displacement of the cerebellar tonsils into the spinal area. This fact, combined with the risk of slumping of the cerebellum if too much bone is removed, led Dr. Lazareff to explore whether a tonsillectomy alone would be a good alternative to the more standard bony decompression.

Lazareff's study involved 15 pediatric patients, ranging in age from 2 to 18 years, who all suffered from symptomatic Chiari malformations, while 8 had syringomyelia as well.

All of the children underwent surgery to remove the cerebellar tonsils with minimal (if any) bone removal. Dr. Lazareff and his colleagues first exposed the tonsils, then cauterized them to create more space. In cases where this was insufficient, they would resect the tonsils.

After the surgery, symptoms improved for all patients; with headaches disappearing 1 week to 2 months post-operatively, significant weight gain for the children who were not thriving before surgery, and a syrinx reduction in 7 out of 8 patients.

On the other hand, opponents of tonsillar manipulation believe that it is risky to remove brain tissue, and that it is a neurosurgeon's duty to preserve as much brain tissue as possible. They believe that it is better to remove bone than a part of the brain.

However, proponents counter that the tissue being removed was compressed and likely damaged. In fact, follow-on work by Lazareff appears to show just that. In a published study, microscopic analysis of cerebellar tonsil tissue removed during Chiari surgery from 43 patients, showed that 38 of the samples were abnormal. The damage included the loss of a specific type of cell and more general neuron damage.

Interestingly, the function of the cerebellar tonsils is not known, which makes the question of whether to remove them even more difficult.

Comparing Techniques

While the somewhat confused situation regarding Chiari surgery may be overwhelming to patients, some surgeons have expressed to Conquer Chiari (off the record) that they feel the controversies in Chiari surgery are no worse, and in fact in many ways not as bad, as those involving other diseases. In many ways it is simply the by-product of the way surgery is; as a profession. New surgeons are trained by mentors who pass on their individual preferences, techniques and tricks. As surgeons become more established, they develop their own experience base and their own styles based on those experiences. Surgeons defend this approach by pointing out that the resources are simply not available to perform rigorous, scientific outcome studies comparing each and every possible surgical technique for every conceivable procedure.

While there is not a lot of data directly comparing surgical techniques, on report from surgeons at the Children's Hospital of Michigan did find that duraplasty and tonsillar resection resulted in better outcomes than bony decompression alone.

Specifically, the surgeons reviewed 60 pediatric patients operated on between 1997 and 2002 (this sample represents a subset of the total Chiari patients seen during that time). For their surgery, all children underwent a craniectomy and 56 underwent some level of laminectomy. After the bony decompression, the dura was not opened in 20 patients, while a duraplasty with bovine graft was performed in 21 patients. For 19 patients, a tonsillectomy was also performed with part or all of the tonsil(s) being removed (Figure 4-10).

Figure 4-10: Surgical Techniques Used In Study (60 Total Patients)

Technique	# of Patients
Bony Decompression	20
Decompression w/ duraplasty	21
Decompression w/ tonsillectomy	19

Overall, 28 of the children experienced what the authors termed complete clinical improvement (47%), while 14 experienced partial improvement (23%), and 18 did not improve at all (30%).

Given the lack of definitive research, surgeons tend to base their approach to Chiari surgery on their own experiences with Chiari patients.

When the surgeons compared the outcomes based on the surgical technique used, they found that for children with Chiari and syringomyelia, the tonsillar resection was much more effective than the duraplasty or bony decompression (Figure 4-11). In fact for the CM/SM children, all 10 who had their tonsils removed improved, while only 4 out of the 7 who had a duraplasty improved. For the children with Chiari only, it turned out that both the tonsillar resection and duraplasty techniques resulted in significantly better outcomes than the bony decompression.

The results from this study are limited by the fact that it was performed retrospectively, meaning looking back in time, and because the surgical procedure used was at the discretion of the surgeon. Unfortunately, the authors did not expand on what criteria the surgeon used to make such decisions.

Figure 4-11: Results By Surgical Technique, CM & CM/SM

	CM/SM		**CM Only**	
	Imp	Not	Imp	Not
BD	5	2	4	8
Dur	4	3	11	4
TR	10	0	8	1
Total	19	5	23	13

Note: BD = bony decompression; Dur = duraplasty; TR = tonsillar resection

Using Imaging During Surgery

In the past several years, some surgeons have begun to use a type of imaging during surgery to help guide the decompression procedure. Color Doppler Ultrasound utilizes sound waves to create an image and can be used to assess CSF flow and tonsillar position and provide surgeons with information on whether the area around the tonsils has been sufficiently decompressed. Some surgeons will use the ultrasound after the bony part of the decompression to decide whether opening the dura is necessary.

While the use of ultrasound during surgery certainly seems like a good idea, to date no data has been published to show if it results in better outcomes.

Complications

For anyone facing the prospect of surgery, it is important to understand the risks involved. Any surgery involves risk and Chiari is no exception; complications can, and do, occur. In looking at the research, complication rates for Chiari surgery vary from less than 5% in some very large patient series, to more than 15% in others.

As mentioned earlier, complication rates are much higher when the dura is opened than when it is not. Some published reports have shown absolutely no complications using just bony decompressions, which is one reason more surgeons are beginning to consider this option.

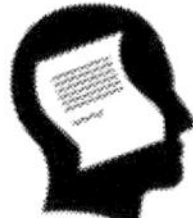

Personal Experience: I am happy to report that I did not experience any complications with the surgery.

Although the complication rate with Chiari surgery can be high, many of the most common complications are manageable and not considered to be serious (although the patient may not think so at the time). While life-threatening complications have been reported in the literature, they are not that common.

Some of the more common things that can go wrong are:

- **CSF Leak** – It can be difficult to get a watertight seal when placing the dural patch and CSF can leak out of the subarachnoid space where it is supposed to be contained. However, as grafts and surgical techniques have evolved, some surgeons have reported experiencing fewer CSF leaks than in the past.
- **Infection** – As with any surgery, infection is always a possibility with Chiari surgery. Obviously, doctors and hospitals take every precaution possible to try to prevent infection, including preventive antibiotics. Unfortunately, they are not always successful and infections are reported in the research literature. In addition, there have been anecdotal reports from patients (or parents) who have struggled to fight infections for weeks after the surgery.
- **Pseudomeningocele** – This occurs when the subarachnoid space (where the CSF circulates) bulges into the surrounding tissue. The size of Pseudomeningoceles can range from small ones which do not require any intervention, to large ones which may require surgery.
- **Graft Problems** – If the dural graft used is not taken from the patient's own tissue, then the patient's immune system may fight the graft and cause inflammation and scarring. These problems do not always come to light right away, but may surface down the road and if bad enough require another surgery to remove and replace the graft.
- **Cerebellar Slumping** – Also known as ptosis, this is one of the more serious complications and involves the cerebellum slumping down even further into the spinal area after surgery because its bony support was

removed. Ptosis can be difficult to treat, but recently surgeons from UCLA published a technique which involves rebuilding bony support for the cerebellum while still maintaining an adequate decompression.

- **Altered CSF** – Although not always listed as a complication in published patient series, there are indications that in some patients the decompression surgery may alter the CSF dynamics. For example, this may result in the development of intracranial hypertension, where the pressure inside the brain is chronically elevated, or post-surgical hydrocephalus. However, it is important to keep in mind that it is not always clear that this occurs from the surgery itself, as opposed to the condition going undiagnosed until after surgery.
- **Other Complications** – The complications listed above are just some of the more common ones and depending on what procedures a Chiari patient is facing, other complications are a possibility. For example, shunts introduce a whole new set of complications, such as the shunt becoming blocked or infected.

The complications detailed above are categorized as surgical morbidity. When medical professionals talk about surgical risks, they refer to morbidity (an undesired result or complication) and mortality (death) rates. While the medical literature does contain isolated reports of mortality associated with Chiari surgery, they are few and far between, especially in the US. Although it has not been established with precision, the mortality rate for Chiari surgery is generally thought to be very low.

Obviously factors specific to an individual patient, such as overall health and other chronic conditions, can influence the risk of complications. This is why it is important for every patient to review, and understand, their specific situation with their doctor before consenting to surgery.

Other Surgeries

While decompression surgery (in whatever form) is considered the standard treatment for Chiari, it is not the only surgery Chiari patients may face. Oftentimes, Chiari patients may have other problems which dictate additional procedures. Although detailed examinations of these procedures are beyond the scope of this book, following is a brief description of some of the other types of surgeries Chiari patients may undergo.

Shunts– A shunt is a tube-like medical device which is surgically implanted to divert CSF from one place to another. A significant number of Chiari patients also have hydrocephalus (excess CSF in the brain) which requires a shunt to divert the extra CSF. There are several types of shunts, but in general the surgeon will program (or adjust) the shunt to achieve an optimal balance of

CSF. Shunts can also used to treat intracranial hypertension (elevated pressure in the head) which is also related to Chiari.

Fusion/Stabilization– As part of a decompression, or at a later date, a Chiari patient may require surgery to stabilize their neck. This can be required when a laminectomy is extensive, when a patient has inherent instability due to their anatomy, or more recently for some patients due to a concurrent condition such as EDS. Stabilization usually involves fusing several vertebrae together and results in a reduced range of neck motion for the patient.

Tethered Cord– The specifics of tethered cord surgery depend on what the cause of the tethering is. For example, in spina bifida patients the defect is closed and the spinal cord released. For tethering due to scar tissue, the binding tissue is removed. If it is believed the filum terminale is pulling down on the cord then the filum is sectioned, or cut.

Scoliosis– Research has shown that decompression surgery can effectively stop the progression of scoliosis related to Chiari; however in cases where it doesn't, further surgery may be required. Scoliosis surgery involves the placement of rods and screws in an effort to stop the curve from getting worse.

Transoral decompression– The surgery for basilar invagination is called transoral decompression, because the surgeon goes in through the mouth. It is an extremely traumatic surgery which involves breaking the jaw and fusion of vertebrae.

Acquired Chiari– For acquired Chiari, the underlying cause of the herniation is addressed, possibly in conjunction with a decompression. For example if a tumor or cyst is pushing the cerebellar tonsils down, then the mass will be removed.

The Surgical Experience

This part of the chapter will deal with the surgical experience from a patient's point of view, mine and others. This section is not based on published research and science, but rather is meant to give a feel for what some of the more mundane aspects of the experience are like, provide some practical tips, and if you're the type that finds humor everywhere, some funny anecdotes.

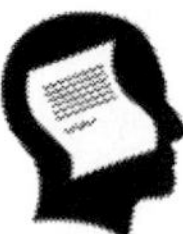

Waiting Is the Hardest Part

Although I was diagnosed in September, I waited until January of the next year to have surgery. My wife had just given birth to our first child and she wanted very much to take her to Florida, where her parents lived, for Christmas. I ended up staying home and barely moved from the couch during the time she was gone.

Anyway, it was difficult to wait such a long time to have the surgery. I remember sitting at work thinking about what it was going to be like and wondering if I was going to be ok. It was maddening and each day seemed to take forever. On the one hand I didn't want to go through with it, and on the other I just wanted to get it done.

Today, I tell people (when asked) that in my opinion it is best to have the surgery as soon as possible once the decision is made.

Pre-op Tests

I'm sure this varies from hospital to hospital and patient to patient, but my pre-op tests included blood work, an EKG and a chest X-ray.

The Night Before and Morning Of

The night before the surgery, my nerves started getting to me. I remember becoming somewhat detached as I paid some bills and went through other preparations. I didn't think I'd be able to sleep, but I did.

I don't remember exactly what time I had to be at the hospital, but I remember it was really, really early. There was no traffic as we drove through the city. When we got to the hospital I was taken to a dingy room to change and I remember thinking what a dump the hospital was. However, my surgeon insisted on doing the surgery there because it was the only hospital which had an attending physician on duty at the ICU 24 hours per day.

In the Operating Room

I said goodbye to my wife and they wheeled me into the operating room where it was absolutely freezing. I pretty much moved myself over to the table and they put some warm blankets on. Then it was lights out and when I woke up I was in the ICU.

ICU

For me, the ICU was the worst part of the experience. It was one large room with a lot of patients and it was difficult to rest. The nurses were incredible, but there was an elderly woman next to me who had had a stroke and her family was struggling with deciding what to do. I found the sheer magnitude of sickness and death in the room overwhelming. The ICU is also where I learned an important lesson about staying ahead of the pain. I had heard the phrase before, but experienced its meaning first hand. I thought I was doing well and asked my nurse to reduce my painkillers (I don't remember what they were). Big mistake. By the time I got a headache it was too late and I had one of the worst headaches of my life for a couple of hours until the pain meds were able to get it under control.

Hospital Room

Once I was transferred to a regular hospital room, things were much better. I got lucky and was put in a private room, so it was quiet, but it was still difficult to sleep because the nurses kept coming in to check things. One of the highlights was when two friends I hadn't seen in a couple of years surprised me by stopping by for a visit. It was a tremendous boost to my spirits.

Discharge & the Ride Home

One thing I hate about being in the hospital is that you never really know when you are going to go home or when the doctor is going to stop by. The day I was expecting to be discharged we ended up waiting and waiting for the surgeon to come and tell me I could leave. It was very frustrating.

When I was finally allowed to leave, the ride home became a memorable experience. Although my wife is an outstanding driver, every bump and pothole in the road was agony. And since it was January in Pittsburgh, there were quite a few. Even though there was nothing she could do about it, I still bring it up if she happens to be driving me somewhere, or if I'm defending my own driving skills.

My other memory of going home was when we got to the front door. At the time we lived in a townhouse, which meant there was a flight of steps as soon as I went in. I was completely exhausted after laboriously working my way up the stairs and collapsed on the couch. Luckily we only had a young baby at the time, because I can't imagine what it would have been like to have the three kids and large dog we now have swarming around me.

The first couple of days I rested quite a bit, but started taking short walks to get the blood flowing. My incision was healing quickly and the staples were getting really tight. It was a big relief to finally get them out. After that, the long road to recovery began.

Plan Ahead

Chiari surgery is a big deal, so you should plan accordingly. Get your affairs in order before the surgery, including:

- No one wants to think about the worst, but it is best to have a will, an advanced directive, and someone selected with the authority to make decisions on your behalf.
- Pay bills ahead of time and do whatever chores you can. You may not be able to do these things for a few weeks after the surgery.
- Make sure you have arranged for help during your recovery, including childcare if necessary.
- Notify the appropriate people where you work and establish expectations that you will likely be off work for a few weeks.
- Think about what you want to take to the hospital. While as a patient you should not have anything with you, someone else can bring you things for your hospital stay after surgery. Consider taking slippers, a robe, sweat pants, some toiletries, etc.
- Make sure you understand your pre-op instructions and follow them carefully.
- If you have any questions make sure you ask them before the surgery.
- Don't be afraid to speak up when you're at the hospital. If you are getting medication, ask what it is and what the dose is. If it doesn't make sense ask if they are sure it is correct. This is where it is important to have an advocate helping watch for potential mistakes.

Hair Tips For Women

Women seem to find the hair situation more daunting than men, so here are a few quick tips from a female Chiari patient:

- Approach the whole issue positively and with a bit of humor. It really isn't a big deal since the hair grows back quickly. Instead of obsessing, make a joke about it.
- Most surgeries are planned many weeks in advance, giving you time to grow out your hair. My hair is short and layered, so I used those weeks to grow out the hair on the upper part of the back of my head.

- After the surgery, I borrowed the "comb over" concept used by bald men, and did a "comb down." The hat I had bought to hide the incision was returned to the store unworn.
- Just for fun, take a picture. The surgery is a big event in your life, and the photo will be a memory.

Visitors

While visitors can be very uplifting, they also can very tiring. Don't be afraid to tell a visitor that you need to rest. Or tell the person that you would really appreciate if they would just sit quietly with you.

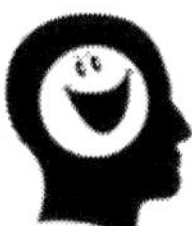

Chiari is a serious subject, but many people use humor as a coping mechanism. If you're one of those people, don't be afraid to laugh! Following are a couple of anecdotes from people who were able to find humor in their experience.

When I was just coming out of surgery, I was still very sedated. The nurses were asking me the standard questions, "Do you know where you are? Do you know why you are here?"

Then, one nurse asked me, "Who is the President of the United States?"

"Hillary Clinton," I replied.

The nurses started looking at each other concerned, but my wife started crying tears of joy.

"He's Ok!" she said. She explained that I always thought that Hillary was really in charge. ~Jerry~

"On June 18, 2001, I underwent surgery to correct my Chiari Malformation. At the time I was only 15 years old, and I am a girl. So while my entire family was in the pre-op room, everyone was crying except me. All I was worried about was how much of my gorgeous brown hair was going to get cut off!" ~Meghan~

When It's Your Child

Although the information in this chapter generally applies to both adults and children, when children are undergoing surgery for Chiari, there are several issues that arise because of their age. The prospect of surgery on a young child can place a tremendous amount of stress on a parents and the family as a whole. Parents will almost always say they wish they could have the surgery instead of their child.

While this is understandable, of course it is not possible. However, parents do play a critically important role in the experience their child has. They must take on the role of advocate during the entire process, essentially provide nursing services once the child is home, and give the kind of love, comfort and assurance that only moms and dads can give, all while trying to maintain work and other family responsibilities. Although it can be overwhelming at times, in the end parents don't have a choice precisely because they are parents.

What to Tell Them

Conquer Chiari is often asked by parents what to tell their child about a diagnosis or the prospect of surgery. Our response is always the same, namely that there is no right answer and to trust yourself as a parent. Children handle things differently depending on their age, maturity, personality and temperament. Some children may want to know all the details of the surgery, while others may just want to be told that they will feel better when it's over and it won't hurt too badly.

Although it can seem like a difficult problem at first, it really boils down to Parenting 101. Parents know their children and, hopefully, how to communicate with them. One thing to remember, however, is that it may take time for a child (or anyone for that matter) to process what they are going through. The questions and resulting emotions may not come all at once and may pop up at unexpected times. Take your time and let your child work things through in their mind, and most importantly trust yourself.

Unfortunately, even confident, skilled parents can run into a difficult problem when it comes time to talk to their child about Chiari. What if they disagree on how to do it? Conquer Chiari has also heard from parents where the mom and dad disagree on how much information to share with their child. Obviously, this can add even more stress to an already stressful situation. Of course there is no right answer in a situation like this, it is simply something the parents must work through for the sake of their family.

You Gotta Laugh!
"My six year old daughter, who has Chiari and syringomyelia was getting ready for surgery in a few days and she had recently overheard us explaining her surgery to some friends. We explained how the doctor would cut out part of her skull and part of her C1 spine. From hearing all this my daughter formed her own explanation of what was going to happen. She was overheard telling her peers how the doctor was going to cut her head off so she would feel better! The funny thing was that she was okay with that...just as long as she would feel better." ~Melissa~

Plan Ahead & Use Your Support System

With Chiari surgery it is good to hope for the best, but plan for complications. As discussed earlier, planning for the time spent at the hospital is important, but it is also important to think about what if things don't go smoothly. This is especially true for parents whose child is going into surgery. While no one wants to think about it, if there are complications proper planning can go a long way during a difficult time. Once something goes wrong, an already stressful situation can quickly become overwhelming and push normally calm, cool, and collected parents to the breaking point.

Before the surgery, think about what would be required if there are complications after the surgery and your child is in the hospital for more than a few days. Chances are you and your spouse will be there as much as possible, so try to arrange for who would drive any siblings around, cook meals, etc.

Discuss with your spouse ahead of time whether both of you would want to be at the hospital at the same time or if you would take shifts. Tell your relatives, neighbors and friends what is going on and ask if they can pitch in if needed. If you're super-organized, line up the tasks ahead of time, pick one person to be in charge of all the helpers, and make a chart of responsibilities. Picking one person to be in charge gives everyone else someone to ask questions of without bothering you, and that person knows it is ok to check in with you now and then.

Most of all, rely on your support system. Whether it's family that lives nearby, good friends, or neighbors, a strong support system can make a world of difference.

The Important Role of Nurses

With a strong support system established to cover the home front, parents can turn their full attention to their child's hospital experience. However, even here, parents should rely on the long-standing, well established hospital support system, nurses. Research (not specific to Chiari) has shown that nurses can have a significant positive impact on the experience of the entire family during a pediatric hospital stay.

Nurses can help explain to parents what is going on, they can provide comfort to the child during times when parents are not allowed to be there, and they can answer questions and solve problems. Most nurses are very nurturing and compassionate and can be a valuable resource for parents. As parents, it is in your best interest to develop and utilize this resource. Ask questions, find out how you can help (it can be difficult to sit around with nothing to do and feeling like you are helpless) and develop a rapport with the nursing staff. Lean on them if you have to for emotional support and don't be afraid to ask for help.

If someone does something you don't like, don't be afraid to speak up, but do it in a way that won't spin the situation out of control. Remember your child is the one going through the surgery and needs the support of the hospital staff.

Post-Operative Pain

Children are not always able to verbalize how much pain they are in and in fact sometimes become quiet when in extreme pain instead of speaking up. If this happens, not enough pain medicines are given and the children suffer needlessly. Narcotics which are routinely used for adults can also be used for pediatric patients, but the side effects - including nausea and vomiting - can be severe. Thus the issue of managing pain in young children after Chiari surgery can be difficult.

However a 2004 study from the University of Alabama-Birmingham found that giving children regularly scheduled doses of pain medicine was more effective than waiting for the children to ask for them.

Specifically, the research team looked at the maximum post-operative pain, amount of narcotics used, amount of anti-nausea drugs used, and length of stay in the hospital in a series of 50 Chiari patients under the age of 21. The patients were divided into two groups (25 in each group). The first group, Group A, received regularly scheduled doses of acetaminophen and ibuprofen alternately every two hours. The second group, Group B, received the same kind of medicines only when they asked for them. Both groups were given narcotics upon request to treat episodes of extreme pain.

As the patients were recovering in the hospital, their pain was recorded using a common 0-5 scale (point to the face that best describes your pain, 5 is severe pain) and the highest pain number per 8 hour nursing shift was entered into a database. In addition, the nurses entered how much narcotics and anti-nausea drugs were required, and lastly, how long each person stayed in the hospital was entered.

The doctors found that Group A - the children who received regularly scheduled doses of medicine - fared better (in every way) than their Group B counterparts. The average highest pain experienced by Group B patients was 3 out of 5, whereas Group A's pain peaked on average at less than 2.

The results were just as dramatic in looking at the use of narcotics and anti-nausea medicine. The Group A children averaged only 1.5 and .5 doses of narcotics and anti-nausea meds per patient respectively, whereas the Group B children needed close to 6 doses of narcotics and over 2 doses of anti-nausea medicine on average per patient. Finally, the average time spent in the hospital was over half a day lower for Group A than Group B (2.2 vs 2.8 days).

Patients should proactively discuss post-operative pain control with their child's surgeon, and these results strongly suggest that regularly scheduled doses are the approach to take.

Have Faith

Chiari surgery is a major, traumatic event, but with a thorough understanding of what is going on and with proper planning and preparation, a patient (or parent) can minimize the impact it has and increase the chances of a successful outcome. Educate yourself, pick a surgeon you trust and establish good lines of communication; plan for the surgery and the recovery afterwards.

These are all good things to do, but having said this, Chiari surgery is also a leap of faith. You are letting someone cut you open and do things near your brain (or to your brain in some cases). While it is important to do everything you can to prepare for this as a patient, at some point – like just before the anesthesia hits – you have to give up control and put it into your surgeon's hands both literally and figuratively. If you are a person of faith, then you may think of it as putting it into God's hands, but either way there is only so much you can do being cast as the patient. In the end, the best thing you can do is have faith, in your surgeon, in yourself, in a higher power, or all three. That is your last, and very important, job as a patient.

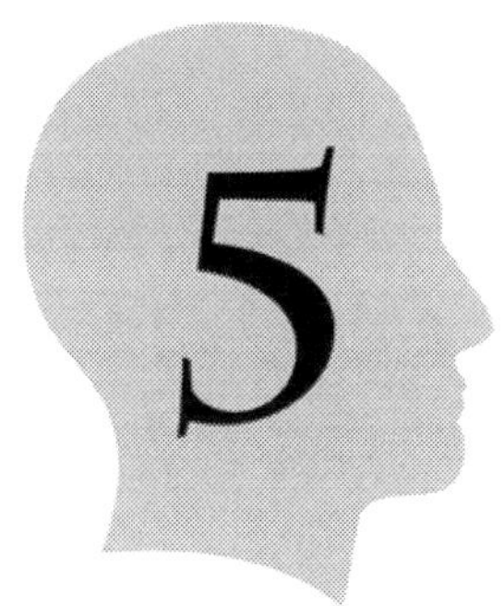

5 Outcomes

"When I asked the surgeon how it went,
he said, "The brain just popped back up!"

~Ann...just after decompression surgery~

Wait & See Outcomes

As discussed in the last chapter, there are essentially two options for treating Chiari. First is the wait and see approach, which may involve some lifestyle changes or medication to treat specific symptoms, but essentially is a monitoring program to make sure the situation does not get worse. Second, of course is surgery, to try to directly alleviate symptoms by reducing crowding and restoring the natural flow of CSF.

While there is not an overwhelming amount of quality research on outcomes in general, the majority of research that does exist tends to focus on surgical outcomes. Therefore, despite the fact that only about 25%-30% of people with tonsillar herniations end up having surgery (meaning most people are in the wait and see treatment category), very little is known about the natural progression of Chiari.

Incidental Chiari with No Symptoms

When a tonsillar herniation is found on an MRI by accident – meaning that the MRI was not ordered to look for Chiari – it is often referred to as an incidental finding. Chances are, people with incidental Chiari have no symptoms that can be attributed to Chiari, which presents a challenging situation for the patient. The medical community generally agrees that surgery should not be performed if there are no symptoms, so by default those incidentally diagnosed are "treated" using the wait and see approach.

Unfortunately for patients, it is impossible to say for a given individual whether symptoms will ever develop or how severe they may become. On the one hand, because of the large number of people with some level of tonsillar herniation compared to the number of Chiari surgeries each year, it seems likely that many people with tonsillar herniation will never develop symptoms.

On the other hand, sudden onset of symptoms, especially after a trauma such as a car accident or fall, is also well recognized. What is not known is whether trauma can spark symptoms in anyone with tonsillar herniation, or only in certain people who for unknown reasons are prone to developing symptoms.

One research study out of Japan did suggest that for the majority of people with no symptoms, surgery may never be required. Dr. Shigeru Nishizawa and his colleagues from Hamamatsu University, followed nine people with Chiari and a syrinx, with no symptoms, for more than 10 years. The results of their work were published in 2001 in *"Journal of Neurosurgery"*.

The nine patients were initially seen for reasons other than Chiari. Three went in because of headaches (but not the kind usually associated with Chiari), three went in for brain check-ups, two were seen for head injuries, and one for sinus problems. Initial MRIs revealed a Chiari malformation in every patient, and follow-up scans revealed syrinxes as well. Neurological exams showed that some patients had abnormal reflexes in their arms and legs, but overall were fairly normal. Because of the lack of symptoms and neurological signs, the subjects decided against surgery and opted for careful observation.

For the next 10+ years, the subjects were evaluated every six months with MRIs and neurological exams. One patient developed some problems with his hand seven years later and decided to undergo surgery. The remaining eight were completely stable and did not develop any symptoms or neurological problems. In addition, the MRIs showed that the syrinxes and Chiari malformations - for all nine patients - did not change over the ten year period.

In an attempt to identify parameters that could be used to indicate surgery is necessary, the researchers used the MRIs to measure the width of the syrinx (at its widest point), the length of the syrinx, and the length of the tonsillar herniation. They then compared these results with data taken from a control group of 11 patients with symptomatic Chiari and syringomyelia who underwent surgery because of their condition.

Surprisingly, there was no significant difference, for any of the parameters, between the groups. In fact, the average width of the syrinx and the average length of herniation were remarkably similar for the two groups. The researchers concluded these parameters were not useful for making a surgical decision and instead suggest focusing on whether there is progression of symptoms, neurological problems, or MRI findings.

The Japanese doctors also stressed that in their view this does not mean that every asymptomatic syrinx will stay that way. In fact, they point out that rapid deterioration and sudden onset of symptoms is well documented with large syrinxes and that careful observation is required, especially for people with syrinxes.

Chiari with Some Symptoms

While there is near universal agreement that Chiari with no symptoms should only be observed, as soon as symptoms enter the picture, consensus breaks down. As discussed in the last chapter, there are no clear-cut criteria for when to have surgery and in many cases it is essentially a judgment call by the surgeon, the patient, or both. In effect everyone is different.

Symptoms that may be intolerable for one person, and end up leading to surgery, may be tolerable to someone else who dreads the idea of surgery. In other words, one person may be willing to trade off a certain amount of quality of life to avoid having surgery, while someone else may not be willing to give up certain activities and will aggressively pursue surgery.

Unfortunately, as has been stressed several times already, the medical literature offers little in terms of guidance in this area. In particular, there is a dearth of research on the outcomes of people with mild to moderate symptoms who choose not to have surgery. How many end up having surgery years later?

Do their symptoms get worse or stay the same? How is their quality of life affected? At this point in time, we simply don't know.

One of the most common questions people who are reluctant to have surgery ask is, can it get better on its own? It turns out that this is actually one area that has been studied and published in the literature.

Spontaneous Resolution

When a syrinx reduces in size without intervention or cerebellar tonsils return to a normal position, it is called spontaneous resolution. Given the nature of corrective surgery, it may be tempting to hold out hope for this type of mini-miracle, but the important question is, is this hope realistic? There is no disputing there are well documented cases of spontaneous resolution, but how often does it occur and is it a realistic option to hope for?

Dr. Kazuhiko Kyoshima from Shinshu University in Japan, and Dr. Enver Bogdanov from the Kazan State Medical University in Russia, studied this issue, reported two cases of spontaneous resolution, and provided a comprehensive overview of the subject in a 2003 publication in *"Journal of Neurosurgery."*

The researchers' first case involved a 10-year old Japanese girl with a history of scoliosis and facial palsy who had developed neck pain over the prior 6 months. With an MRI, the doctors found a syrinx that extended from C4 - T11 and a tight cisterna magna; although the fluid flow at the foramen magnum was not completely blocked. Decompression surgery was planned, but never happened because of problems intubating the young girl. MRI scans 22 months later revealed that the syrinx was smaller and the girl reported her neck pain was not as severe. A follow-up MRI 10 months later showed a further reduction in syrinx size and the girl's neck pain had completely disappeared along with an improvement in other symptoms. A third MRI follow-up, 21 months later, showed no further change in syrinx size.

The second reported case involved a 39-year old Russian man. He was an agricultural worker who was suffering from progressive weakness in his legs. A neurological exam revealed some sensory deficits and an MRI showed a malformation with crowding at the foramen magnum and a syrinx from C2-T2. The man did not want surgery and suffered through worsening symptoms for a month. His symptoms stabilized over the next month and then slowly began to improve. Six months later, the man reported a substantial improvement in his symptoms and an MRI revealed that the cerebellar tonsils had actually moved up - so there was less crowding - and the syrinx was smaller.

In addition to their two cases, the authors reviewed 37 cases of spontaneous resolution that have been well documented since 1990. While most of the cases were Chiari related Syringomyelia; spontaneous improvement has been documented in cases of trauma, Multiple Sclerosis, and syrinxes of unknown origin as well. Interestingly, in the cases involving Chiari related syringomyelia, children were much more likely to show improvement in the actual Chiari malformation as well, compared to adults.

So what is a patient to make of all this? Clearly there are well documented cases where syringomyelia, and even Chiari malformations, stop progressing or improve on their own; however there is no clear understanding of how or why this occurs. In addition, noted Chiari expert Dr. Thomas Milhorat points out in a comment published in the same issue that very long-term follow up of these types of cases would be required to determine if the improvement is permanent or just temporary. In another comment, Dr. Edward Benzel points out that relative to the total number of Chiari and syringomyelia cases, the number of spontaneous resolutions is very low.

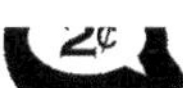

Editorial Analysis: These comments are important to understand, especially about how often spontaneous resolution, or improvement, may occur. Over the course of about 10 years, the researchers found 37 documented cases of spontaneous resolution, but how does this relate to the total number of Chiari cases? In the US alone, it is estimated that there are between 3,000 and 5,000 Chiari decompression surgeries performed annually. Taking the more conservative number of 3,000, that means that over the same 10 years, there were 30,000 surgical cases of Chiari in the US. Again conservatively, there were likely the same number of cases in the European Union, Japan and the rest of the world. This would mean that for the 37 cases of spontaneous resolution, there were 60,000 *surgical* Chiari cases. Now, we have to consider over that same time period how many non-surgical, but symptomatic cases of Chiari there were. Assuming that 1 in 3 people diagnosed with tonsillar herniation have surgery, implies there were 120,000 non-surgical Chiari cases during that time. However, it is likely that many of these were asymptomatic, so for the sake of analysis, we will assume that 25% of these were symptomatic to some degree, which would give us an additional 30,000 non-surgical, symptomatic Chiari cases. This brings the total Chiari cases over the ten year period to 90,000. This means that spontaneous resolution (as reported in the medical literature) occurred approximately once for every 2,500 cases of Chiari (37/90,000).

Obviously, this is not a precise analysis but is only intended to put into perspective how often spontaneous resolution occurs. Also, the number of spontaneous resolution cases could be higher for two reasons. First, it is likely not all cases are reported. While it is an unusual event and would seem likely to be reported, there may be cases with mild symptoms which go away and would not warrant any type of publication. Second, since 60,000 patients had surgery, we don't know if any of them would have gotten better on their own. Despite these issues, it seems clear that spontaneous resolution is probably a rare event.

Can Children Grow Out Of It?

An extension of the spontaneous resolution question is the idea that some children can actually grow out of a Chiari malformation. Recall that it is believed that Chiari is due to a small posterior fossa region of the skull which results in crowding of the brain tissue. Obviously, children are growing constantly, so this leads to the question can Chiari in some children be a temporary condition due to mismatched growth?

In other words, in certain cases, is there a period of time where a child's skull has not grown sufficiently and is causing crowding, but then at a later time the skull growth will essentially catch up and the crowding, and symptoms, will be relieved?

This is obviously an intriguing idea, and there are in fact some case reports of this occurring. In addition, there is anecdotal evidence that some doctors are telling parents that their children with mild symptoms may grow out of it in a few years. However, as with the natural progression of Chiari in general, there have been no large studies examining how often this might occur or how to identify which children this may actually happen to.

Further, the whole situation is complicated by the fact that for children who appear to grow out of it, one has to wonder whether the symptoms were originally due to Chiari or were they related to something else of a transient nature? Here again we run into the problem of not having a simple, objective definition of Chiari.

Syrinx Progression

Interestingly, one aspect of the natural history of Chiari and syringomyelia that has actually been studied in a large number of patients is what happens to syrinxes that are left alone. In the US, many surgeons consider the presence of a syrinx to be enough reason to operate, so the natural progression of a syrinx has not been studied; but in other parts of the world this is not necessarily the case. In fact, throughout the years, there have been indications that for at least a subset of syringomyelia patients, if syrinxes are left alone for many years, they will eventually begin to shrink and even collapse on their own.

Supporting this notion are reports of groups of patients who exhibit the neurological signs and symptoms associated with syringomyelia (as opposed to symptoms caused by Chiari) but do not appear to have a syrinx when examined with MRI. An example of this is Milhorat's landmark study which found a significant group of people who fit this category.

One group who has studied the natural progression of syringomyelia directly is Bogdanov and Mendelevich of Kazan State Medical University, in Russia. In a specific rural area of Russia, there appears to be an unusually high rate of syringomyelia, especially among men. In one publication, Bogdanov and

Mendelevich reviewed over 100 cases of syringomyelia which were not operated on, but from which people had been suffering from for as long as 46 years. Interestingly, they found that the size of a syrinx tended to decrease at the later stages of the disease. This supports other research findings which have shown that symptom progression stabilizes after 10 years in about one-third to one-half of patients (again, this doesn't mean they got better, just that symptoms stopped getting worse).

In a second report (2006), Bogdanov and Mendelevich - along with Heiss at NIH - extended their work and proposed that patients who have signs and symptoms of syringomeylia but no syrinx, may actually be in a post-syrinx state. In other words, they hypothesized that in some cases, syrinxes eventually collapse on their own.

To support their theory, the team looked at 168 Russian Chiari/syringomyelia patients who were seen between 1997-2001. Each patient underwent a neurological evaluation and an MRI. From this, the researchers identified two separate groups of patients. The first group (Group A) was comprised of 14 patients who exhibited signs and symptoms of SM, but did not show a syrinx on MRI. The second group (Group B) was comprised of 15 patients who also had signs and symptoms of SM, but who showed flat, collapsed syrinxes on MRI.

When the authors compared the two groups, they found they were very similar clinically (Figure 5-1). Neurological deficits were comparable between the two groups and characteristic of Chiari related SM. In addition, several patients in each group had noticeable atrophy of the spinal cord (their cord was narrower than 8mm). Finally, for the patients in both groups, the progression of symptoms had stabilized for at least 3 years.

The Russian team believes that since the clinical findings of Group A were similar to those patients with collapsed syrinxes which were still visible, it is likely that the patients in Group A had syrinxes which spontaneously resolved at some point in the past. They were, in effect, post-syrinx.

Why would syrinxes resolve on their own in some people? It is important to realize that syrinx growth is a dynamic process and while there are several theories as to its underlying mechanism, none have yet been proven conclusively. One of the current leading theories of syrinx formation is called the piston theory and was developed by researchers at the US National Institutes of Health. The piston theory proposes that with each heartbeat, the cerebellar tonsils are driven down into the crowded spinal area like a piston. This in turn creates a pressure wave in the cerebrospinal fluid, which forces the fluid into the spinal cord, forming a syrinx.

The scientists in this study propose two possible mechanisms for syrinx resolution. First, the natural flow of CSF is somehow restored at the level of the Chiari malformation which results in the syrinx resolving. Second, after an extended period of expansion, the tissue around a syrinx becomes so thin that it eventually ruptures and allows the syrinx to drain into the CSF in the subarachnoid space. In support of this idea, the team identified three patients in whom there was clear communication of fluid - on MRI - between the syrinx and the subarachnoid space.

Based on their findings, the authors define the post-syrinx state as characterized by:

1. Stable signs and symptoms of central myelopathy (spinal disease)
2. MRI evidence of Chiari and either an absent or collapsed syrinx
3. No evidence of other diseases which can mimic syringomyelia

While the idea is intriguing, it is also important to note (as the authors do) that the post-syrinx state is just one possible natural outcome of syringomyelia. The damage that a syrinx causes can be permanent and can lead to paralysis for some people. It is also important to note that the symptoms for the patients in the study above did not resolve just because the syrinx collapsed. Today, there is no way to predict for an individual how a syrinx will progress and the cost of not taking action may be extremely high. How to treat syringomyelia is an issue that should be discussed at length with medical professionals.

Figure 5-1:
Clinical Features of Post-Syrinx Group (A) vs Flat Syrinx Group (B)

	A (14)	B (15)
Avg. Age	44	55
Symptom Duration (Yrs)	21	28
# w/ dysesthetic pain	3	10
# w/ sensory loss	13	13
# w/ muscle atrophy	4	6
# w/ weakness	13	14
# w/ spinal atrophy	4	6

Note: Group A did not have syrinx on MRI, but did have syrinx related symptoms; Group B had flat, collapsed syrinx on MRI

Practical Tip: Monitoring Symptoms
For those following the wait and see approach it is important to realize that monitoring whether symptoms are getting worse is the key. To this end, and because sometimes it can be difficult to compare how you feel today versus a year ago, consider keeping a symptom journal. It doesn't have to be on a daily basis, but perhaps once a week write down how

your symptoms were that week. Were there any new symptoms? Did any go away? How would you rate them on a scale from 0-100?

If you're only seeing the doctor every six months or once a year, this type of journal can help you decide what to tell him during your visit.

And of course, remember to get your MRIs!

Surgical Outcomes

How Do You Define Success?

The first step in talking about outcomes for Chiari surgery is to define what is meant by success. Unfortunately, this is not as easy as it sounds. Certainly from a patient's perspective success means not having any symptoms and a return to a healthy life with no limitations or restrictions.

However, lining up a patient focused definition of success with the published research can be challenging. Basically, there are three problems with the current research as it relates to definitively establishing the long term success of Chiari surgery:

1. **Surgical Techniques Vary** – As discussed in the last chapter, there are many variations to the standard Chiari surgery. Because of this, comparing results from different research articles is difficult. For example, if in one report of 20 patients the dura was always opened and in a different report of 15 patients the dura was only opened in a few, how do you combine, or even compare the results? Further, since most published Chiari research involves only a small number of patients, it is difficult to generalize the findings of any one publication and so it becomes critical to find a way to look at the results of many publications in aggregate.
2. **There Is No Standard Definition Of Success** – The second big problem is that every surgeon uses different criteria when reporting surgical outcomes. In addition, the criteria used are often vague and fail to take into account the real world of the patient. It is common in research publications to see statements such as "the MRI showed adequate decompression", "the syrinx stabilized or reduced in size", or "most symptoms had resolved by final follow-up". Besides being vague, these types of measures fail to take into account whether the patient has returned to his/her former lifestyle. Not only does this again make it difficult to combine the results of different studies, but the bar is set too low by defining success this way. While a syrinx shrinking is certainly a good thing, does it mean that the patient has returned to their job, or is able to be an active parent? What is needed is a standard outcome

measure which takes into account objective medical findings such as MRI results and neurological exam results, but also factors in issues such as whether a person can still work, has to work at a different job, their emotional state (are they depressed?), any residual physical limitations, and whether any life plans were altered such as marriage, children, etc.

3. **The Follow-Up Period In Most Outcome Studies Is Too Short** – There is significant anecdotal evidence that long-term recurrence of symptoms is a real problem. Whether due to some type of trauma or the natural effects of aging, some patients report symptoms coming back five, ten or even fifteen years after surgery, yet the follow-up period for most studies is 2 yrs or less. Given this, one has to wonder if the research is presenting an accurate picture of the long-term success of surgery. Some surgeons counter this by saying that they would report if any patients experienced problems down the line. That's all well and good except that if a person has problems 5-10 years later, what are the chances they will return to the same surgeon? In one study, the authors reported an 89% "success" rate one month after the surgery, but this dropped to just 67% at the two year mark. A procedure with an 89% success rate may be considered good, but the fact that this dropped to just 67% in two years is troubling. At one month post-op, most patients have not yet tried to resume what would be considered a normal life, with work, school, family responsibilities, social activities, etc. Fortunately, as Chiari surgeries become more common, it is likely that there will be some true long-term studies published.

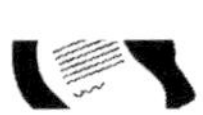

Personal Experience: As is true with many things in life, expectations can influence how patients perceive the success, or failure of surgery. My wife accompanied me to my pre-operative consultation and heard everything I did, but as I would find out later she interpreted what we heard much differently than I did. Whether it was because I had done research and understood how serious syringomyelia can be, or for some other reason, my wife's expectation going into the surgery was that I would be completely, 100% better afterwards. While the surgery did reduce the size of my syrinxes and restore some CSF flow, it became apparent very quickly that I was not going to be magically cured. As the reality set in, my wife expressed that she thought the surgeon had misled us and minimized the situation. While I understand why she thinks this (and she may be right), I tend to have a different view. With the realization that I could have been paralyzed, or forced to go on disability right away, I was pretty happy with the outcome and thought the surgeon was very direct and open about what to expect. Thus, I think expectations can have a strong influence on a person's perceptions of the success of surgery.

Practical Tip: Another lesson from the story above is to be very specific in communicating with your surgeon and be careful not to hear what you want to hear. If a doctor says something such as, "You'll be ok." This can be interpreted in a number of different ways. He may mean that the surgery will stop the progression of the disease, while you may think it means you will be 100% better.

There are four specific, important questions to ask a surgeon before undergoing decompression surgery:

1. Given your experience, what do you think the chances are that I will be asymptomatic (symptom free) after surgery?
2. What do you think the chances are that my worst symptoms will improve, but that I will still have some symptoms?
3. What do you think the chances are that the surgery will fail and I would need additional surgery?
4. What has been the complication rate among patients you've operated on using this technique?

Don't let the surgeon respond with vague generalities, push for specifics. That way, you will know going in what to expect. However, it's also important to keep in mind that there is no way to predict for any given individual whether surgery will work or not, so in the end you should be prepared for any outcome.

What the Research Says

In General

Despite the limitations noted above, quite a bit can be learned about surgical outcomes from the published medical literature. There are numerous reports of the outcomes of patient series, both large and small, from surgeons all over the world. Naturally, some of these publications report success rates higher than average and some lower than average (although one has to wonder how many surgeons would publish results which show a lower than average success rate). While it is difficult to combine the reports in a scientific way, when taken in totality they do present a general picture of the success rate of surgery for Chiari.

Thus, keeping in mind that there are numerous techniques which are referred to as decompression surgery, that success is poorly defined, patient follow-ups tend to be too short, and perhaps most importantly, that for an individual patient there is no way to objectively predict whether surgery will be successful.

In general the Chiari research reveals the following:

1. Between 30%-50% of people become essentially symptom free after surgery.
2. An additional 30% will experience a significant improvement in their symptoms and quality of life. This means that surgery is "successful" about 80% of the time.
3. For approximately twenty percent of people, surgery will not provide any real symptoms relief, meaning that surgery will have failed.
4. In general complication rates are less than 5%, with most complications being minor and manageable (although they can seem like quite an ordeal for the patient and their family).
5. While it has not been examined specifically, there are very few mortalities reported associated with the actual decompression surgery (for Chiari I), especially in the US.
6. While the data is not conclusive, there are indications that young children have better outcomes than older children, and that children in general may have better outcomes than adults.
7. Again while not conclusive, complex anatomy, long duration of symptoms, syringomyelia and severe scoliosis may negatively effect outcomes.
8. Interestingly, the research is overwhelming that the size of the Chiari malformation – meaning how many mm's the cerebellar tonsils are herniated – is NOT related to patient outcomes.

Thus, in general surgery is successful (whatever that means) about 80% of the time. However, currently there is no effective way to determine in advance who will benefit from surgery and by how much.

Surgical Outcomes for Adults

Additional insight into surgical outcomes can be gained by looking more closely at certain studies which are representative of the general research.

For adults, one such study was published in 2005, by Dr. Diane Mueller a PhD neurosurgical nurse practitioner at the University of Missouri-Columbia, and a Director of the C&S Patient Education Foundation, and Dr. John Oro, a neurosurgeon (now at the Chiari Treatment Center in Colorado, www.chiaricare.com). In it, they reported the results of a study which examined the change in the self-perceived quality of life of 112 Chiari patients after surgery.

To measure quality of life, Dr. Mueller chose to use the Sickness Impact Profile (SIP). The SIP has been in wide use since 1976 and measures quality of life dimensions such as physical, psychosocial, recreation, sleep, work, and social interaction. The profile is a self-report questionnaire with 127 questions related to activities such as sleep, balance, movement, hygiene, home maintenance, concentration and social interactions, etc. The survey is scored such that the higher the score, the more impaired the perceived quality of life is. In other words, a score of 0 represents a good quality of life with no impairments.

One hundred seventy two Chiari patients were given the opportunity to participate in the study. One hundred fifty two agreed and completed the SIP survey before their surgery. The participants were asked to complete the same survey one year after undergoing their decompression surgery. In addition, the post-op survey included open-ended questions asking people their perception of their quality of life since surgery, their general health status, and activity level. Forty people failed to return the one year follow-up survey, leaving 112 patients as participants in the study.

The study group was comprised mainly of women, with only 8 men versus 104 women. The average age of the group was 40 and almost 20% of the group had syringomyelia in addition to Chiari. The size of herniations ranged from 3mm to 30mm, with an average of 9.4mm. The group endured the usual range of symptoms, with 97% reporting headaches. Other common symptoms included dizziness, neck pain, and weakness and numbness in the extremities. Each patient underwent a decompression surgery which included a craniectomy, laminectomy, and duraplasty. There were very few complications, with only one patient requiring additional surgery for a cyst which had developed.

One year after surgery, the survey showed 84% patients had experienced a significant improvement in their quality of life (Figure 5-2). All of the dimensions of the survey showed improvement with the total physical scale improving by 77% and the total psychosocial scale improving by 79%. While the number of patients who became asymptomatic was not explicitly reported, it can be inferred from graphs in the publication that at least half of the patients had an overall post-op score of 10 or less. Interestingly, neither syringomyelia, the size of the Chiari herniation, nor age were related to quality of life after surgery.

The open-ended questions included in the follow-up survey yielded slightly different results, with 75% of the people reporting their quality of life had improved after surgery, 15% reported no change, and 10% said it is was worse. Among the improved group, patients included statements such as, "I have my life back", "I wish I had done the surgery sooner", and "I did not realize how sick I was before". When the authors dug deeper into the responses of those who reported worsening of their quality of life and general health, they found that many reported adverse events and incidents outside the scope of their Chiari experience.

Finally, in an attempt to account for the 40 patients who did not respond to the follow-up survey, the researchers used their own notes and anecdotal reports from follow-up visits to classify the change in quality of life of as many of these people as they could. They were able to rate 35 of the 40 and found that in this group 71% had improved, 20% were unchanged, and 9% had gotten worse. It is interesting to note that the improved rate for the group who did not return the form is lower than for the group who did. When the results of the two groups were combined, 79% of patients showed improvement in their quality of life one year after surgery, which of course is very close to the generalization that surgery is successful for 80% of patients.

Figure 5-2:
Change In Quality Of Life 1 Year After Surgery (112 Patients)

Measure	Better	Same	Worse
Survey	84%	Not Available	Not Available
Open-ended questions	75%	15%	10%

Note: When survey results are combined with verbal assessment of 35 patients who did not return post-op survey, 79% showed improvement.

Surgical Outcomes for Children

Similar to the Mueller/Oro study, there are several publications which are representative of what is seen for pediatric cases. In particular, Greenlee and Menezes published a report in 2002 detailing the surgical results for 25 children under the age of six and went the extra step of categorizing their results as resolved, improved, and unchanged for both subjective symptoms and objective neurological findings.

All the children underwent surgery, which entailed a craniectomy, laminectomy, duraplasty, and shrinkage of the tonsils. In addition, 4 of the syringomyelia patients had shunts placed to help with CSF flow. There were only minor complications from the surgery and overall results were very good (Figure 5-3). Symptomatically, 92% of the children improved, with 46% experiencing complete symptom resolution. With regard to neurological findings, 73% of the patients experienced improvement while 27% remained unchanged. For the children with syrinxes, 1 resolved completely, 10 improved, and there was no change in 1 (MRIs were not available for 4). Unfortunately, 3 of the children had to undergo additional surgery due to recurring symptoms, for an overall failure rate of 12%.

It is interesting that the improvement rate for symptoms was significantly higher than for neurological findings (meaning abnormalities found during a neurological exam). It could be that in addition to a real improvement, there is an inherent placebo, or psychological effect of undergoing surgery which makes symptoms seem better but does not influence objective findings. Following this line of speculation (and that's all that it is), it could also be that immediately following surgery there is an overall improvement in most symptoms above and beyond the underlying physiological improvement, which is why some people tend to have symptoms come back over time, as is often noted in the research. In other words a placebo effect makes people feel better than they really are, but the placebo effect wears off over time.

Figure 5-3: Surgical Outcomes in Children Under Six

Category	Outcome	%
Symptoms	Resolved	46%
	Improved	46%
	Unchanged	8%
Neuro Findings	Resolved	31%
	Improved	42%
	Unchanged	27%

Source: Dr. Greenlee, Dr. Menezes, et al. Chiari I Malformation in the Very Young Child. Pediatrics. 2002 Dec;110(6):1212-9.

A much larger outcomes study, involving 130 children of all ages, was published in 2003 by Tubbs, McGirt and Oakes. The article reviewed their experience in treating Chiari over the past twenty plus years and detailed their overall success and complication rates. The average age at time of surgery was 11 years, with the most common presenting symptoms being head/neck/back pain and scoliosis. Fifty-eight percent of the children also had a syrinx.

The overall success rate was good, with 83% of the patients experiencing some level of relief (unfortunately, this study is a prime example of a fairly vague definition of success). It should be noted that the surgeons' operative technique changed over time as they started using shunts less frequently, which improved their success rate.

Of the primary symptoms, headache and neck pain did not resolve in 12% of the cases and scoliosis did not improve in 17% of the cases. The doctors noted that scoliosis with an initial curve of greater than 40 degrees was less likely to improve than more mild curves.

Of the entire group, surgical complications occurred in only 2.3% of the patients and included hydrocephalus and one case of severe, life-threatening brainstem compression which was treated immediately with surgery. Overall, nine patients (7%) had to undergo additional surgeries; eight for syrinxes that didn't reduce in size and one for persistent headaches. The patient who had persistent headaches had not received a duraplasty in the initial operation and the headaches went away after a duraplasty was performed in a second operation. For the group with persistent syrinxes, only one required the insertion of a shunt and the rest responded well to re-operation. The doctors noted that in every case of re-operation for persistent syrinx, it was later found that CSF was not flowing freely out of the fourth ventricle. It is also interesting to note that in this large series of patients, no correlation between the amount of tonsillar herniation and clinical outcome was found.

Factors That Influence Outcome

While general statements about the effectiveness of surgery are encouraging, what every patient wants to know is whether it will work for them. Unfortunately, there is currently no way to objectively, definitively say who will benefit from surgery and by how much. There is no way to determine, beforehand, whether crippling headaches will disappear completely, whether strength will return in full, whether balance will improve, etc.

However, doctors and researchers have been looking for predictors of surgical success for years now with mixed results. So while we don't yet know enough to make individual predictions, there are indications that certain factors – such as CSF flow, scoliosis, duration of symptoms and age - may play a role, in varying degrees, in influencing surgical outcomes. These factors, and the sometimes mixed research behind them, are discussed below. It will be interesting to see if in the next 3-5 years someone is able to put together a quantitative combination of factors which can be used to predict surgical outcomes and in effect say who is a good candidate for surgery.

CSF Flow Blockage

Since Chiari is so intimately entwined with the natural flow of cerebrospinal fluid, it is perhaps not surprising that researchers have looked at whether the amount of CSF blockage caused by Chiari can be used to predict surgical outcomes. What may be counterintuitive however is that the limited evidence that exists suggests that people with more, or even complete, blockage may actually benefit more from decompressions surgery.

In fact, in the summer of 2006, McGirt et al. published a study in *"Journal of Neurosurgery"*, which seemed to indicate just that. The study looked at 130 Chiari patients treated at Duke University between 1997 - 2003. All patients had tonsillar herniations of at least 5 mm, and in fact the average herniation was a sizeable 11 mm. The average age of the patients was 16, but the group included both children and adults. There were slightly more females than males, and 35% of the group also had syrinxes. The most common symptom was occipital headache (back of the head), but sensory deficits, frontal headaches, and neck pain were also prevalent.

Figure 5-4: Factors Affecting Surgical Outcome

Predictor	Increased Risk Of Failure
Normal CSF Flow	4.8X
Frontal Headache	4X
Scoliosis	9X

Prior to surgery, patients were given a cine MRI to look at their CSF flow at the craniovertebral junction and based upon that were classified as having either normal or abnormal CSF flow. Not surprisingly, 81% of the group had abnormal flow, with 43% (of the total) showing complete blockage, and 38% showing some reduction. Conversely, despite a minimum of 5mm of tonsillar herniation, 19% of the patients were classified as having normal CSF flow preoperatively.

All patients underwent decompression surgery and were evaluated one month, one year, and if possible, two years after surgery. At the one month follow-up, 89% of the patients were considered to have had successful treatment, but this dropped to 67% at the two year mark (highlighting the need for repeated, long-term follow-ups in outcomes research).

When the researchers applied statistical analysis to their database of information, they found that patients with normal CSF flow prior to surgery were actually 4.8 times more likely to have a failed outcome after surgery than patients with blocked or restricted flow (Figure 5-4). Similarly, patients without CSF flow improvement after surgery were twice as likely to have poor surgical outcomes.

In addition to CSF flow, they also found that frontal headaches (as opposed to the classic back of the head Chiari headache) and scoliosis were significant predictors of outcome. Specifically, patients with a frontal headache as a primary symptom were four times more likely to have a poor surgical outcome than patients without this symptom and patients with scoliosis were nine times more likely to have a poor, or failed, outcome.

These results build on an earlier study out of India which used a different imaging technique, radionuclide cisternography, to look at CSF flow and outcomes.

Radionuclide cisternography involves injecting a tracer agent into the CSF system. As the tracer agent disperses, images taken at different times clearly show where the tracer is, and thus reveal how the CSF is flowing. The Indian research team used this technique on 17 patients with both Chiari and Syringomyelia, treated between 2000-2002.

Prior to treatment, each person was given a disability score using a modified scoring system. The researchers began with a system developed to measure disability due to spinal disease and added components specific to Chiari and SM. The final system had 8 categories: sensory, paresis, gait, urinary/bowel, muscle control in the arms/legs, neck pain, respiratory problems, and cranial nerve signs. The first four categories were scored 1-5, with a 5 representing no disability, and a 1 representing total disability. The latter categories were scored similarly, but with a range of 1-3. When combined, the total possible score, which represented no disability, was 32.

Also before surgery, each patient underwent the radionuclide cisternography. The tracer was injected into the lumbar region, and an image taken immediately after. Follow-up images were taken 1, 2, 4, 6, and 24 hours after the injection.

From these images, the researchers identified three categories of CSF flow, which they termed rapid, delayed and blocked. In the rapid group, which consisted of 7 patients, the tracer element quickly moved up the spinal cord and crossed the foramen magnum into the brain region in less than an hour. Here it quickly dispersed as it would in a healthy person.

In the delayed group, which also consisted of 7 patients, the tracer crossed the foramen magnum in the usual amount of time, but then it was delayed and took nearly 24 hours to disperse throughout the brain area. Finally, in the blocked group, which consisted of 3 patients, the tracer never crossed the foramen magnum, indicating that the CSF flow was completely blocked by the Chiari malformation.

All the patients underwent decompression surgery and then were reevaluated at follow-up (3 months to 1 year after surgery) using the disability scoring system. In addition, 10 patients underwent the radionuclide cisternography for a second time and 11 patients underwent a standard MRI.

Before the surgery, the patients in the rapid flow group had the highest average score on the disability scale (27 out of 32), meaning they were the least affected by the CM/SM (Figure 5-5). Both the delayed and blocked group of patients had lower scores, with the blocked group suffering the most (20 out of 32).

After surgery, the groups scored at about the same level, however the improvement in the blocked group was dramatically higher than the delayed and the rapid group. In fact, the patients in the rapid group only improved on average by 0.7 from before surgery, compared to an average increase of 8.3 in the blocked group.

The follow-up radionuclide cisternography showed that all 10 patients who took the test demonstrated normal CSF flow (they would be categorized as rapid). In addition, the MRIs showed that the syrinxes collapsed in 4 of the patients.

Figure 5-5: Pre and Post Disability by Flow Type

Flow Group	# of Patients	PreOp Disability Score	PostOp Disability Score
Rapid	7	27.0	27.7
Delay	7	23.1	27.3
Block	3	20.3	28.6

While this type of imaging is not practical for everyday use, in this study it effectively demonstrated that what some people refer to as borderline Chiari cases, may not respond well to surgery. Since the goal of decompression surgery is to create more space around the cerebellar tonsils and restore the normal flow of CSF, it is a validation of this approach that people with blocked flow tend to improve.

The question with CSF flow as a predictor becomes why do people with normal, or near normal, CSF flow but who exhibit Chiari like symptoms and herniation not respond as well to surgery? One possibility is that while these people do have tonsillar herniations, their symptoms are not actually due to compression in this area or disrupted CSF flow. Thus, expanding the posterior fossa provides little to no relief.

Cine MRI and CSF flow receive a lot of attention in the Chiari community, and while there is some evidence of its usefulness based on private communications with Conquer Chiari, it is clear that more than a few neurosurgeons remain unconvinced about the importance of cine MRI in either diagnosing Chiari or evaluating the success of surgery.

Scoliosis

Scoliosis, an abnormal curvature of the spine, is most often thought of as affecting children. Indeed, the relationship between scoliosis and Chiari/SM in children actually receives a good deal of attention from the research community. Such research has established criteria for what types of scoliosis indicate an MRI should be done and has shown the effectiveness of performing decompression surgery to halt the progression of the scoliosis.

While these are positive steps, another aspect of the scoliosis/Chiari research, is that it is becoming clear that the presence of scoliosis, especially if severe, has a negative influence on patient outcomes. The McGirt study referenced above found that the presence of scoliosis translated into nine times increased risk of surgical failure.

More recently, in 2007, a study out of Japan looked at how scoliosis affected outcomes in adults and found pretty convincing evidence that patients with scoliosis fare worse than those without scoliosis.

Figure 5-6: Impact of Scoliosis

	W/Scol	W/out Scol
Avg Length of Syrinx	12.8	7.2
Duration of Symptoms	14 yrs	7 yrs
UE Muscle Atrophy	73%	8%
Abnormal Leg Reflex	93%	42%
Avg. Preop JOA Score	10.1	14.4
Avg Postop JOA Score	11.9	15.8

Notes: syrinx length is measured in vertebral segments; JOA stands for Japanese Orthopedic Association scale; UE=upper extremity; significant refers to the difference being statistically significant and likely to be due to chance

Specifically, the study looked at 27 adult CM/SM patients treated between 1995-2002. To study the role of scoliosis, the patients were divided into two groups based on whether they had 10 degrees or more of abnormal spine curvature. Using this method, 15 patients were placed in the scoliosis group and 12 in the no scoliosis group. In the scoliosis group, the average curve was a sizeable 23 degrees, with 10 of the patients exhibiting a single curve, four a double curve, and one a triple curve.

All the patients underwent a similar surgical procedure which involved a C1 laminectomy and removal of the outer layers of the dura. The researchers then compared the two groups across a number of parameters, including:

- length, width and shape of the syrinx
- degree of tonsillar herniation
- duration of symptoms
- muscle atrophy in the upper extremities
- abnormal leg reflexes
- cranial nerve symptoms
- pre-op and post-op clinical status as measured by the Japanes Orthopedic Association (JOA) scale
- calculated recovery rate

Their analysis revealed a number of significant differences between the groups (Figure 5-6). Specifically, the average length of the syrinx in the scoliosis group was almost 13 vertebral segments long compared to 7 in the no-scoliosis group. Perhaps most strikingly, nearly three-fourths of the scoliosis group suffered from upper extremity muscle atrophy, but only 8% of the no-scoliosis group did. Similarly, a whopping 93% of the patients with scoliosis also exhibited abnormal leg reflexes, while less than half of the patients without scoliosis did. Both pre and post-op clinical scores, along with the calculated recovery rate, were significantly worse for the scoliosis group as well.

The researchers also found that the length of the syrinx and the duration of symptoms were correlated to the degree of scoliosis. In other words, patients with longer syrinxes, or who had suffered from symptoms for longer, tended to have worse cases of scoliosis. Interestingly, neither the width of the syrinx, nor the amount of tonsillar herniation was found to be related to the amount of scoliosis or the clinical scores.

Finally, the authors built a statistical model to determine which factors influenced the final JOA score (at the last follow-up). While the primary factor was the pre-op JOA score - meaning how bad symptoms were prior to surgery - they also found that the degree of scoliosis and the duration of symptoms significantly influenced outcomes.

Based on their findings, the doctors concluded that adults with CM/SM related scoliosis tend to have poorer outcomes. One possible reason for this is that scoliosis may essentially be a symptom of syringomyelia and represent an advanced state of the syrinx when significant, possibly irreversible damage has been done.

Duration of Symptoms

Duration of symptoms is one of the most common factors studied in trying to determine what influences outcomes, but to date the research on it has been mixed. In 2003, Asgari reported finding no correlation between duration of symptoms and clinical outcome in a group of 31 patients. However, in 2004 Arora reported a study which found that duration of symptoms (grouped as less than 6 months, between 6 months and 3 years, and greater than 3 years), was in fact strongly related to the surgical outcomes. Namely, a longer duration of symptoms prior to diagnosis and surgery resulted in poorer outcomes.

One reason for the confusing results may be that duration of symptoms is important in some cases but not others. For example, maybe people who endure symptoms associated with a syrinx for years tend to have worse outcomes, but maybe in people with Chiari only; it doesn't matter. Or perhaps it is not a Chiari versus syringomyelia issue, but rather for reasons not yet known, a subset of patients tend to get worse over time while others don't.

A study by Attal in 2004 lends some credence to the Chiari versus syringomyelia idea. Specifically, this group found that in 16 syringomyelia patients both temperature sensory deficits and the presence of neuropathic pain after surgery were associated with duration of symptoms prior to surgery. Similarly, Nakamura found that in 25 CM/SM patients, duration of symptoms was related to whether pain improved after surgery. In other words, people whose pain did not improve after surgery had been suffering from symptoms longer than those whose pain did improve.

Interestingly, Nakamura found that duration of symptoms was related to pain both before and after surgery. Specifically, prior to surgery the average duration of symptoms for those suffering from pain was more than 30 months. In contrast, the average duration for the - no pain - group was only 15 months. After surgery, the difference was just as striking. The average duration of symptoms for the - improved - group was about 20 months, while the average for the no improvement group was much higher at about 40 months.

Practical Tip: Despite the fact that not all research has shown a connection between the duration of symptoms and outcomes, based upon research such as Nakamura's, Conquer Chiari has adopted as part of its Research Agenda a goal that the average time between onset of symptoms and diagnosis be reduced to two years or less. There are indications that for those patients whose outcomes may be sensitive to duration of symptoms that two years may be an important time point.

Syrinxes

While it is logical to assume that people with both Chiari and syringomyelia will do worse after surgery than people with Chiari only, the research has not always shown this to be the case. For example, a study of nearly one hundred children found that while children with Chiari only improved after surgery 79% of the time, only 59% of the children with both Chiari and syringomyelia improved. Yet the large quality of life study by Mueller, (cited earlier) failed to find any connection between the presence of syringomyelia and outcomes.

One possibility is that the presence of a syrinx in and of itself does not dictate a poor outcome because not all syrinxes are the same. Some syrinxes are long and thin, some are round and some bulge out to one side, and as the study discussed at the beginning of the chapter highlighted, not all syrinxes cause symptoms.

In a study of 25 syringomyelia patients, Nakamura examined whether the shape of the syrinx was related to residual pain after surgery. To do this, patients were categorized as having either a central syrinx contained entirely within the central canal, an enlarged syrinx which in turn enlarged the central canal, or a deviated syrinx which bulged in one direction (often into what is known as the dorsal horn of the spinal cord).

Fig 5-7: Syrinx Classification

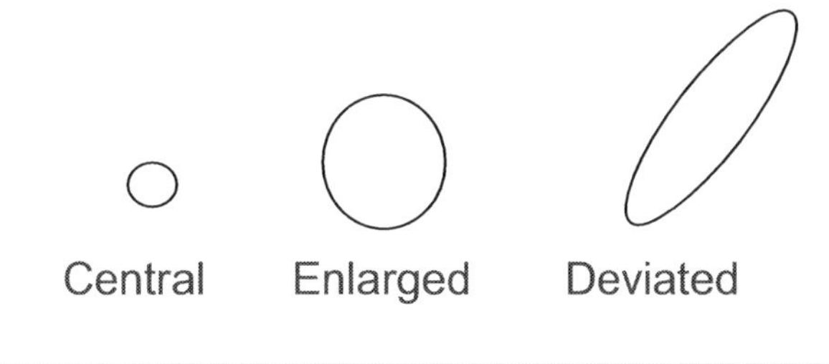

Central Syrinx - Contained within the central canal

Enlarged Syrinx - One that enlarges the central canal

Deviated Syrinx- A syrinx that bulges in one direction more than others; often into the dorsal horn area of the spine

The study found that not only was syrinx shape related to post-surgical, residual pain, but it was related to the presence of pain prior to surgery as well. Specifically, all 8 patients with deviated syrinxes had pain, while only 9 of the 15 enlarged syrinxes, and neither of the two central syrinxes caused pain. Post-surgically, only 1 out of the 8 patients with a deviated syrinx showed any pain improvement (a very poor outcome). In addition, in 3 patients, an enlarged syrinx transformed into a deviated syrinx, and in all three cases the patients showed no pain improvement. In total, 10 out of 11 patients who had deviated syrinxes either before or after surgery still suffered from pain after surgery.

Based upon these findings, it is likely that certain syrinxes – which penetrate the dorsal horn where nerve fibers run – cause permanent damage which decompression surgery can not help. It is also likely that other syrinxes cause symptoms that are reversible once the CSF dynamics are restored and the syrinx is no longer active.

Personal Experience: When I was discussing with my surgeon whether to have surgery right away (my older daughter had just been born) he told me that I could wait but that you can never tell when the damage from a syrinx will become permanent. At the time he was right, but there is now a research group looking at whether an advanced imaging technique can be used to identify whether individual nerve fibers have been damaged by a syrinx.

One complicating factor in studying how syrinxes affect outcomes is the fact that syrinxes change size and shape over time, but the damage they cause may not. There is actually some evidence that once syrinxes reach a certain size, they will begin to shrink on their own (although this does not mean the patient gets better, but they may stop getting worse). Thus at any given point in time, the size and shape of a syrinx may not match the symptoms it has caused over time. This makes correlating the physical characteristics of a syrinx with symptoms or neurological findings at a single point in time very difficult.

Herniation Size

As has been discussed throughout this book, despite being the basis for the original findings of Hans Chiari, research has shown time and again that the amount of tonsillar herniation (as measured in mm) does *NOT* correlate with symptom severity or clinical outcome. In other words, someone with a 3mm herniation is not guaranteed to have a better outcome than someone with a 20mm herniation.

This is very important to keep in mind as a patient facing surgery, a large herniation does not necessarily mean a poorer outcome and vice versa. This has been demonstrated clearly in many research studies involving hundreds of patients of all ages and with a variety of symptoms.

Complex Anatomy/Other Diseases

The anatomy of the craniovertebral junction can vary among Chiari patients. Some people have tonsillar herniation but no other significant problems, while others seem to have a variety of abnormalities in the region, such as congenitally fused vertebra, bone pushing on the brainstem, or even a kinked brainstem. While there has been little to no research directly comparing the outcomes of patients with "simple" anatomies versus complex ones, it seems logical to assume that in general people with more complex anatomical problems may tend to have poorer outcomes.

Theoretically, this could be for a couple of reasons. For one, such patients may require additional procedures to provide stability, etc.

Second, some of these abnormalities may be difficult to treat and thus go uncorrected (see Personal Experience below).

Personal Experience: When reviewing my MRI with me, my surgeon had trouble finding the precise words to use to describe my anatomy around the brainstem and top of the spine. He kept saying it was kind of like this, and kind of like that, but the point was that there were a number of abnormalities, not all of which could be fixed using a posterior fossa decompression. The standard surgical approach to basilar invagination, (which I have to some degree) is through the mouth and is even more traumatic than the posterior fossa decompression. Because of this, my surgeon recommended waiting to see how I felt after the standard decompression before deciding whether the remaining symptoms were worth doing anything else.

Similarly, Chiari has been linked in the medical literature with numerous genetic conditions which can further complicate the situation. Common sense says that if Chiari is just one of several underlying problems that it may be more difficult to treat and outcomes may not be as favorable even though this has not been reported in the medical literature.

Age

There is a general feeling in the Chiari community that children on average tend to have better outcomes than adults after surgery. However, this is completely unscientific and in fact, similar to duration of symptoms, the research is not conclusive on whether age at time of surgery plays a role in outcomes.

A 2004 study by Navarro of 96 children found that those operated on when they were younger than eight were three times more likely to improve than children older than eight. The quality of life study by Mueller however found no correlation between age and outcome after surgery for the adults they treated. In addition, a study by Scott, (discussed in more detail later in this chapter) actually found that children under five were more likely to require additional surgery than older children.

It is possible that age is a factor in outcomes only up to a certain point after which it doesn't matter, but it is also possible, and perhaps more likely, that there simply has not been enough research focused on studying this issue to determine whether age at time of surgery is indeed important.

Putting It All Together

While there are indications that in general a number of factors play a role in outcomes after surgery, it is important for patients to keep in mind that there is no way to predict for any given person whether surgery will work or not. So while an adult with syringomyelia who has suffered with pain for years and has progressive scoliosis on average may fare worse than someone with Chiari only, whose symptoms came on suddenly and was diagnosed right away, it does not mean that surgery will fail for any specific individual. Research has a long way to go in building a model that will be able to accurately predict who will benefit from surgery and by how much.

Therefore, if you are facing surgery, it is very important to discuss this topic in depth with your surgeon.

Objectively Measuring Success

Just as researchers are trying to find a way to objectively define Chiari in general, researchers are also trying to find objective indicators of a successful surgical outcome. Almost by definition, any parameter or test that effectively measures Chiari before surgery, is likely to also be useful as an indicator after surgery, so many of the same candidates discussed earlier in regards to finding a new definition of Chiari are also leading contenders for measures of surgical success.

Specifically, research has been published recently on CSF flow patterns and compliance before and after decompression surgery.

CSF Flow

One such candidate for measuring the success of surgery is quantifying the flow of CSF. While clinicians may use their judgment and cine MRIs to evaluate whether there is sufficient CSF flow, some researchers are taking a more detailed, and mathematical, approach to the subject.

Anyone who's played with a garden hose in the summertime understands the concept that the water will flow out faster if you partially cover the end of the hose with your thumb. There is evidence that a similar thing happens when a Chiari malformation blocks the flow of cerebrospinal fluid (CSF), and a group from the University of Wisconsin has shown that decompression surgery actually reverses that effect and can reduce the velocity of CSF as it flows around the cerebellar tonsils.

In a healthy person, CSF flows from the brain to the spinal cord and back again with every heartbeat. When the heart beats, it pumps blood into the brain. Since the skull is rigid, the increased blood in the brain creates pressure which sends CSF from the brain, through the foramen magnum, and into the spinal area (this is referred to as the caudal direction). As the heart retracts, the process is reversed and some CSF flows back into the brain (this is referred to as the cephalad direction).

With the development of phase-contrast MRI, scientists have been able to begin quantifying how CSF flows into and out of the spinal area. Unfortunately, this is not an easy process. Analyzing the data from the MRI is not straightforward and several techniques have been developed, which don't necessarily produce the same results. In addition, the flow of CSF itself appears to be very complicated and varies from person to person. Despite these obstacles, there are early indications that like a garden hose, the tonsils of a Chiari malformation do create abnormal CSF flow and create high-speed jets that are not found in healthy people.

To study this effect, Haughton and Iskandar examined 8 Chiari patients who underwent surgery between 1999 and 2001 and who had phase-contrast MRI studies done both before and after surgery. They used a technique they developed to measure the maximum velocity of every voxel - a 3-dimensional pixel - in the foramen magnum area 14 times during the cardiac cycle. From this, they identified the maximum velocity for each patient in both the caudal and cephalad directions. In addition, they reviewed clinical symptom data on whether the subjects suffered (before and after surgery) from:

- occipital headaches
- Valsalva (strain induced) headaches
- motor deficiencies
- sensory deficiencies
- vertigo
- cranial nerve dysfunction

The surgical technique used was similar for all patients and included a craniectomy, C1 laminectomy, and duraplasty. The group published their results in the January, 2004 issue of "*American Journal of Neuroradiology*".

Overall, the researchers found that the CSF velocity in the caudal direction did decrease for 6 out of the 8 patients. For the group as a whole, the average maximum velocity dropped significantly from 3.4 cm/s to 2.4 cm/s. In the cephalad direction, the maximum velocity also decreased for 6 out of 8 patients, but the decrease was more pronounced than the other direction. On average, the maximum cephalad velocity decreased from 6.9 cm/s to 3.9 cm/s, a finding that is on the verge of being statistically significant.

Surprisingly - given the growing popularity of CSF flow studies - the researchers did not find a correlation between clinical outcome and a reduction in CSF velocity. In addition, for three patients, either one or both velocities actually increased after surgery.

Mathematically studying fluid flow is a complicated and difficult undertaking where many assumptions are often made in an attempt to get a handle on the problem. The failure of this study to find a connection between symptoms and CSF velocity may indicate that CSF analysis needs to look beyond simple velocity, or it may indicate that there really is no connection between the two. Either way, the researchers are continuing to actively look at CSF flow patterns as an indication of surgical success and are refining their techniques.

Compliance

Also using advanced imaging techniques, a group of researchers out of Chicago has demonstrated that a parameter known as compliance may be a useful measure of surgical outcome in Chiari patients. Anusha Sivaramakrishnan, Dr. Noam Alperin, and Sushma Surapaneni from the University of Illinois, Chicago, along with Dr. Terry Lichtor, a neurosurgeon at Rush-Presbyterian Medical Center, examined the effects of decompression surgery on a number of MRI derived parameters - including compliance - in 12 Chiari patients.

The Chiari patients included 8 women and 4 men with herniations ranging from 5mm -17mm. Four had Chiari only, 5 had Chiari plus syringomyelia, and 3 had Chiari plus hydrocephalus Each patient underwent a similar surgery which included a sub-occipital craniectomy, laminectomy, and duraplasty. Eleven of the twelve patients improved symptomatically after surgery, while one person continued to suffer from symptoms.

Using phase contrast MRI, the research team measured - both before and after surgery - the amount of spinal cord displacement, the maximum CSF velocity, maximum CSF flow rate (how quickly a volume of CSF moves), the amount of CSF which flowed back and forth between the skull and spine, and the intracranial compliance.

As discussed earlier, compliance is a measure of a vessel or container's, stiffness. It is measured as the change in volume of a vessel in response to a change in pressure. A highly compliant container, like a balloon, can be expanded by blowing air into it. A low compliance container, like a glass jar, will not expand much as the pressure inside it is increased.

Recall that with every heartbeat, blood rushes into the brain/cranium via arteries, blood flows out through veins, and CSF flows from the skull to the spinal area. Thus, intracranial compliance is a measure of how the cranium/brain area responds to the inrush of blood during a heartbeat. To measure compliance, the research team quantified the total amount of blood and CSF flowing into and out of the skull area during a heartbeat, quantified the pressure of the CSF, and then mathematically derived a Compliance Index for each subject.

Of all the parameters measured, the team found that only the Compliance Index significantly changed on average after surgery (Figure 5-8). It increased an average of 64 % for the group and increased in 10 of the 12 patients. In one person, it remained unchanged, and it actually decreased in one person. Interestingly, the person in whom compliance decreased after surgery was the person who continued to suffer from symptoms after surgery. During surgery, this patient was noted to have a significant amount of dural scarring and adhesions, which may explain why the operation did not work.

Figure 5-8: Compliance Index Pre and Post Surgery

Measurement	Before Surgery	After Surgery
Max Spinal Cord Displacement (mm)	.32	.25
Max CSF Velocity (cm/s)	1.6	1.56
Max CSF Volumetric Flow Rate (ml/min)	180.5	153.5
Compliance Index	6.9	11.3

Note: Only Compliance demonstrated a statistically significant change from before to after surgery

While the compliance finding is the most significant, it is also noteworthy that this study did not find that simply measuring CSF velocity was a useful parameter. This is in contrast to the work of Haughton/Iskandar and highlights the complexity of research in this area.

Although this work is preliminary, Dr. Alperin was recently awarded a large NIH grant to study how compliance relates to Chiari and compliance remains a promising candidate for an objective measure of success.

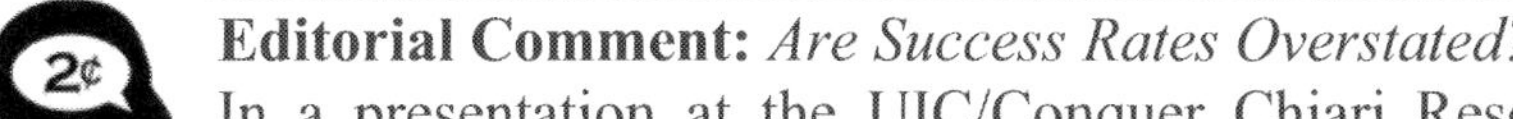

Editorial Comment: *Are Success Rates Overstated?*
In a presentation at the UIC/Conquer Chiari Research Symposium 2007, I stated that I believe that success rates are overstated in the medical literature. What I meant by this is that I think the medical community has an overly optimistic view of the outcomes of decompression surgery. However, this is my opinion and I very well could be wrong.

I don't think it is drastically overstated and I do think it's safe to say that surgery, especially if patients are carefully selected, will help a majority of people. But the question is, how much does it help and do people really return to a completely normal life? Or, do they just learn to live with the limitations that Chiari imposes? How many people change careers because of Chiari, or choose to forego having children, or give up activities they truly enjoyed? We don't know the answer to these questions.

Further, as outlined in the beginning of this chapter measuring success is difficult. If a surgery does not work, or if symptoms return 2 years after surgery, will the patient return to their original doctor, or will they seek out someone new?

Unfortunately, whether surgery will work remains one of the great unknowns that Chiari patients must face.

Residual Symptoms

Whether the overall success rate of Chiari is overstated or not, the reality is that a significant percentage of patients, especially those with syrinxes, will continue to experience at least some residual symptoms after surgery. At what point residual symptoms cross the line to become a failed surgery is purely a matter of opinion.

Residual symptoms also tend to be dynamic, waxing and waning over time, aggravated by certain activities (or the weather) and relieved by other activities. We will discuss coping with residual symptoms in more detail later in the book, but some of the most common problems people continue to have are:

Pain

A survey by the American Syringomyelia Alliance Project (ASAP) found that pain is the number one problem people have to deal with after decompression surgery. Often, Chiari and syringomyelia patients end up facing different kinds of pain as well; burning neuropathic pain, allodynia (where a light touch is interpreted as pain), and musculo-skeletal pain to name a few. Different types of pain and ways of coping with them are discussed in much more detail later in the book.

Heachaches

Sometimes people can feel like the surgery was a success because overall they feel much better, but they may still suffer from occasional headaches. This can be especially true for someone whose CSF flow may have improved but was not completely restored, or someone who continues to have chronically elevated intracranial pressure.

In addition, the type of headache can change. For adult men especially, it can take a long time for the thick muscles of the neck to heal after the trauma of surgery and can leave them prone to tension headaches. Also, if a plate was not used during surgery, the muscles of the neck can attach directly to the dura which can lead to headaches.

Muscle Weakness

Weakness of the neck and shoulder girdle is a common problem for CM/SM patients, even after surgery, as can be weakness in the legs. If the weakness is due to nerve damage from a syrinx it can be difficult to overcome and regain strength. However, even over the long-term nerve function can improve and it is important to continue to try to regain strength with the help of a qualified professional.

Loss of Sensation

Research has shown that for people with a syrinx, loss of sensation – to touch or temperature – in a specific area is one of the least likely symptoms to improve with surgery. This is likely due to nerve damage from the syrinx to the nerve fibers which communicate sensation information to the brain.

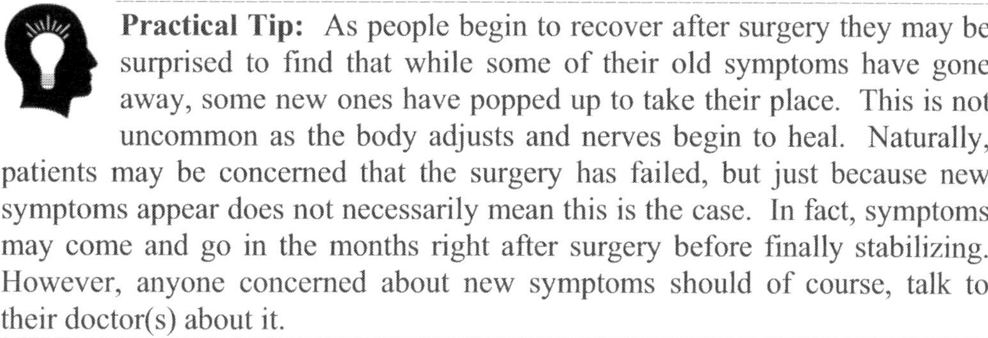

Practical Tip: As people begin to recover after surgery they may be surprised to find that while some of their old symptoms have gone away, some new ones have popped up to take their place. This is not uncommon as the body adjusts and nerves begin to heal. Naturally, patients may be concerned that the surgery has failed, but just because new symptoms appear does not necessarily mean this is the case. In fact, symptoms may come and go in the months right after surgery before finally stabilizing. However, anyone concerned about new symptoms should of course, talk to their doctor(s) about it.

Personal Experience: My residual symptoms change with the seasons. During the winter, I feel really good…strong, no headaches, little pain, high energy. However, during the dog days of summer in July and August I start to get headaches, my neck hurts, my whole body aches and my energy level plummets. I literally count the days until September when I can feel good. Maybe the heat of the summer causes just enough swelling to trigger the symptoms or maybe it has to do with atmospheric pressure, but whatever the case may be it is literally like night and day.

However, no matter the time of year, my biggest residual symptom is muscle weakness on the right side of my neck and right shoulder.

Even after years of physical therapy and exercise, the right side of my upper body is noticeable smaller than my left and this weakness causes me many difficulties, such as with reading, working on the computer, and sitting or standing for long periods of time.

When Surgery Fails

At the 2007 Conquer Chiari Research Symposium, Dr. Ghassan Bejjani, of the University of Pittsburgh and a Scientific Advisor to Conquer Chiari, presented a concise but thorough overview of the different reasons that decompression surgery can fail in adults. His analysis was based on his own experience, in addition to published medical literature. While there are not really any large scale reports on failed surgery in adults, Dr. Bejjani was able to piece together different causes from references in smaller patient series.

While his presentation was focused mostly on adults, it is clear that most, if not all, of the reasons he cited apply equally to children as well. The following is a summary of his analysis.

Possible Reasons for Failed Decompression Surgery

1. **Inadequate Decompression**
   a. No Duraplasty – In an effort to reduce trauma during surgery, there is a growing trend to leave the dura intact, especially for children. If a patient did not receive a duraplasty during the initial surgery and symptoms did not improve, many surgeons will reoperate and open the dura.
   b. Not Enough Bone Removed – If not enough bone is removed during decompression then the brain tissue can still be compressed and CSF flow blocked. Essentially, the decompression was not big enough and a reoperation is likely necessary.
2. **Recurrent CSF Obstruction**
   a. Scarring – Sometimes scarring and adhesions even if removed during the initial surgery can redevelop and obstruct CSF flow leading to problems.
   b. Retethering of the Spinal Cord – An extension of the scarring problem above, if the spinal cord becomes abnormally anchored and tethered, symptoms are likely to result.
   c. Regrowth of Bone at the Foramen Magnum – There have actually been several case reports, documented with MRIs, of children in whom the bone that was removed around the cerebellar tonsils actually regrows and recompresses the area, necessitating additional surgery.

3. **Surgical Complications**
    a. Pseudomeningocele – One of the more common complications associated with decompression surgery, pseudomeningoceles can range from asymptomatic to requiring surgical repair.
    b. Cerebellar Sag (Ptosis) – One of the most serious complications, cerebellar sag is where the cerebellum slumps down after surgery because its bony support has been removed. Although it can be difficult to treat, Lazareff recently published a surgical technique which involves rebuilding the support for the brain while maintaining an adequate decompression.
    c. Altered Neural Hydrodynamics – Neural Hydrodynamics refers to how CSF flows in the brain and spine. Some patients can develop hydrocephalus or chronically elevated intracranial pressure (IIH) after decompression surgery (or it was undiagnosed before the surgery, see below). Naturally, these conditions cause symptoms, often similar to Chiari, and are usually treated surgically by implanting a shunt to divert CSF.
    d. Cranio-Cervical Instability – Chiari patients tend to have an unusual anatomy at the junction of the head and neck. This, combined with removing bone during decompression surgery, can lead to instability in some people and cause problems. If the neck is not stabilized during the initial surgery, additional surgery may be necessary to do so.
    e. Muscle Adheres to the Dura – Since part of the skull is removed during surgery, and if nothing is put back in its place, certain muscles of the neck have nothing solid to attach to and may attach directly to the dura. If this occurs, then when the neck muscles are used, they can pull on the dura (thus lowering compliance) and cause problems, such as headaches. This is why surgical manufacturers are working with neurosurgeons to develop Chiari plates that are put in where the skull pieces were removed. A plate provides the muscles with something to attach to and can greatly reduce this problem.
4. **Concurrent Conditions**
    a. Idiopathic Intracranial Hypertension – The link between chronically elevated intracranial pressure (also known as pseudotumor cerebri) and Chiari is not completely understood. As discussed in more detail later in this chapter some patients appear to develop PTC after surgery, but it is also likely that some patients have PTC prior to surgery, which means that decompression surgery will only provide temporary relief of their symptoms.
    b. Basilar Invagination – A significant percentage of Chiari patients also have some degree of basilar invagination or impression (where the second vertebrae is moved up and pushes on the brainstem). In general, this is not directly treated by a posterior fossa decompression,

so a patient whose symptoms are due mostly to basilar invagination may not get relief from a standard Chiari decompression.

c. Other – Chiari has been linked with numerous genetic conditions which obviously can bring their own complications and problems to a Chiari surgery.

5. **Symptoms Not Due To Chiari**
   a. Asymptomatic Tonsillar Ectopia – Because of its many manifestations, Chiari is often misdiagnosed as other diseases and problems. However, there is a flip-side to this phenomenon as well. Namely, because there is not a good, objective definition of Chiari and not everyone with herniated cerebellar tonsils has symptomatic Chiari, a person's symptoms may not always be due to the tonsillar herniation. When this is the case, then of course decompression surgery will do nothing to help the patients.

What the Research Says (Pediatric)

While in general there are not many studies focused on failed surgery, a noticeable exception came from Harvard pediatric neurosurgeon, Dr. R Michael Scott, and his colleague, Dr. David Sacco. In a 2003 study, the surgeons reviewed the hospital records, medical imaging, operative reports, and follow-up data of patients who were undergoing a reoperation for Chiari malformation during the past 14 years and compared the data to patients who were undergoing their first operation. The researchers specifically were trying to determine if age at time of first surgery, type of Chiari malformation (I vs. II), bony abnormalities, and/or initial operative technique contribute to the need for reoperation.

Of 133 operations for Chiari I or II that were performed, 22 (17%) represented reoperations. Interestingly, the reoperation rates for Chiari I and Chiari II were almost identical, with 16 out of 100 Chiari I surgeries being reoperations and 6 out of 33 Chiari II surgeries being reoperations. Also of note is the fact that exactly half of the reoperations (11) were required within 1 year of the initial surgery and half (11) were not performed until more than a year from the time of the initial surgery. Reasons for reoperation included a persistent syrinx in 11 patients, continued neurological symptoms in 9 patients, and problems with stent placement in 2 patients.

In looking at patient age at time of initial surgery, the researchers found that of the 43 patients whose initial surgery occurred when they were younger than 5 years old, 11 required reoperation (26%). In contrast, of the 90 patients who were older than 5, only 10 required additional surgery (11%).

The researchers also found an apparent association between skull anomalies - craniosynostosis - and the need for reoperation. There is an established link between abnormal skull shape and Chiari malformation, but this study also found that out of 9 patients with craniosynostosis, 5 were undergoing a reoperation. The authors speculated that a complicated - and confusing - bone structure around the foramen magnum can lead to an inadequate decompression unless it is carefully studied and understood by the neurosurgeon. In addition, craniosynostosis likely leads to abnormal CSF dynamics and may cause persistent problems that are difficult to resolve with decompression surgery.

The final factor the researchers examined as a cause of surgical failure was operative technique. Five of the reoperations that were performed were necessitated by problems with a fourth ventricle catheter - or stent. While the authors believe in using a catheter in patients with syringomyelia, they acknowledge that problems can develop if the tubing is too long or is not placed properly.

Although the study involved a significant number of patients, because of its design it is difficult to draw strong conclusions based on this data alone.

What the Research Says (The PTC Link)

Another notable exception is research exploring the link between Idiopathic Intracranial Hypertension (aka pseudotumor cerebri, PTC) and Chiari. According to Dr. Bejjani, this is what actually got him interested in looking at failed surgery. Basically, he noticed that some of his patients would initially experience symptom relief after decompression surgery, but then symptoms would come back about six months after surgery. When one patient reported feeling better after a lumbar puncture (a procedure where a needle is injected into the CSF filled space of the spine in the lumbar region), he realized that she might be suffering from PTC and felt better because the lumbar puncture (LP) drained CSF and reduced the patient's intracranial pressure.

Some time later, Dr. Bejjani published a report on his experience with six patients whom he believed showed signs of PTC after decompression surgery. Four of the patients were treated with shunts, while two chose to undergo regular lumbar punctures to drain CSF and take medication to help control their ICP.

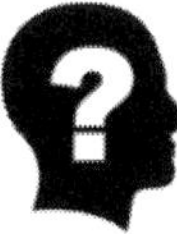

What Is Idiopathic Intracranial Hypertension (IIH)?

- Condition where intracranial pressure (ICP) is abnormally high for unknown reasons; normal ICP is considered <20cmH2O (water)
- Also called pseudotumor cerebri; first identified in the late 19th century
- Most common symptoms are severe headache and visual disturbances

- Can lead to blindness from pressure on the optic nerve
- Diagnosed when an MRI is normal and lumbar puncture shows elevated ICP
- Eye exam may reveal papilledema, a sign of increased ICP
- Number of people affected is not well established, but some estimates are as high as 1 in 100,000
- More common among overweight women of childbearing age
- Usually treated medically with drugs that lower ICP
- Some patients require surgery around the optic nerve to prevent blindness
- In some patients, a shunt is placed to drain CSF out of the brain

---

In a larger study, Dr. Frim, from the University of Chicago, looked back at failed surgeries to see if PTC could account for some of them. Specifically, they reviewed 192 surgeries they had performed (they excluded patients with abnormal skull shapes and hydrocephalus) and found that surgery had failed in 36 cases (19%). They then identified PTC among the 36 failures using the following criteria:

1. Cine MRI showed adequate CSF flow out of the 4th ventricle and across the skull-spine junction
2. Chiari-like symptoms came back after decompression surgery
3. Elevated CSF pressure as measured by a lumbar puncture
4. Symptoms were temporarily relieved after draining a large amount of CSF (through the lumbar puncture) and reducing the CSF pressure in half

Using these criteria, the researchers found 15 patients, 6 adults and 9 children, who were classified as having PTC after their decompression surgery. The symptoms they suffered from included head pain, body aches, balance problems, and visual disturbances. The fifteen PTC-Chiari patients accounted for nearly half of the failed surgeries (42%) and 8% of the entire surgical group.

Five of the six adults and all of the children underwent a second operation to insert a shunt in order to drain CSF and lower their intracranial pressure. Unfortunately, only one of the adults showed any improvement after this procedure. However, 7 of the 9 children did improve significantly with the shunting. These results are not as good as those from Bejjani's study, but the number of patients in each study is too small to draw any conclusions from regarding treatment.

While there is strong evidence of a link between Chiari and PTC, what exactly that link is remains a mystery. Does Chiari, or even decompression surgery lead to PTC; does PTC cause Chiari; or could it be both? At the moment it seems likely that it is both as there is evidence both that PTC can lead to Chiari and there is also evidence that decompression surgery can somehow change the CSF hydrodynamics and cause PTC.

Further Treatment Options

In general how patients are treated after a failed decompression surgery depends largely on the reason the surgery failed. If the decompression was inadequate then more bone can be removed or the dura can be opened and expanded to provide more space. If the spinal cord has become tethered in one or more spots, then it will likely need to be released surgically. If there are indications of PTC, than a shunt or regular LP's to drain CSF would be the treatment options to consider.

The key from the patient's point of view is to make sure there is a good understanding of why the surgery failed so that the proper treatment can be pursued. From an outcomes point of view, there is very little data available on the success of reoperations, but the meager data that is there suggests that the percentage of successful surgeries is even lower than with initial decompressions.

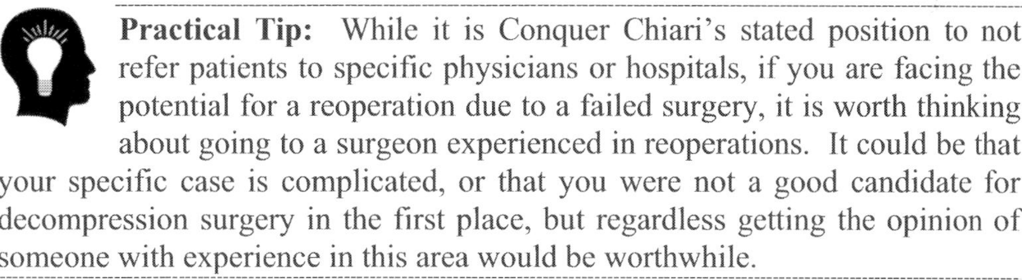

Practical Tip: While it is Conquer Chiari's stated position to not refer patients to specific physicians or hospitals, if you are facing the potential for a reoperation due to a failed surgery, it is worth thinking about going to a surgeon experienced in reoperations. It could be that your specific case is complicated, or that you were not a good candidate for decompression surgery in the first place, but regardless getting the opinion of someone with experience in this area would be worthwhile.

Long Term

Symptom Recurrence

Most of the outcomes data that does exist follows patients for only 1-2 years. This begs the question, what can Chiari patients expect 5, 10 or 15 years after surgery? While the topic has not been systematically studied, there is substantial anecdotal evidence, and many neurosurgeons will acknowledge, that long term symptoms recurrence is a real issue.

Conquer Chiari has heard from many people who were doing well, for years, and then began to experience symptoms again. The problem with anecdotal reports is that it is difficult to put them into perspective. Chances are that someone who experiences symptoms after 5 good years will look on the internet for reasons why and is likely to ask an organization like Conquer Chiari if it is common. Whereas someone at the 5 year mark with no symptoms is very *unlikely* to contact Conquer Chiari. In other words, we are much more likely to hear about the cases of symptoms coming back than the ones where everything is fine. This makes it impossible to determine, from this type of anecdotal reporting, how frequently symptoms recur in the long term.

Despite this, theoretically there are two major reasons that long term symptom recurrence could be more common than we think. First, as everyone knows our body changes as we age. What is not as well known is that as people age their dura tends to thicken naturally and develop scarring and adhesions. These are all bad things for Chiari patients as a thick dura can restrict CSF flow and lower compliance, which we know may be related to symptoms.

The second major factor in long term symptoms recurrence is trauma. Again turning to the anecdotal evidence, it appears that many Chiari patients can be doing quite well and then they undergo some type of trauma, such as a car accident or fall. We know that a significant percentage of patients report trauma as a precipitating factor in their original symptoms, so it seems logical that a trauma after surgery could cause problems as well.

In fact, research not directly focused on Chiari suggests that Chiari patients may be more susceptible to head trauma than the average person.

Trauma

In 2006, an international team led by Konstantin Salci of Uppsals University, Sweden, showed that low intracranial compliance may leave the brain vulnerable to traumatic injury. While the thrust of the work related mainly to the management of traumatic brain injuries, since compliance may play a big role in Chiari symptoms, the findings should be of interest to the Chiari community as well.

Recall that intracranial compliance represents, in one sense, how well the brain handles the cyclic inflow of blood driven by the heart. With Chiari, the herniated tonsils block the natural outlet for CSF and studies have shown that Chiari patients tend to have lower intracranial compliance than normal. In addition, it has been shown that successful decompression surgery results in an increase in intracranial compliance.

In this study, Salci and his colleagues used a rat model to demonstrate that rats with lower intracranial compliance suffered greater effects from subsequent brain insults (physical insults, not the verbal kind). Specifically, the researchers took a number of rats, removed parts of the skull and exposed their dura. Next, in some of the rats, they dropped a weight on to the exposed dura to cause swelling. They then replaced the skull pieces but on some of them glued layers of rubber on the inside of the bone. The rats randomly received 0,1,2, or 3 layers of rubber, which incrementally reduced the space available for the brain to expand. The goal of all this work was to reduce the intracranial compliance of some of the rats by varying degrees.

After the compliance lowering work, some of the rats were chosen to get repeated injections of saline which were infused into their brain compartments. This infusion of fluid into the brain was intended to test the effect of the reduced compliance (which recall is the ability to handle an increase in volume). Finally all the rats were euthanized and their brains examined to measure the levels of specific substances known as metabolites. Metabolites are by-products of the body's natural metabolism and abnormal levels in the brain can indicate disease or damage.

The researchers found that the rats with the lowest compliance (three layers of rubber) had the most significant metabolic changes in their brains. While this was purely a chemical change, in other words the real-world effects of these changes were not evaluated, it is interesting that when the brain loses its natural compliance it loses its cushion, so to speak, to absorb certain events.

While the results from studying rats do not always apply to people, it may be that the lower compliance of Chiari patients leaves them vulnerable to head traumas, which in turn spark symptom recurrence.

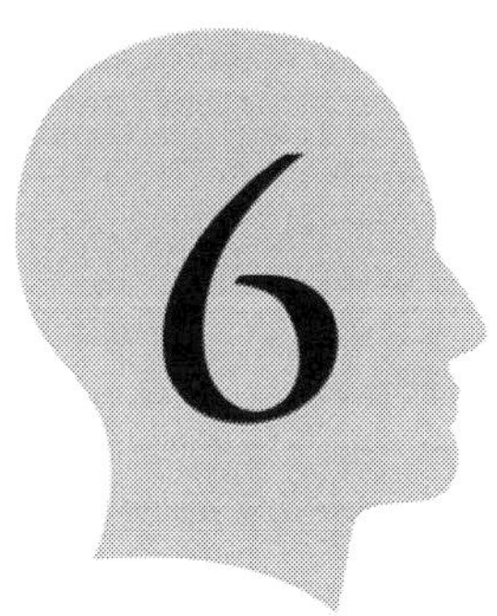

6 Recovery

"Recovery is brought about not by the physician, but by the sick man himself. He heals himself, by his own power, exactly as he walks by means of his power, or eats, or thinks, breathes or sleeps"

~George Groddeck (1866-1934)~
German Physician from
"The Book of It"

In General

This is by far the shortest chapter in the book. Not because the topic of recovery is not important, but rather because there is essentially no published research on the subject. Even by Chiari standards, the issue of recovering from surgery has been poorly researched and it seems like every surgeon has a different approach: some recommend physical therapy, some don't; some put strict limits on activities, some don't; some encourage people to return to work quickly, others advise waiting; some follow up with patients, others refer them to a neurologist.

Because of this, in addition to being very short, this chapter is based more on logic, practical thinking, and patient experiences than the results of research studies.

Everyone Is Different

For a patient entering the recovery period after decompression surgery, it is important to understand that everyone is different. While it is useful for patients to trade tips and talk about how long it took them to do certain things, remember there is no set standard. Each person recovers in their own time and in their own way. The following quotes from two Chiari patients highlight the extremes of the recovery phase:

"I was home in 5 days and up to the full activities of a mom and mom's taxi within 14. I did my chores slower and it was awhile before I could actually see what was on my dinner plate because my neck was so stiff!"~ Susan~

"Recovery was an adventure in and of itself. I had to ask for help in doing the simplest things. I had to rely on everyone to carry me through."~Anonymous~

Susan jumped right back into her role as an active mom, while the other patient seemed incapable of doing anything for an extended period of time. These quotes are the norm, not the exception. Some people recover very quickly, and are back to almost full strength in a matter of weeks. Others may take years to recover, and their recovery may come in fits and starts as they struggle to advance and then run into multiple setbacks.

Some factors that can affect how long (and easily) a person recovers from surgery include:

- **Surgical Complications** – Obviously, if a person has direct complications from the surgery, such as an infection or CSF leak, their recovery will be not be as smooth.

- **Success of Decompression** – For some people, Chiari symptoms disappear almost immediately after surgery, and when that occurs recovery from the surgery itself is usually much easier. For people whose symptoms take time to go away (or don't go away at all) recovery can be more difficult, especially if those symptoms continue to limit physical activity.
- **Duration of Symptoms/Physical Condition** – If a person has suffered for years from Chiari and syringomyelia related symptoms, then there's a good chance they have become very weak and their overall health may have deteriorated. For these people, the recovery process is starting at a different level and more time may be needed to feel good and be strong enough to engage in physical activities. In other words, recovery can be not just from the surgical trauma itself, but from the effects of symptoms as well. For a patient with muscle atrophy due to a syrinx, it can take a long time to rebuild strength.
- **Other Diseases** – Clearly a person with multiple health problems, such as heart disease, high blood pressure, or diabetes may have a harder time recovering from surgery than an otherwise healthy person. Similarly, as has been discussed previously in this book, Chiari is sometimes accompanied by related conditions, such as intracranial hypertension, which if not identified and addressed can impact recovery. Probably the most striking example of this is syringomyelia. Recovering from the effects of a syrinx can take a year or more, as compared to recovering from the trauma of surgery itself.
- **Lifestyle** – There may not be research to back this up, but it is logical to assume that a person's lifestyle will impact their recovery. Eating right, getting plenty of rest, drinking plenty of fluids and avoiding alcohol and tobacco are likely to help in the recovery process. One reason professional athletes can recover so quickly from injuries is because many of them tightly control what they eat and drink, how much rest they get, etc.
- **Mental Attitude** – Similar to lifestyle, it seems logical to assume that a person's mental attitude can have a strong effect on their recovery. A person with a positive approach is more likely to engage in activities that encourage recovery and thus will likely heal quicker. This in turn feeds back into their attitude resulting in a positive feedback loop. In contrast, someone with low expectations, or a negative approach, will be looking for reasons to not engage in activities that help recovery and will magnify small setbacks. This in turn feeds back into their mental view and creates a negative feedback loop.

Find Your Own Way, Common Sense & Work

Since there is no research, and since everyone is different, patients must find their own way when it comes to recovery. Each person must go at his or her own pace and find what works for them. Obviously it is important to listen to your doctors, especially if they restrict your activities, but it is also important to use common sense. It's important not to be too aggressive in recovering, but it's equally important to push when you have too.

Finally, it is important to recognize that recovery and healing is hard work. Chiari is not a sprained ankle; it is a serious disease and a traumatic surgery. A methodical, disciplined approach to recovery will pay off in the end.

The Recovery Process

As stated previously, there is no research in this area, so the following sections contain personal experiences and practical tips for the different phases of recovery.

The First Week

From a medical point of view, in the first week or two of recovery, the patient is recovering from the acute trauma of surgery. Recall that surgery can include cutting through a lot of muscle, removing bone, and manipulation underneath the dura. It is a traumatic surgery and takes time to recover from. Most patients will go back to the doctor 7-10 days after the surgery to get staples and/or stitches removed.

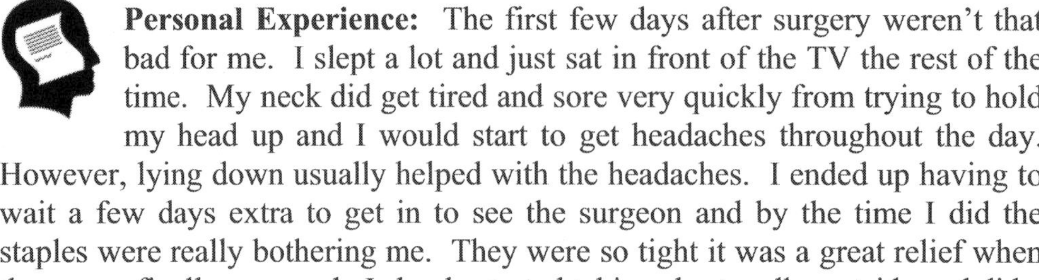

Personal Experience: The first few days after surgery weren't that bad for me. I slept a lot and just sat in front of the TV the rest of the time. My neck did get tired and sore very quickly from trying to hold my head up and I would start to get headaches throughout the day. However, lying down usually helped with the headaches. I ended up having to wait a few days extra to get in to see the surgeon and by the time I did the staples were really bothering me. They were so tight it was a great relief when they were finally removed. I slowly started taking short walks outside and did a few neck exercises the surgeon recommended (but these didn't feel too good).

Practical Tip: Many patients are given a high dose of steroid at the hospital. This can mask a lot of pain and make people think that things aren't going to be too bad, then when the steroids wear off it can be quite a shock. In other words, some people feel pretty good immediately after surgery, but then a week later feel a lot worse.

3 Months Post-Op

By the three month mark, many people feel the need to try to return to their previous activities and responsibilities. This is understandable as it is difficult for anyone to take that amount of time away from work and family. However, this is also a risky time when patients can push too hard and suffer significant setbacks. The best approach in returning to activities is to slowly push the envelope. Don't try to do everything all at once.

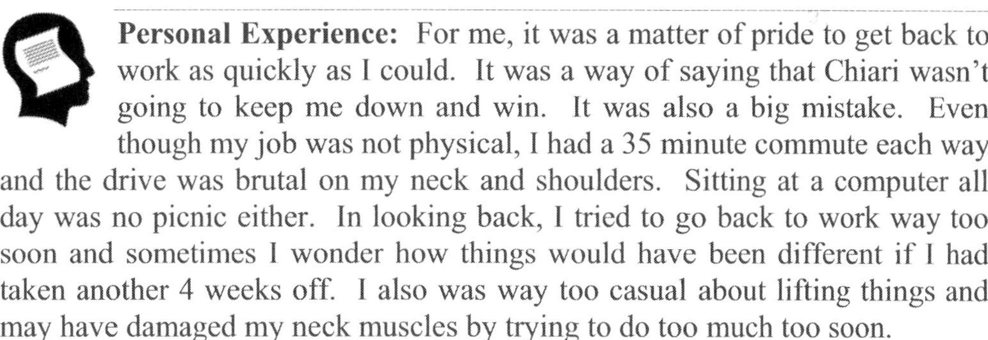

Personal Experience: For me, it was a matter of pride to get back to work as quickly as I could. It was a way of saying that Chiari wasn't going to keep me down and win. It was also a big mistake. Even though my job was not physical, I had a 35 minute commute each way and the drive was brutal on my neck and shoulders. Sitting at a computer all day was no picnic either. In looking back, I tried to go back to work way too soon and sometimes I wonder how things would have been different if I had taken another 4 weeks off. I also was way too casual about lifting things and may have damaged my neck muscles by trying to do too much too soon.

Practical Tip: If possible, consider returning to work part time at first, or if your job permits it work at home. This way you can slowly build up your endurance and slowly take on more responsibilities. Similarly, go very slowly when it comes to using your neck muscles for lifting things. Try to remember that these muscles were cut as part of the surgery and need time to heal.

One Year Post-Op

"Six months later, and the hair has grown back over the surgical scar on the back of my head. I had to teach my right side how to work again. It is amazing to actually feel my right hand and foot again after so many months of numbness and unresponsiveness."~Shelley~

By the one year mark, many people are back into the full swing of their lives. They may get tired a little more easily or they may get an occasional headache, but for the most part they have recovered not only from surgery, but from their symptoms as well.

However, many people do not feel that good even a full year after surgery. They may still feel very weak or just in general not feel good. The reality is that nerve tissue can take a long time to heal (if it heals at all), so people whose nervous systems were under stress can take a long time recover. Also, people who have suffered for years are starting their recovery from a very weak position and it takes time to regain strength.

Personal Experience: One year after surgery I was very frustrated with my progress. My neck hurt constantly, I still got headaches, and my whole body was just stiff. When I look at videos from that time I can't believe how slowly and stiffly I moved (compared to today). I kept going back to my surgeon asking what was wrong and he kept saying that I was adequately decompressed. I tried physical therapy once with terrible results and was tired of taking Celebrex all the time. At this point, I was questioning whether the surgery was worth it. What I didn't realize at the time was that I wasn't allowing myself the time to heal. I hadn't focused on recovering the way I should have and I also had unrealistic expectations. I failed to realize how incredibly weak I had become before surgery and I also failed to realize the damage that a syrinx can do.

Practical Tip: It can take more than a year to feel better after Chiari surgery. The problem many patients have is trying to figure out whether the surgery "worked" since they still feel so bad. Unfortunately this is a difficult question to answer. There is not really an objective test after surgery to evaluate whether it worked, rather a patient must rely on doctors' opinions. If you still feel bad a year after surgery, consider getting a couple of opinions from surgeons, especially ones familiar with Chiari. If everyone agrees the decompression was adequate, then you know you are dealing with recovery issues. If someone finds another problem, such as intracranial hypertension, then again you know what you're dealing with.

"One year after my surgery, I was wondering if this was as good as it was going to get" ~ Rick Labuda ~

Three Years Post-Op

"Everything was not wonderful at once though. It took 18 months to get all the strength back in my right arm (nerves heal slowly), I had really annoying myoclonus for several months afterward, I had tinnitus for about one year, I had problems with balance and confused speech for about 3 months, I still have episodes of dizziness but they are few and far between."~Pam~

Although published research usually doesn't go out this far, as the quote above demonstrates, 2-3 years is usually long enough for people to recover. However, this is not always the case. Anecdotally, some people have reported that they are still getting stronger five years or more after surgery. It is not exactly clear why this is the case, but often there will be a triggering event that sparks a delayed recovery. For example, a person may change jobs, find the right mix of medications, or finally find a way to control pain which was interfering with the recovery process.

Personal Experience – I muddled through the first few years after surgery. I tried different medications, acupuncture, physical therapy, and a number of other things in an attempt to get better. My neck hurt constantly and it seemed like a hundred times a day something happened that flared it up. In addition I just didn't feel good in general. Finally, I decided I needed to change some things. I had been thinking about the newsletter and Conquer Chiari, so I decided to leave my career and focus on this and my recovery. Working at home allowed me to lie down when I needed to and avoid situations which were difficult and painful. At the same time, I began exercising in a heated pool. I found the warm pool very effective in loosening up my muscles and providing a good way to increase my strength. When I first started, I couldn't even swim one length of the pool and now at least once a week I swim laps for 20-30 minutes. The gains have been amazing. My strength and endurance have improved dramatically and I'm able to do so many other things I wasn't able to do before. There were many setbacks along the way, but once I focused on my recovery and gave it the attention it needed, I was on the path to success.

Practical Tip – While many people will recover without a concentrated effort, if you're not recovering, at some point you need to make the decision to make your recovery a priority. This can be difficult with the demands of work and family, but if you make the commitment to yourself, you will likely find you will be in a better position to handle your other responsibilities. It's similar to the instructions given on an airplane regarding the oxygen…take care of yourself first, so that you can help others.

Symptoms

During the time period right after surgery, it is quite common for patients to experience a variety of symptoms. As the body adjusts and begins to heal, some symptoms go away, others can become worse, and new symptoms can appear and disappear in an apparently random fashion. This can be a very frustrating and confusing experience for a patient, as it can be difficult to tell if the surgery was successful.

During this time it is important not to overreact, but rather be observant and stay in communication with the doctors providing follow-up care. Even if some symptoms get worse, try to evaluate whether the major symptoms which drove the decision to have surgery are getting better. And remember it can take time for things to settle down symptom wise.

Use Your Support System

Now is the time to call in all the favors you may have accrued over the years. Chiari surgery is a major event and having a strong support system can be a real benefit. If friends and family offer help, take it, don't be proud and try to act as if it's no big deal.

Cooking dinner, driving kids around, cleaning the house, mowing the lawn, shoveling the driveway, all these things not only can be difficult, but can negatively impact recovery. So if people don't offer, ask for help. Ask your family and your friends. Use the materials on the Conquer Chiari website to help them understand what you can and can not do and how they can help.

A strong support system can enable a person to focus on their healing and also give them the peace of mind that they don't have to worry about things that they can't do. This of course can help speed up the recovery process.

7

Living with Chiari

My Brain is a Mess

My brain is a mess,
Looking around as I must,
My life is full of stress,

I spend everyday trying to fix,
Straighten and organizing all my things,
Adding more and less to the mix,

The doctors all say it is all in my head,
The evidence is clear in the pictures,
This is mixed up I dread,

The films they have taken do not lie,
So what is this problem,
It is all in my head I cry,

My brain is a mess,
The pictures all show,
Can we fix this more or less?

~Andrea Oliver~

Chiari Can Affect Every Aspect of Life

For some, the Chiari experience ends after recovering from surgery. For these people the surgery works, their symptoms resolve, and they return – more or less – to the life they once had. For others however, Chiari is a chronic disease which they will battle daily, even after surgery. For these people, some symptoms may persist – especially pain – and their lives will be inexorably altered. They will struggle to work, to maintain relationships, and to regain some type of "normal" life.

For these people, Chiari can affect every aspect of their life: physical, mental, emotional, economic, spiritual, and perhaps most hurtfully, their personal relationships. This is where the true, ugly impact of Chiari can be seen, in marriages that fall apart, in children who must bear the burden of unending pain, in moms unable to care for their children the way they would like to and in dads unable to work and provide for their families.

The next three chapters are for the people, and families, who fight against Chiari in their daily lives. This chapter provides an overview of a topic very important to many in the Chiari community, pain. While a thorough, in-depth look at pain could easily comprise an entire book on its own, what follows touches on the most important and relevant aspects of what pain is, its impact on daily life, and treatment options. This chapter also touches on the impact that Chiari can have on a family and some issues specific to women and children.

While this chapter focuses mostly on the negative impact that Chiari can have, Chapters 8 & 9 focus more on the positive and what people can do to fight Chiari. Specifically Chapter 8 looks to the future and why there are reasons for hope in our battle. Finally, Chapter 9 presents a view (the author's view) of how an individual can confront and conquer Chiari.

Pain

According to the International Association for the Study of Pain, pain can be defined as:

An unpleasant sensory and emotional experience associated with actual or potential tissue damage, or described in terms of such damage.

It may seem silly to try to define pain, after all everyone knows what pain is, but pain is one of those concepts that is difficult to pin down. While a person knows when they are in pain, describing the intensity and feelings associated with the pain can be difficult. Because pain is inherently subjective, it can be difficult to study, diagnose and treat.

However, pain is a vitally important subject to the Chiari community. In fact, surveys have shown that pain is the single most common, and likely most difficult problem CM/SM patients face after surgery. It is likely that many reading this right now may be experiencing some type of pain, be it a burning pain for no reason, or painful muscle spasms in the neck and shoulders. For many in the Chiari community, pain is a way of life. And while everyone has felt pain at some point in their lives, unless you have experienced severe, chronic pain, it is nearly impossible to understand how it can affect a person over time, and how it can lead to a myriad of other problems.

There are several reasons why chronic pain in general, and the pain associated with Chiari and syringomyelia in particular, is much worse than an everyday scrape or bruise:

1. **Chronic vs Acute** – The cut-off between acute and chronic pain is generally considered to be three months. In other words, pain that lasts longer than three months is said to be chronic in nature, while pain that lasts a week or two is thought of as acute. However, the difference between chronic and acute pain goes well beyond a point in time. Chronic pain actually becomes a medical condition unto itself. While it is not completely understood why some pain becomes chronic, many leading theories believe that actual, physical changes occur over time and that nerves can be become sensitized to pain. This means that a person may perceive pain more easily over time when exposed to a long-term painful stimulus.
2. **Chronic Pain Is Complex** – Chronic pain is a complex phenomenon and people often suffer from more than one type of pain. One published pain study put it this way, "Patients who have chronic neuropathic pain [often] have more than one type of pain. For example, a man who has post-herpetic neuralgia at high and mid thorax may have constant ongoing pain that keeps him awake all night; mechanical allodynia and hyperalgesia that prevent him from wearing any clothing so he cannot be active and socialize; secondary myofascial pain in the shoulder so that use of that arm is limited; and after a few short weeks of his pain, the patient is by now sleep deprived, depressed, anxious, and very irritable." (Backonja and Galer, Neurol Clin 1998;16).

   One could easily substitute Chiari or syringomyelia for post-herpetic neuralgia in the above quote and still have an accurate description. Chronic pain can trigger a cascade of events and lead to a downward spiral for the person on the receiving end.

   In addition, as the definition by the International Association for the Study of Pain indicates, pain is all about the experience, and research has indicated that how people experience pain is influenced by many things, including the higher thinking centers of the brain. This is illustrated by the Gate Theory of chronic pain, which states that as pain signals travel from the peripheral nerves through the spine and to the brain, they pass through a series of gates. Different factors, such as thoughts and emotions, can control these gates and either allow pain signals to pass through freely or restrict their passage.

So, for example, if a person is intensely concentrating on work - like writing a book chapter on pain - their chronic pain level may be low because the brain has closed some of the pain gates in order to concentrate on the task. However, when they take a break, or are done for the day, the pain may increase markedly, because there is nothing closing the pain gates and the pain signals on the nerves can pass through to the pain centers in the brain.

3. **Pain Is Subjective -** Since pain involves perception, that also means that pain, by definition, is a subjective experience. In other words, there is no way to know how much pain a person is feeling (or even what that feeling is like) other than how they describe it. Unfortunately, this can lead to problems of believability for people suffering from chronic pain. Because the pain is internal, other people may not believe they are in pain or think they are exaggerating how much pain they are in. In fact, one pain study found just that, namely that it is a common experience with the early stages of chronic pain that no one else believes the pain is real. Since the pain is often hidden, it can be difficult for other people to understand what someone is going through and this lack of validation can lead to emotional and social problems and even a loss of identity as the pain sufferer begins to doubt themselves.
4. **Chronic Pain Has a Wide Ranging Impact** – This will be discussed more thoroughly later in this chapter, but research has shown that chronic pain has an impact on overall health, commonly leads to depression, can fundamentally affect the structure of the brain, lead to economic hardship for families, and even alter people's spiritual beliefs. In other words, as opposed to acute pain, chronic pain can become an overwhelming problem which seeps into many aspects of a person's life.
5. **Chronic Pain Is Linked to Depression** – Research has shown time and again that people in chronic pain suffer from depression and anxiety at a high rate. In addition, the link appears to go beyond an intellectual type connection where people become sad because they are in pain and can't do certain activities. While this is likely a factor, it also appears that chronic pain can actually deplete the levels of key neurotransmitters in the brain which are known to affect mood. In other words, pain and emotion share some of the same chemical messengers in the brain. So pain influences mood at the most basic level and vice versa. This is probably why some anti-depressants can be used to treat pain.

6. **Lack of Effective Treatments** – While there are plenty of over the counter medicines to treat everyday aches and pains, treating chronic pain is a whole different ballgame. Despite millions and millions of dollars of research, some types of chronic pain, such as neuropathic pain due to nerve damage, remain very difficult to treat, leaving patients with few options for relief.

Neuropathic Pain

One of the main reasons that the pain of CM/SM patients is so difficult to deal with is because it is often what is called neuropathic pain. In general, neuropathic pain refers to pain due to nerve damage, but as is often the case, the devil is in the details. It turns out there are actually many different types of neuropathic pain. At the highest level, neuropathic pain is a result of damage to either the central nervous system (meaning the spinal cord and brain) or peripheral nerves (the actual nerve fibers which run throughout the body). In addition, the pain can be in response to a stimulus (such as touch or temperature) or arise on its own (spontaneous pain).

Stimulus driven pain is often referred to as hyperalgesia, which is an exaggerated response to a painful stimulus; or allodynia, which is pain from something which normally does not cause pain. An example of hyperalgesia is when a small pinprick results in a sharp, stabbing pain, or when the touch of a cold object causes a painful burning. An example of allodynia is when something as innocuous as the light touch of clothing is painful and unbearable.

Spontaneous pain, which can be either constant or intermittent, is often described as shooting or burning pain, and happens for no apparent reason. Of course, in the world of neuropathic pain, nothing is simple and many people suffer from a mix of both stimulus driven and spontaneous pain. Paresthesia, which is an abnormal sensation such as a tingle, and dysesthesia, which is an unpleasant, abnormal sensation are good examples of this complexity, as they can arise either spontaneously, or from stimulus.

Underlying Mechanisms

Although the exact mechanisms behind neuropathic pain are not completely understood, there are several theories on how different types of pain can develop. In looking at the peripheral nervous system, tissue damage to a certain part of the body results in a complicated series of actions centered around the inflammation process. As the body releases different chemicals to deal with the damage, the presence of these chemicals can make the nerves which carry pain signals back to the spine and brain extra sensitive. Once sensitized in this fashion, the nerves do not go back to their natural state. This type of sensitization often results in hyperalgesia, or the exaggerated response to a painful stimulus.

The spinal cord itself can also be the source of pain problems. It is thought that certain cells in the spinal cord (the pain receptors) are fundamentally altered when exposed for too long to a true, painful stimulus. Thus, once the nerves in the spinal cord are altered, even if the original source of the pain is alleviated, problems can occur. This can lead to allodynia, or the painful response to something that shouldn't be painful. When a person with allodynia "feels" the touch of a shirt, for example, the signal is carried properly from the nerve endings to the spine, but then it is misinterpreted as pain. How the nervous system changes over time in response to pain is extremely complicated and is just beginning to be understood.

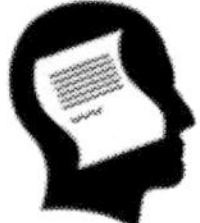

Personal Experience: Of the several types of pain I try to put up with, allodynia in my neck, shoulders and upper back is particularly troublesome. This is because there are very few shirts I can wear which don't become extremely uncomfortable – and even painful – after just a few minutes. I just can't stand the weight of something in that area. While this might be fine if I lived in Hawaii, living in Pittsburgh pretty much requires a shirt for most of the year. But in all seriousness, it makes it very difficult to be professional outside of my home. If I meet with someone and have to put on a real shirt (I always wear tank tops around the house) then I know I will feel lousy by the end of the meeting just from the shirt. If the occasion requires a jacket, it is just that much worse, and I have not worn a tie in years, even in times when it was proper to do so.

Spontaneous pain, often described as burning in nature, is thought to occur when nerve fibers send extraneous signals. This can be from nerves losing their protective covering, or from chemical-electrical imbalances that develop, causing improper firing of the nerve cells.

The damage that a syrinx does to the spine can lead to any or all of the types of neuropathic pain listed above. And as the next section details, the price paid for living with that type of pain is very high indeed.

High Cost of Pain

Unlike Chiari, there is an abundance of research into all aspects of chronic pain. While this is good, it has also revealed that living in chronic pain can have a negative effect on a person's overall health, blood pressure, mental state, economic viability and spiritual beliefs.

Overall Health

The cost of living in pain was highlighted by a 2004 study (Berger et al.) which utilized a large healthcare insurance database to show that people suffering from what the researchers termed a Painful Neuropathic Disorder (PND) are much more likely to suffer from additional health problems and incur much higher healthcare costs.

The database used, housed information on more than 3 million people, and from this, the researchers identified over 50,000 people who had been to the doctor at least twice in the year 2000 and suffered from a PND, such as back/neck pain due to neuropathy, diabetic neuropathy, post-herpetic neuralgia, etc. The researchers also created an age and gender matched control group - meaning the average age and male/female ratio was identical - of the same number of people who did not have a PND (Figure 7-1).

Figure 7-1: Effects Of Living With A Painful Neuropathic Disorder

	PND	Control
# of subjects	55,686	55,686
Avg. age	57.8	57.8
% female	58.5	58.5
% with one PND	88.9	0
% with two PNDs	9.8	0
% w/ no other chronic disease	6.1	69
% w/ 1 other chronic disease	23.5	18.2
% w/ 2 or more other chronic diseases	70.4	12.8
% taking antiseizure drugs	11.1	1.2
% taking antidepressants	11.3	2.4
% taking NSAIDs	39.7	13.8
Avg. annual healthcare costs in $	17,355	5,715

The database analysis revealed that over 70% of the PND group also suffered from two or more other chronic conditions. This is in stark contrast to only 13% of the control group with two or more chronic conditions. At the other end, only 6% of the PND group did not have another chronic condition, whereas the majority (69%) of the control subjects had no other chronic disease. This is a staggering result which essentially says that nearly everyone living with neuropathic pain also suffers from at least one other chronic health problem.

As to be expected given its impact on overall health, having a PND also proved to be very expensive as well. Specifically, subjects in the PND group incurred an average of over $17,000 in medical costs annually. In comparison, subjects in the control group only rang up an average of $5,700 in medical costs per year. This means that people with neuropathic pain have almost three times the health costs as people not living in pain.

Depression/Anxiety

There is significant anecdotal evidence that depression and other mood disorders affect a significant percentage of Chiari patients. What is not known is whether Chiari causes this directly – for example the pressure affects the production of certain neurochemicals – or if the high rate of depression is secondary to living with pain and disability. Although it may take years to answer that question, research has clearly demonstrated that mood disorders like depression are common among people living in chronic pain and with disability due to a wide range of causes, not just Chiari.

For example, in a study of a problem close in nature to CM/SM, researchers (Dersh et al) found that more than half of people with a disabling spine problem suffer from major depression. The 2006 study represented one of the largest, most detailed examinations of the subject to date. Specifically, the research group studied 1,323 patients with disabling spinal problems who had been admitted to a rehabilitation program designed to increase and restore functionality.

To be eligible for the study, patients had to have been partially or totally work disabled for four months, suffered from a work-related spine injury, surgery either didn't work or was not an option, non-operative treatments were ineffective, and severe functional limitations were present. As mentioned previously, over 1,300 patients met the criteria and were enrolled in the study.

For each patient, a medical history was taken, as well as a physical exam, psychological intake interview, disability assessment interview, and a quantitative functional evaluation. The treatment program they were enrolled in included activities such as supervised exercise programs, vocational rehabilitation, group therapy, and disability education and management.

Specific to this study, the patients were also administered structured clinical interviews according to the Diagnostic and Statistical Manual for Mental Disorders (DSM). These interviews are designed to identify the presence of current (or recent) major psychiatric problems, such as mood, anxiety, substance, and personality disorders.

What the study found was a staggeringly high rate of problems among the disabled patients. Specifically, the study patients were 10 times more likely to have a major mood, anxiety, or substance disorder than the general population, and 13 times more likely to suffer from a personality disorder than average (Figure 7-2).

Problems included high rates of major depression (56%), anxiety disorder (11%), substance use/abuse problems (14%) and a host of personality disorders (70%), such as paranoid, avoidant, and dependent personalities. Interestingly, the location of the injury on the spine (high, low, or multiple) did not appear to play a major role in the presence of psychiatric problems, implying the specific type of injury may not be as important as the injury's disabling effects.

Figure 7-2:
Prevalence of Psychiatric Disorders among Spinal Disabled Patients

Disorder	% of Study Patients With	% of General Population
Any	64.9	15.4
Major Depression	56.2	2.2
Anxiety	10.6	7.3
Any Substance	14.1	7.0
Any Personality	69.6	14.8
Paranoid	30.8	4.4
Avoidant	12.7	2.4
Dependent	7.3	0.5

Obviously, these results highlight the critical need to address underlying psychiatric problems when dealing with a disabling spinal injury (and likely other disabling conditions). Not doing so, can severely limit functional recovery and quality of life.

Although this research was not specific to Chiari, and it is not always easy to generalize results, it is important to realize that Chiari, and especially syringomyelia, patients essentially suffer from an upper spinal cord injury. So while a similar study, using the DSM criteria, among Chiari patients would be valuable, given that this research found that the location of the injury was not important, it seems likely that Chiari patients suffer from a similar high rate of mood and personality problems.

Brain Shrinkage

One of the most disturbing findings regarding the impact of chronic pain is a 2004 study out of Northwestern University (Apkarian) which found that chronic pain prematurely ages the brain. In the research, Dr. Apkarian and his team used MRIs to measure the volume and density of the brains of 26 people with chronic back pain (CBP) and compared them to the brains of 26 healthy volunteers.

Each of the 26 members of the pain group had experienced unrelenting pain for more than a year in their lower back. In some, the pain radiated down into the legs, in others it didn't. In addition to the brain MRIs, the CBP subjects reported their pain intensity and how long they had been in pain. To aid in the analysis, members of the pain group were also classified as having neuropathic pain - due to nerve damage - or non-neuropathic pain. The 26 volunteers that composed the control group were recruited to match the age and gender makeup of the CBP group as closely as possible.

The researchers used two different techniques to measure the volume of the neocortical gray matter (the part of the brain responsible for most higher order functions) from the MRIs. Overall, they found that the subjects in the pain group had 5%-11% less gray matter volume than the control subjects, a statistically significant finding. People normally lose about 0.5% of their gray matter each year as they age, so this result translates to the pain patients experiencing 10-20 years of aging compared to the control group.

In looking at neuropathic versus non-neuropathic pain, the team found that in the neuropathic pain group, the volume loss was related to pain duration. In fact, in the neuropathic group, each year of pain equated to a 0.2% loss in gray matter ($1.3cm^3$). In the non-neuropathic group, pain duration was not related to volume loss.

The neuropathic pain group also fared worse when the team measured the density of the gray matter in specific regions of the brain. In the prefrontal cortex - responsible for high level functions - they found that people in neuropathic pain had gray matter that was 27% less dense than the control group, and people with non-neuropathic pain had gray matter that was 14% less dense. They also found that the thalamus - a region of the brain which relays pain and other sensations - was significantly less dense in the pain group as compared to the control group.

Although this study can not prove it conclusively, the researchers believe the results show that chronic back pain causes brain tissue to atrophy in certain areas. If proven to be true, this would mean that chronic pain not only alters the neurons of the spine, but has a structural effect all the way to the brain as well. Although these findings have troubling implications for the Chiari community, it is important to keep in mind that this research was specific to low back pain and that the results may not be the same for people suffering from other types of pain.

Blood Pressure

Researchers have known for some time that the systems that regulate blood pressure and pain are linked in some way. In healthy people, a higher resting blood pressure is associated with a decreased sensitivity to acute pain. In other words, if you're blood pressure is high, you wouldn't feel as much pain if someone stuck you with a pin. Scientists speculate that the link between the two systems is a way to restore normal arousal levels after a painful stimulus. The body responds, or is aroused, initially by pain, but then the pain signals are turned down so that the rest of the body's systems can return to normal.

In people with chronic pain however, the relationship between the two systems is reversed. For a chronic pain sufferer, higher blood pressure levels have been associated with an increased, or higher sensitivity to pain, as opposed to a decreased, or lower sensitivity in healthy people. In people with chronic pain, the increased sensitivity extends beyond acute pain as well, with higher blood pressure also being linked to an increased sensitivity to chronic pain.

In addition, a 2005 study (Bruehl) found that the relationship goes both ways and that chronic pain can lead to higher blood pressure (which we all know is bad). Specifically, the research study retrospectively examined the medical records of 300 chronic pain patients and compared them to the records of 300 medical patients who were not in chronic pain.

The medical records for the pain group yielded information on demographics, cause of pain, pain duration, pain intensity, history of hypertension, family history of hypertension, and history of medication use. For the non-pain group, records were examined to exclude people who had reported either chronic pain or chronic headaches. Information on demographics, history of hypertension, and history of medicine use was collected for those subjects identified as not suffering from chronic pain.

Both the pain and non-pain groups were comprised of people between the ages of 18-65. The most common types of pain in the pain group were myofascial (62%), and neuropathic (25%). The pain sufferers reported an average pain intensity of 2.7 out of 5 and had been in pain on average for 37 months.

In analyzing the data, Bruehl and his team found that the pain group had a significantly higher prevalence of hypertension (high blood pressure) than the non-pain group. Specifically, 39% of the pain group had been clinically diagnosed with hypertension, versus only 21% for the non-pain group. The pain group rate of hypertension was also significantly higher than the national norm (matched for age and race) of 23% in men and 14% in women. The non-pain group, in contrast, was not different from the national norm for either men or women.

The researchers also found significant sex differences in the pain group. Although in general men have a higher rate of hypertension than women, in the pain group a higher percentage of women (41%) were diagnosed with hypertension than men (36%). Interestingly, people in the pain group who also had hypertension were much more likely to be taking antidepressants and anxiolytics (anxiety medicine) than those with chronic pain but without hypertension. Finally, statistical analysis revealed pain intensity was the strongest predictor of hypertension, even more so than common risk factors such as age, sex and family history.

Based on their results, the researchers believe that chronic pain somehow fundamentally alters the relationship between the cardiovascular and pain regulatory systems. For example, one hypothesis is that a common substance modulates both blood pressure and pain pathways. Thus, chronic pain may exhaust this substance and reduce its regulatory effect on blood pressure.

Economic

In addition to the physical and mental toll that chronic pain inflicts on a person, research has also shown that dealing with a chronic medical condition can have a large economic impact as well. In a study published in 2005, Himmelstein found that nearly half of personal bankruptcies are due to major medical problems.

To arrive at this conclusion, the researcher used questionnaires during bankruptcy proceedings and follow-up interviews to see what role major medical problems played in the need to file bankruptcy. In addition to finding that almost half of bankruptcies are prompted by medical issues, the study found that many families went without food, utilities and access to medical care prior to filing for bankruptcy (Figure 7-3). The data also showed that losing health insurance was a predictor of future bankruptcy due to a medical condition. Finally, the surveys showed that the average out of pocket medical costs for people who were filing bankruptcy due to medical problems was more than $11,000.

Figure 7-3: Effects of Medical Driven Bankruptcies

Privation	% of Medical Bank.	% of Non-Medical Bank.
Went without food	21.8	17.0
Water, electric shut off	29.6	26.4
Lost phone	43.6	35.9
Moved due to financial reasons	17.8	14.3
Lost insurance	46.7	34.6
Went without medical visits	60.7	45.0
Failed to fill a prescription	49.6	37.6
Changed care arrangements	6.7	2.7

Spiritual Beliefs

The effects of living with chronic pain are so pervasive, they can even alter a person's spiritual beliefs. Research has indicated that religion and spiritual beliefs can have a positive effect of general health and recovery from illness, but in a 2005 study Rippentrop showed that the relationship goes both ways and that chronic pain can influence spiritual beliefs. The study involved surveying 122 chronic pain patients on their pain and beliefs.

The research found that pain patients had less desire to reduce pain and suffering in the world and felt more abandoned by God than well-established norms (the survey they used is endorsed by the National Institute of Aging and is commonly used in research). In addition, the study found that the longer someone was in pain the less forgiving they felt and the less support they felt they received from organized religion. Possibly as an extension of feeling that organized religion was failing to support them, the study also found that the poorer a patient's physical health was, the more they engaged in private religious activities, such as prayer.

Perhaps more than any other research, this study reflects the true burden chronic pain can place on a person. A burden so heavy it can affect someone's fundamental beliefs.

Importance of Seeking Treatment

Because chronic pain can have such a negative impact on a person's life it is very important for patients to seek treatment for their pain. While many doctors are not properly trained, and do not want to treat pain, pain specialists are equipped to deal with such patients. Recently, multi-disciplinary pain clinics have become more popular and Chiari patients in pain should utilize this emerging resource.

Dr. Mark Gorchesky spent years as a anesthesiologist and pain medicine specialist, treating over 100,000 patients before his career was cut short by a chronic, debilitating, and painful condition. After treating pain patients for so many years, Dr. Gorchesky got a first-hand look at what it's like to navigate today's healthcare system. As both pain specialist and pain patient, Dr. Gorchesky enjoys a unique perspective when it comes to pain, and in March 2004 he shared some of his insights on seeking treatment for pain with Chiari & Syringomyelia News. The following is excerpted from that interview:

> **Should anyone with chronic pain seek treatment from experts?**
> **Dr. Gorchesky:** Resoundingly YES! In medicine today we've graduated into very significant and highly technical and specialized areas and fields. We all see and are treated by primary medical doctors, but if things don't tend to go well, we're often referred to other doctors. For

example, if you have a rash, you are seen by a specialist in dermatology. If you have bone disorders you are seen by doctors of orthopedics and bone specialists. So, if someone were suffering with pain for longer than six weeks to six months, it would be a natural progression to be seen by experts in the field, and those are pain medicine physicians.

What is a pain clinic?
Dr. Gorchesky: There are a number of different types of centers the words - pain clinic - have been used to describe. Sometimes it refers to a single modality-like a place where either it's a doctor practicing, using shots, blocks or injections; or a chiropractor just using manipulation. A pain center may have one or two different modalities but the ideal setting is a multidisciplinary pain management center or institute where the individuals are board certified in pain medicine. They use multiple modalities including physical medicine, physical therapy, psychology, biofeedback, pharmacology, regional anesthetics and a whole combination of alternative and complementary means. Treating the mind, body and spirit appears to be the best approach in the long-term with the best long-term plausible results.

What should a patient expect at a Pain Center?
Dr. Gorchesky: When one enters a multidisciplinary pain evaluation center, one should expect a very thorough evaluation towards finding an accurate and correct diagnosis. If you don't have an accurate diagnosis, treatment plans will fail. In the beginning, the most important thing is supplying your medical records. They would also want to see if there are legal issues, scenes of accidents and anything written about that. They will also look at the objective data that you have had taken before, such as x-rays, CT scans, MRIs, previous procedures and surgeries, and medicines you have used. A very thorough history will be taken on all of your general medical issues, then a particular pain history will be taken, about when your particular pain started, how did it get started, what makes it worse, what makes it better, does the timing of it appear to be in relation to anything, do meds make it better or worse, and your own particular opinion of why you think this is going on. Observing all of the things that have been done in the past and creating an opinion is very important. Ninety-nine percent of the decision-making in a diagnosis is often made with a very specific and thorough history. After that's completed, a very thorough physical examination will be used, a broad physical examination of all of the systems and then a focused exam on your particular problems. They should look very carefully at how you walk, how you sit, the duration of your ability to sit or stand or move if there are limb disorders. If there are problems with moving or

musculature, they may look at different lengths of your legs and pelvis, the length of your legs to the length of your arms, your spine and if there are any curvatures, muscle spasms, nervous disorders, movement disorders, even reflex changes or neurosensory changes. Once there is an accurate diagnosis, the doctor should impart a plan and a program for you in a multidisciplinary way. He should use additional disciplines to his own to help improve your situation. Goals should be to improve your function, aid in your coping through this disorder, decreasing your need and dependence on the health care system, reducing your need and dependence on habitual medications, and lastly to reduce your pain and pain perceptions. He should reassess with each visit, whether or not these goals are being reached.

How People Deal with Pain

Before diving into the details of different pain treatment options, it is worth taking a look at how people in general combat chronic pain. This book has mentioned several times that spinal cord injury (SCI) can be used as a substitute when research directly on Chiari is not available. So while, there is no published information on how CM/SM patient deal with chronic pain (although one such study is underway), there is research on how people with an SCI deal with their pain.

In 2003, Dr. Widerstrom-Noga and Dr. Turk, researchers with the Miami Project to Cure Paralysis, used an extensive postal survey to collect demographic information, pain characteristics, pain impact on daily life, and the type and effectiveness of pain treatments used from 120 people with SCI related pain.

Overall, close to 60% of the respondents had tried some type of pain treatment in the previous 18 months, with massage being the most common treatment (Figure 7-4).

Figure 7-4:
Common Pain Treatments Used

Treatment	%
Massage	26.7
Heat	16.7
Other Physiotherapy	15.0
Ice	13.3
Medication	10.0

Ten percent had used some type of medication, with opioids and NSAID's being the most commonly used (Figure 7-5). Interestingly, none of the factors surveyed were statistically related to who would use either the non-drug treatments, or over the counter medications.

Figure 7-5:
Common Pain Medications Used

Medication	%
Opioids	22.5
NSAID's	20.0
Acetaminophen	18.3
Anticonvulsants	17.5
Antispasticity	16.7
Sedatives	15.0
Antidepressants	12.5

In contrast, people who chose prescription medication as their pain treatment stood out in a number of ways. The prescription medication users reported more intense pain, used more adjectives to describe their pain, more pain locations, more allodynia, and greater difficulty in dealing with pain than people who used other types of treatments. Based on this, the researchers performed a sophisticated statistical analysis to see if they could identify a set of predictors for who is most likely to use prescription medications. They found that a combination of more intense pain, presence of evoked pain, greater difficulty in dealing with pain, perceived support from a significant other, and being married predicted prescription medication use.

As for the perceived effectiveness of the different treatments, overall the physical therapies were perceived to be the most effective with 50% of the respondents reporting their pain to be considerably better or even being pain free. Among the medications used, opioids were somewhat effective with 33% reporting considerably better or pain free. For the other common type of drug, NSAIDs, only 21% reported their pain to be considerably better (no one reported to be pain free using NSAIDs) but, 50% did report their pain to be slightly better.

The fact that the most successful treatments only scored a 50% or less effectiveness rate clearly shows that treating chronic spinal pain can be problematic. This may be one reason that not everyone sought treatment.

According to Dr. Widerstrom-Noga, "We were surprised to find that such a large group of people [40%] did not use treatments despite experiencing significant chronic pain. We do not know why this is the case. It may be that people who have had pain for a long time and have previously tried a number of treatments and not found them helpful assume that nothing will help,"

Although it can be frustrating trying to find ways to relieve pain, it is important for those suffering to keep looking and to not give up.

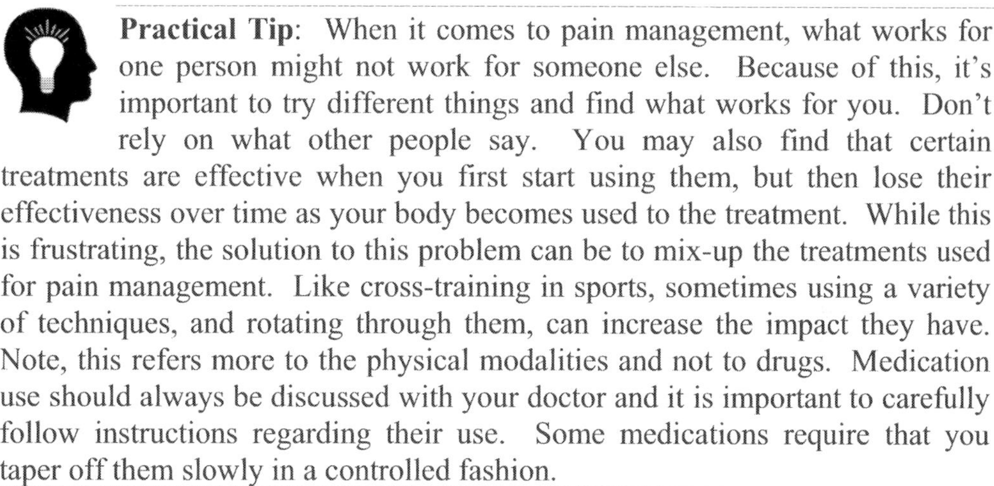

Practical Tip: When it comes to pain management, what works for one person might not work for someone else. Because of this, it's important to try different things and find what works for you. Don't rely on what other people say. You may also find that certain treatments are effective when you first start using them, but then lose their effectiveness over time as your body becomes used to the treatment. While this is frustrating, the solution to this problem can be to mix-up the treatments used for pain management. Like cross-training in sports, sometimes using a variety of techniques, and rotating through them, can increase the impact they have. Note, this refers more to the physical modalities and not to drugs. Medication use should always be discussed with your doctor and it is important to carefully follow instructions regarding their use. Some medications require that you taper off them slowly in a controlled fashion.

Physical Modalities

The simplest type of pain treatments are physical modalities, such as heat, ice and massage. Obviously, techniques such as heat and ice can easily be used at home and are relatively cheap. This is likely why they are among the most commonly used as referenced in the study above. However, their long-term effectiveness is somewhat questionable. While heat and ice can provide temporary relief, and can and should be used frequently, by themselves they are not likely to provide significant, long-term relief.

Beyond simple heat and ice, techniques which use electricity and sound are available to help loosen muscles and calm down overactive nerves. TENS stands for transcutaneous electrical nerve stimulator; it is a small battery powered device which generates a weak electrical signal. Patches are placed on the skin near the problem area(s) and the patches are attached to the TENS unit by cords. When the unit is turned on, an electrical signal passes through the body; both the intensity and frequency of the signal can be controlled. Depending on the intensity, the patient may feel anything from a slight tingle to strong, repeated muscle contractions. The electrical stimulation can relax tense muscles and, in theory, calm down overactive nerves. Although using electricity for pain relief is a very old practice, the research on its effectiveness is mixed.

Ultrasound is a device which uses sound waves to deliver energy deep into muscles, which heats them up and relaxes them. Basically, a trained practitioner rubs a wand type device – which is attached to the unit – over the affected area. By changing the frequency of the sound waves, the energy can be directed for maximum relief. Although it is commonly used to relax tense muscles, ultrasound can not be used at home.

Massage, for obvious reasons, is a very popular method to relieve muscle pain. Although massage usually does not address the underlying problems, it can be very beneficial and helps restore the proper biomechanics. When muscles become tense they start to work against each other instead of working together. This becomes painful, and massage, by a skilled therapist, can help bring back the natural balance.

One technique which Chiari patients sometimes shy away from is exercise. Although it is important to discuss any limitations with a physician, exercise can be a very effective way to reduce secondary pain. As mentioned earlier in the chapter, Chiari patients often suffer from several types of pain and one of those types is often musculo-skeletal. Whether from inactivity or nerve damage, Chiari patients may be weak in the shoulder/upper back area which can lead to further problems. A physiatrist or physical therapist can work out a program to rebuild that strength and improve flexibility and ease of motion.

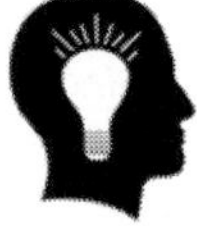

Practical Tip: If you find that a TENS unit works for you, many insurance companies will pay for one that you can use at home. Ask your doctor for a prescription and ask a medical supply company if your insurance will cover the costs.

If you're suffering from chronic neck, shoulder and back pain, a physical therapist can be your best friend. Ask your doctor for a prescription and then find a physical therapist who is willing to listen to you about Chiari and syringomyelia. The physical therapist can use TENS, ultrasound, massage and exercise to try to rebalance and retrain your muscles. In addition, they can help in establishing a home exercise program to improve strength, flexibility and endurance.

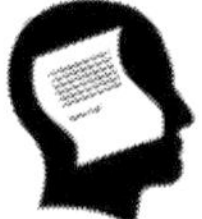

Personal Experience: The muscles in my neck, shoulders and upper back become tense very easily and go into spasm at the drop of a hat. Because of this, I have tried all of the techniques described above and still employ them as needed. Sometimes TENS helps to calm things down (I have a unit at home), and sometimes I need to go to the physical therapist (I'm a frequent customer) to get back on track. One thing I try to do is get a lot of exercise and keep my strength up. It seems like the strength in my right shoulder disappears very quickly if I don't exercise regularly. Inevitably this leads to neck pain as my shoulder becomes out of position and tugs on my neck muscles. One thing I have found that works pretty well is to exercise in a heated, indoor pool. The water minimizes the impact of the exercises and makes for a very good, smooth workout. You don't have to swim (although swimming is a great way to build strength), many YMCAs and fitness clubs offer exercise classes in their pools. I also try to walk as much as I can. Walking is a great way to keep a healthy weight and increase the blood flow which keeps muscles loose. Inactivity can make muscles which are prone to being stiff even worse.

Did You Know: A physiatrist is a doctor (MD) of physical and rehabilitative medicine, who specializes in restoring function to people. To become a physiatrist, individuals must successfully complete four years of graduate medical education and four additional years of postdoctoral residency training.

A new physical modality for pain, which was recently approved by the FDA for use in the United States is Low Level Laser Therapy (LLLT). Also known as a cold laser, LLLT has been used for years in Europe and is rapidly gaining popularity among professional athletes as a way to treat muscle related pain. However, the research on the effectiveness of LLLT is somewhat limited. While there have been some well designed studies showing that LLLT offers some benefits, more extensive research is required to validate and quantify its usefulness.

Inactivity can make muscles which are prone to being stiff even worse.

Drugs/Medications

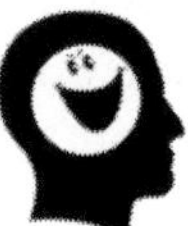

You Gotta Laugh!! My 13 year old daughter was just home from the hospital after decompression surgery for ACM and had a few visitors.

They asked her how her pain was and she replied, "I wish I had some of that methamphetamine they gave me in the hospital!"

Believe me a few of the adult visitors were quite wide-eyed for a moment and then we all laughed.

She really meant morphine! *~Karen~*

NSAIDs

NSAIDs (non-steroidal anti-inflammatory) are widely used class of drugs, sold both over the counter and by prescription which offer pain relief, anti-inflammatory and anti-fever qualities. Common brand names include Motrin (Ibuprofen), Aleve (Naproxen) and Celebrex (Cox-2 inhibitor). NSAIDs are commonly used for pain relief because many are readily available over the counter. They work by affecting certain chemicals in the body – known as prostaglandins – which cause inflammation.

Despite the fact that they can be found in almost every medicine chest in the country, many people don't realize that NSAIDs can cause serious side effects and that thousands of people die each year from complications due to NSAID use. The reality is that NSAIDs can cause severe gastrointestinal problems, especially in high dosages or if used for an extended period of time. Research has shown that peptic ulcers are a common occurrence in people taking an average dose of NSAIDs on a daily basis. In addition, NSAIDS can affect other medical conditions, such as asthma, high blood pressure and liver problems.

Before taking NSAIDs on a daily basis to treat chronic pain, it is important to discuss this topic with a qualified physician, who may recommend taking an antacid along with the NSAID, recommend a specific dosage, and can look out for any problems.

Because ibuprofen and naproxen can be hard on the digestive system, drug companies developed a new type of NSAID, known as Cox-2 inhibitors (Vioxx, Celebrex, Bextra). Unfortunately, these drugs were found to cause heart problems for certain patients and Vioxx was pulled off the market (Celebrex is still available).

In December, 2004 the Food and Drug Administration issued an advisory on the subject:

FDA advisory, December 2004

- Physicians prescribing Celebrex (celecoxib) or Bextra (valdecoxib), should consider this emerging information when weighing the benefits against risks for individual patients. Patients who are at a high risk of gastrointestinal (GI) bleeding, have a history of intolerance to non-selective NSAIDs, or are not doing well on non-selective NSAIDs may be appropriate candidates for Cox-2 selective agents.
- Individual patient risk for cardiovascular events and other risks commonly associated with NSAIDs should be taken into account for each prescribing situation.
- Consumers are advised that all over-the-counter (OTC) pain medications, including NSAIDs, should be used in strict accordance with the label directions. If use of an (OTC) NSAID is needed for longer than ten days, a physician should be consulted.

Non-selective NSAIDs are widely used in both over-the-counter (OTC) and prescription settings. As prescription drugs, many are approved for short-term use in the treatment of pain and primary dysmenorrhea (menstrual discomfort), and for longer-term use to treat the signs and symptoms of osteoarthritis and rheumatoid arthritis. FDA has previously posted extensive NSAID medication information at:

http://www.fda.gov/cder/drug/analgesics/default.htm.

Opioids/Narcotics

Opioids (also known as narcotics) are a powerful family of pain drugs which work by blocking the pain messages from getting to the brain. Narcotics are commonly used to treat acute, post-surgical pain (think morphine), but can also be used to treat chronic pain. Although powerful, this family of drugs carries significant side effects which make them difficult to take for many people. In addition, they are addictive in nature, so careful patient selection is important.

For reasons beyond the scope of this book, in general, society has taken a negative view on using narcotics for pain control and doctors have to walk a fine line in how they prescribe them. There is a tremendous amount of controversy surrounding the use of opioids - or narcotics - to treat chronic pain. On the one hand, some pain experts say that doctors are too stingy in handing out pain medicine and shouldn't worry so much about people becoming addicted. On the other hand, high profile, celebrity addiction cases are fueling a media frenzy and adding to the perception that chronic pain sufferers are really addicts in waiting and that narcotics should be avoided at all costs. Add to this the politics of the decades old War on Drugs, and you get a volatile mix of opinions, hyperbole, and political agendas where the only true losers are the people who continue to suffer on a daily basis.

While it would be nice to turn down the noise and take an objective, scientific look at the use of opioids to treat chronic pain; unfortunately, the results from the scientific community to date have been inconclusive. Clearly, narcotic drugs offer pain relief. However, how much relief they provide to people suffering from chronic, neuropathic pain remains unclear. It *is* clear that opioids have very significant side effects which make taking them unbearable for some people.

A controlled study published in the March 27, 2003 issue of *"New England Journal of Medicine"*, demonstrates that while opioids offer hope to some people, they are not a cure-all. Dr. Rowbotham and his colleagues from the Pain Clinical Research Center, at the University of California, San Francisco, conducted a double-blind, randomized, study to evaluate the effects of an opioid - taken by mouth - on chronic, neuropathic pain.

The study involved 81 adults who suffered from neuropathic pain due to causes such as post-herpetic neuralgia, post-stroke central pain, spinal cord injury, and multiple sclerosis. The participants could not have used opioids before and were screened for drug, alcohol, psychological, and other health problems. In addition, all participants had unsuccessfully tried to control their pain with other types of drugs. Once accepted into the program, the participants were randomly assigned into a group which would receive either a low dose of an opioid (Levorphanol), or a high-dose of the drug. Neither the participants, nor the doctors running the experiment knew which group the participants were assigned to.

In both groups, the pain medicine dosage was ramped up gradually over a period of 4 weeks, after which the participants could control their own dosing - up to pre-set limits - for an additional 4 weeks. During this time period, the participants were encouraged to find a dosage that balanced the pain benefits with any negative side effects. The participants were then tapered off the drug over a third, 4 week period. While taking the drug, the participants recorded their pain levels (0-100) and whether the drug provided relief in a daily pain diary. In addition, their psychological state and quality of life were periodically assessed using the Multidimensional Pain Inventory (MPI) and other assessment tools. The MPI is a well recognized questionnaire which assesses the impact of pain on quality of life, perceived social support, and ability to perform daily activities.

As might be expected, both groups experienced a reduction in pain, with the high-dose group benefiting more than the low dose group. Measured on a scale from 0-100, the high-dose group experienced a 36% reduction in pain on average. The low-dose group, in contrast, experienced a 21% reduction. It should be noted that the pain levels were still significant for both groups (even with the drug benefits), an average of 42 for the high-dose group and 53 for the low-dose group.

In addition to pain relief, both groups reported better sleeping and less interference in their functioning, yet interestingly, there was no difference in these scores between the two groups. Many metrics, such as ability to do chores and outdoor work were not improved in either group.

However, side-effects proved to be a significant problem for many, with 22 people dropping out of the study, mostly due to adverse side-effects. While this seems high, it is actually in-line with other narcotic studies which generally have a drop-out rate near 25%. The high-dose group reported more severe side effects than the low-dose group, including anger, irritability, and mood changes, in addition to general drowsiness and confusion.

This study highlights the mixed bag that opioids offer. For some people with chronic, neuropathic pain, the drugs offer at least some much needed relief. But for others, the side effects are too much and are not worth whatever relief they bring. And unfortunately the specter of addiction continues to cast a pall over the whole subject and interferes with the effort to help those who need it most.

Neurontin

The drug Neurontin - generically known as gabapentin - is one of the most widely prescribed drugs on the market and has been tried by many Chiari patients. Bringing in more than $2 billion in annual revenue for Pfizer, its manufacturer, it is a high-profile drug with a bit of a storied past. Originally designed - and approved - as an anti-epilepsy drug, it has since been FDA approved to treat post-herpetic neuralgia, a painful type of neuropathic pain that some people develop after having shingles. But with billions of dollars of sales, it is clear that Neurontin is being prescribed for more uses than just those two. In fact, a large portion of Neurontin sales are from what are known as off-label uses. Once a drug is approved by the FDA, doctors are allowed to prescribe the drug not only for the approved use, but for other uses for which they think the drug might be effective.

This is an important and necessary part of medicine. Many drug benefits were discovered by prescribing them off-label, including the heart related benefits of aspirin. Unfortunately, as will be discussed later, this is also where Neurontin's checkered past comes into play. Pfizer (actually Parke-Davis, a division of Warner-Lambert, which Pfizer acquired) has been accused of illegally marketing Neurontin and encouraging doctors to prescribe it off-label.

What Is Neurontin?

Neurontin was designed to look like a neurotransmitter known as GABA. GABA is an important neurotransmitter, and several types of drugs, including sedatives, work by affecting how GABA attaches to other chemicals at the molecular level. In addition, the role of GABA in spinal cord injuries is thought to be important and is being investigated by spinal cord injury researchers.

What is surprising is that no one knows how Neurontin works. No one can explain how it offers pain relief or acts as an anti-convulsant. Despite looking like GABA, it does not affect how GABA attaches - or binds - in the brain, it doesn't affect how GABA is processed, and it isn't converted into GABA by the body. In addition, gabapentin does not affect dopamine or serotonin, other common neurotransmitters. The substance was also tested to see if it would bind to many different types of sites at the molecular level, but it does not. In a study involving a rat brain, the drug was found to attach to certain areas, but the connection between those sites and how the drug might work is not clear. Adding to the mystery is the fact that gabapentin itself is barely absorbed by the human body and is fairly quickly eliminated through the kidneys and urine.

Does It Work?

Despite the unknowns, there is growing evidence that Neurontin does indeed offer some level of relief for some types of neuropathic pain. Setting aside the anti-epileptic effects of the drug, Pfizer's literature on Neurontin cites two randomized, double-blind, placebo controlled studies on the use of Neurontin for managing postherpetic neuralgia. The studies involved 563 patients who were experiencing pain at least 3 months after their bout with shingles. The patients were given either Neurontin or a placebo for a several week period (dosage was ramped up to 3600mg/day). Both studies showed a significant reduction in reported pain throughout the treatment for those receiving the drug. In fact, around 30% of the participants receiving the drug reported a 50% or greater improvement in their pain.

The question is, does this apply to syringomyelia related pain? Fortunately, Neurontin has also been shown to help pain associated with spinal cord injuries. In a study published in 2003 (Spine 28(4):341-6), 31 patients with neuropathic pain due to spinal cord injury were given Neurontin over an 8 week period. The patients were divided into two groups based on whether they had been experiencing pain for less than or more than 6 months. Despite the fact that they tried other types of pain medicines to no avail, Neurontin did reduce the pain for both groups. On a scale of 0-10, the average pain score for the less than 6 month group dropped from 7.3 to 3 over the course of the treatment. While the other group also responded to the drug, the average score only dropped from 7.6 to 5. So while this study shows Neurontin can provide relief for SCI related pain, getting started early on the drug may be important.

Another study demonstrating the effects of Neurontin on a wide variety of neuropathic pain was published in the journal, *"Pain"* in 2002 (Pain 99(3):557-66). This double-blind, randomized, placebo controlled study looked at over 300 people suffering from neuropathic pain due to a number of different causes. Over an 8-week period, the participants either received Neurontin or a placebo. The results showed a significant difference in the pain relief between the group receiving the drug and the placebo group.

Of special interest to the CM/SM community is growing evidence which shows that Neurontin can reduce the brutal consequences of allodynia. This type of pain - feeling pain from things that shouldn't be painful - can be especially limiting and difficult to deal with. In well established rat models, gabapentin - along with other, similar drugs - has been shown to dramatically reduce allodynia.

Side Effects

A drug's effectiveness is only half the equation. In order to be useful, any side effects caused by the drug must be minor enough to be tolerated or the drug is essentially worthless. As discussed earlier, narcotics are powerful pain relievers, but also have very strong side effects. In narcotic studies, it is not unusual for more than 20% of participants to drop out because of side effects. In addition, drug tolerance and addiction pose even bigger challenges to the effective use of a narcotic for pain relief. The question is, are the side effects of Neurontin as bad as the other narcotic drugs?

In a postherpetic neuralgia study cited by Pfizer, the most common side effects of Neurontin were sleepiness, dizziness, numbness, and bruising. Twenty-eight percent of participants reported experiencing dizziness and 21% sleepiness. Because of this, more than 3% of participants experienced accidental injuries versus just 1% of the control group. In addition to the most common effects, there are a wide range of less common side effects which nonetheless did not occur in the placebo group. These range from dry mouth to rashes and blurred vision to stomach problems and cognitive impairment.

Similar side effects are listed in other published gabapentin studies but are usually characterized as mild to moderate. Overall, the drug is considered very safe with few and infrequent serious medical side effects. One reason for this is that the body metabolizes very little of the drug itself and the drug doesn't stay in the body for very long. Addiction to the drug has not been studied adequately to make a determination that it is a problem.

Anecdotally, people contacted by Conquer Chiari with experience taking Neurontin present a mixed view. Most encountered some side effects, with sleepiness and cognitive impairment being most prominent. Several people stopped taking the drug because of the side effects, but one person who stayed on it for awhile became used to the side effects and after a period of time was able to function normally.

Pregabalin

Pregabalin (Lyrica) is a follow-on drug to Neurontin which has recently become available in the US to treat neuropathic pain associated with diabetic peripheral neuropathy. It was designed to be more effective than gabapentin with fewer side effects. Although it has not been studied in relation to CM/SM pain, a randomized, controlled, double-blind study of spinal cord injured patients did show that it significantly reduced pain, improved sleep and lowered anxiety compared to a placebo (Figure 7-6). However, many users still reported side effects such as sleepiness, dizziness and lack of energy, although they were classified as only being mild to moderate.

Figure 7-6: Study Results, Pregabalin (69) vs Placebo (67)

	Pregabalin		**Placebo**		**Sig?**
	Start	End	Start	End	
Pain	6.54	4.62	6.73	6.27	Y
Sleep	4.22	2.79	4.98	4.71	Y
Anxiety	6.74	5.16	8.67	7.49	Y
Depression	5.86	5.44	6.61	6.29	N

Note: Sig? refers to whether the difference between the pregabalin group and placebo group was statistically significant, meaning the result is not likely due to chance.

Complementary & Alternative Medicine (CAM)

Due to the limited effectiveness of the pain treatments discussed above, many people end up turning to what can be called complementary and alternative medicine (CAM). In fact, a 2004 survey by the US Government found that 36 percent of adults use some form of CAM. Complementary and alternative medicine is such a large topic that one of the institutes of the National Institutes of Health (NIH) is dedicated to it, namely the National Center for Complementary and Alternative Medicine (NCCAM).

According to NCCAM, complementary and alternative medicine can be defined as:

[CAM is] a group of diverse medical and health care systems, practices, and products that are not presently considered to be part of conventional medicine. Conventional medicine is medicine as practiced by holders of M.D. (medical doctor) or D.O. (doctor of osteopathy) degrees and by their allied health professionals, such as physical therapists, psychologists, and registered nurses. Some health care providers practice both CAM and conventional medicine. While some scientific evidence exists regarding some CAM therapies, for most there are key questions that are yet to be answered through well-designed scientific studies--questions such as whether these therapies are safe and whether they work for the diseases or medical conditions for which they are used.

In addition NCCAM makes a distinction between complementary and alternative medicine:

Complementary medicine is used together with conventional medicine. An example of a complementary therapy is using aromatherapy (a therapy in which the scent of essential oils from flowers, herbs, and trees is inhaled to promote health and well-being) to help lessen a patient's discomfort following surgery.

Alternative medicine is used in place of conventional medicine. An example of an alternative therapy is using a special diet to treat cancer instead of undergoing surgery, radiation, or chemotherapy that has been recommended by a conventional doctor.

There are many types of CAM treatments and therapies, ranging from mind-body relaxation techniques, to spinal manipulation, to touch healing, just to name a few. Because CAM therapies lie at the edge of, or outside, conventional medicine, their use is somewhat controversial. Unfortunately, there is no scientific evidence to support the effectiveness of most of the treatments, and the field is ripe with abuse and scam artists. Unscrupulous practitioners are all to willing to take money from patients desperate for relief.

However, there is also some evidence that certain alternative treatments can be effective in certain situations. The NCCAM website **http://nccam.nih.gov/** reviews which treatments are considered to be scams and which have some evidence to support their use.

Practical Tip: As a patient, it is best to be very careful when evaluating alternative treatments. Beware of the practitioner who says that his technique can not be evaluated scientifically or demands payment for a series of treatments up front.

The discussion below focuses on those treatments which have some scientific evidence to support their use in treating pain. Currently, Conquer Chiari is not aware of any alternative treatments which are directed at correcting the underlying problem of Chiari and/or syringomyelia (see Chapter 4).

Acupuncture

Acupuncture is an ancient Chinese practice which involves the placement of small needles at specific points in the body. It is based on the theories of Traditional Chinese Medicine and, according to the tradition, works by restoring the natural flow of the body's energy along certain pathways.

Acupuncture is one of the most widely studied complementary medicine techniques and, despite its roots in a system that is completely different from Western medicine, is beginning to emerge from the shadows and become mainstream. Acupuncture is regulated at the state level and there is a national accrediting agency, the National Certification Commission for Acupuncture and Oriental Medicine. There are thousands of MD's who are trained in acupuncture and acupuncture as practiced today is likely to be a mix of ancient thought and modern technology.

Most practitioners recognize the ancient thoughts on acupuncture, but also recognize the power of modern medicine. These modern day acupuncturists utilize the best of both systems. While the diagnosis process may involve checking the pulse and the tongue, it is also likely to involve a medical history, a neurological exam, and looking at MRIs and X-rays.

In fact, one of the more intriguing lines of research into acupuncture involves trying to identify the mechanism by which it works. Some people still believe in the traditional ideas of acupuncture, some people think something similar to the energy channels exist but we haven't found them yet, and some people think a different mechanism is at play.

The introduction of functional MRI - used to identify which areas of the brain are active during certain tasks - has shown dramatically that acupuncture has real physical effects. One study demonstrated that an acupuncture point on the little toe associated with correcting vision problems did indeed stimulate the visual cortex in the brain when a needle was inserted. Other studies have shown similar connections between acupoints and corresponding regions of the brain.

Theories for how acupuncture works are varied. One states that acupuncture accelerates the conduction of electromagnetic signals, another that acupuncture triggers the release of natural opioids into the central nervous system, and a third focuses on acupuncture changing the release of neurotransmitters in the brain. While some evidence exists to support each of these, none have been proven conclusively, yet there is still the possibility that some form of channels or meridians exist in the body.

One of the most dramatic advances in acupuncture was the development of electroacupuncture (EA). Electroacupuncture combines traditional acupuncture with an electrical current applied to the needles at a specific frequency and intensity. For pain relief and muscle tension, some acupuncturists use EA exclusively. This technique is based on the recognition that the body's nervous system uses electricity and on research which shows that the body responds to electrical currents at different frequencies.

A second, and equally important advance, has been the adoption of disposable needles. Since about 1980, virtually every acupuncturist in the US has used disposable needles for their treatments. This way there is no chance of passing disease from one patient to another.

As acupuncture has become more common in the US, there is naturally more focus on answering the question of whether it works. Beyond the basic language barrier, one reason acupuncture has been slow to be adopted by the established medical community is that many of the studies on acupuncture lack the methodological rigor required by the Western scientific community. But, as the number of people trained in both acupuncture and the scientific method grows, so too does the amount of rigorous research into the effectiveness of acupuncture.

In 1997, the National Institutes of Health (NIH) addressed this question by convening a panel of non-partisan experts to listen to presentations, ask questions, and try to reach a conclusion. The panel issued a Consensus Statement which essentially stated that despite some limitations on the research, there is evidence that acupuncture is effective in treating some conditions and that more research is warranted.

Since then hundreds of research articles have been published evaluating the effectiveness of acupuncture in treating back pain, cancer pain, and even heart disease. As Federal funds have become available to researchers, more controlled, randomized trials have been conducted, improving the overall quality of the research.

So does acupuncture work? The short answer is that for some conditions, yes, it does work, and the more research is done, the more likely it is to be shown to work in even more cases. For example, one recent study showed that acupuncture was fairly successful in flipping breech babies. There is also pretty strong evidence that acupuncture can help with different types of pain, including dental pain and neck pain.

Most relevant to CM/SM patients was a study involving 153 patients which found acupuncture was effective in treating neck pain. Specifically 68% of the study participants reported that their pain improved by at least 50%. Unfortunately, the treatments were less effective for pain that had been present for a long period of time.

Since acupuncture involves needles penetrating the skin, naturally there have been questions about its safety. However a review of the medical literature found only 715 reports of adverse events out of over one million treatments. The most common problems were trauma and infection.

As more people try acupuncture and as more traditional doctors are trained in its use, it is likely that one day acupuncture will no longer be considered an alternative treatment, and rather will be accepted into the realm of traditional medicine.

Personal Experience: I found a local acupuncturist - who is also a Doctor from China - on the NCCAOM web site (www.nccaom.org) and called for an appointment. The doctor called me back to get some background. Although there was a bit of a language barrier, I was able to determine he wasn't familiar with Chiari and syringomyelia, but he asked to see my MRIs, so I went ahead and set up an appointment. Before my visit, I printed out the Overview presentation from the Conquer Chiari site and gathered my MRIs and medical records.

In the hours leading up to my appointment, I became very nervous. What if it made things worse? What if it actually sparked a recurrence? My mind flipped back and forth between the lure of easing may pain versus the risk of doing anything - especially something as esoteric as acupuncture. In the end, the promise of reducing - or even eliminating - the pain won out and I headed out for my appointment.

When I arrived at his office, it looked much like a regular doctor's office and there were the standard forms to fill out - although I did notice that the doctor evaluation sheet had a section for a tongue evaluation. The doctor introduced himself and took me into a regular looking exam room. He started taking a history and we quickly dove into what Chiari and SM are all about. He was very happy that I had brought the presentation and was eager to learn about the conditions. He then focused on my residual neck and shoulder problems and performed a typical physical exam - strength, range of motion, etc. - that I had had countless times before.

He concluded that my trapezius muscle (the large triangle shaped muscle on the back that connects to the head and shoulder) was incredibly tight and thought that was causing most of my problems. To my surprise, and disappointment, however, he also cautioned me that acupuncture can only do so much. He said that if there were serious nerve damage, the acupuncture probably would not help. He also said that the beneficial effects of the treatments may not last very long, and finally that it may take 5-6 treatments to see any results. He went on to say that his style of acupuncture was different than the ancient technique; he uses electroacupuncture to relax muscles and also heats the area with a light tuned to a specific frequency. Overall the visit was almost identical to seeing a Western style doctor or physical therapist as his exam entailed nothing out of the ordinary.

The doctor then showed me the needles he would be inserting and I took off my shirt and lied face down on the treatment table (the table was like a massage table with a place to put your face and rest your hands). The doctor began inserting needles in my shoulder and neck area. Although there was almost no pain, there was a strange sensation when he twirled the needles. I thought he had hooked up the electricity already, because it felt like there was a charge going through different parts of my body, but when I looked up, I realized the feeling was from just the needles. Only one needle actually hurt - in my neck, right at a nerve root - and he warned me in advance it might hurt, but he removed the needle right away and things seemed ok. Once the needles were inserted, he hooked up the electric device starting with the needles on my trapezius muscle. The current made the muscle twitch, but it wasn't unpleasant. Next he brought over a heat lamp type device and started warming up the muscles on my back and neck. The whole session lasted about an hour and right after I got up, my neck and shoulder were much looser. I paid $60 for the visit - not covered by insurance - and set up an appointment for a week later.

I was feeling pretty good when I left his office, but by the time I got home my neck had stiffened considerably and was actually swollen on the right side. Needless to say, I thought my worst fears had been realized and I began berating myself for taking such a risk. That night was tough sleeping because of my stiff neck, but by morning it was a little better. To my delight, I found that even though my neck was tight, my shoulder felt great. I could move my arm in a way I hadn't been able to for years. I called the doctor to tell him about my swollen neck, and he said that it should go away and that because of the SM I was probably more sensitive to stimulation near the nerve root. He went on to say that if I went back, he would work away from the neck more. At that point I wasn't sure what to do, because my neck felt lousy but my shoulder felt great.

Over the next couple of days however, the swelling in my neck subsided and things really loosened up. I was able to do things I hadn't done in a long time with very little pain. There was still some discomfort, and I could tell my shoulder muscles were weak, but the pain and mobility had definitely improved. The effect did start to taper off the next week as I banged away on the computer all day long, but it still wasn't as bad as it was before. I decided to go to my second appointment the following weekend.

The second appointment was shorter than the first. The doctor reviewed with me what had happened following my first treatment and suggested that he apply the electric stimulation further away from my neck. My wife had reminded me to verify that he uses disposable needles, so he showed me the packages they come in and assured me that's all he uses. As he was inserting the needles, I mentioned to him that the last treatment had really made my right hand feel better, so he focused some attention on that as well. When he hooked up the electrical stimulation, he found a level I was comfortable with - he did mention I was very sensitive to stimulation compared to most people - and the treatment lasted about 20 minutes.

Things felt pretty good this time after the treatment and I continued for several weeks. Unfortunately, over time the effect of the acupuncture began to fade. I think overall the treatments improved my functionality, but it seemed like I built up a tolerance to the treatments over time. Still, I think it was well worth trying and would consider going back for more treatments in the future.

Fish Oil

Fish oil contains what are known as essential fatty acids (specifically omega-3). These substances are important for the body's health, but must be supplied through diet. Certain types of fish, such as salmon, are rich in fatty acids like omega-3, which are thought to promote healthy cellular membranes.

There is a growing body of evidence, with hundreds of published research articles, which points to the benefits of the omega-3 fatty acids found in fish oil. These benefits include a lower risk for coronary disease, and many people believe, natural anti-inflammatory properties and improved nerve functioning. In fact, the FDA has even stated that there is supportive, but not conclusive, evidence that the consumption of omega-3 fatty acid lowers the risk of coronary heart disease.

So everyone should eat a lot of fish, right? Not exactly; while certain types of fish are a great source of omega-3, there is also a growing concern about the levels of toxins, like mercury, in these fish due to polluted waters. This has led to government recommendations to *limit* the amount of these types of fish eaten, especially for children and pregnant women.

This, in turn, has led to an explosion of fish oil supplements on the market. These supplements claim to supply the omega-3 fatty acids necessary for good health, but without the toxins. They do this by extracting the oil from the fish, processing it for purifications, and packaging it into liquids and geltabs.

While the economics of the fish oil supplement industry continue to evolve, so too does the research to evaluate its potential benefits. With the FDA giving a limited nod to its impact on heart disease, other researchers have focused on how it might help their own patients.

Along these lines, in a 2006 study Dr. Joseph Maroon, a neurosurgeon, asked patients he was treating for non-surgical spine pain to try fish oil supplements in place of NSAIDs.

Between March and June, 2004, two hundred fifty patients were seen for non-surgical spine pain, such as degenerative disk disease. Every patient was taking NSAIDs to try to control their pain. For the study, the patients were asked to take a fish oil supplement with omega-3. They were to take 2400 mg a day for two weeks, then lower the amount to 1200 mg a day. At the same time, after the initial two weeks, they were asked to taper off taking NSAIDs.

A questionnaire was sent to each patient approximately a month after they began taking the fish oil supplement. Out of the initial 250 patients, 125 returned the survey. This group had been taking the fish oil for an average of 75 days and reported very positive results.

Specifically, 60% of the patients reported that their joint pain had decreased and their overall pain level had improved. Additionally, 59% were able to completely stop taking NSAIDs and 88% said they would continue to take the fish oil.

A simple study such as this is far from conclusive evidence that fish oil is able to take the place of NSAIDs. However, combined with previous, more rigorous studies of fish oil and arthritis pain it does present a strong case for the benefits of fish oil in treating pain. In addition, there is a sound theoretical basis for how omega-3 can act as an anti-inflammatory at the molecular level. Also, in general, fish oil has few side effects, but it can increase bleeding at very high doses.

For people thinking about taking fish oil supplements it is important to realize that these products are not regulated and that care should be taken in both deciding to take them and the selection of a product. As always, it is best to speak with a trained medical professional to determine if this type of supplement is right for you. Also, it is important to select a supplement which has removed the toxins that are so prevalent in these types of fish. It should be noted that many products use the term pharmaceutical grade (or medical grade) to refer to oils without the toxins, but these terms do not have a standard definition.

Thinking Away Pain

According to NCCAM, mind-body therapies "use a variety of techniques designed to enhance the mind's capacity to affect bodily function and symptoms. Some techniques that were considered CAM in the past have become mainstream (for example, patient support groups and cognitive-behavioral therapy). Other mind-body techniques are still considered CAM, including, prayer, mental healing, and therapies that use creative outlets such as art, music, or dance."

Because the perception of pain is believed to be influenced by the higher order brain function, it is natural to wonder if the conscious brain can proactively influence how pain is felt. Or, in other words, is it possible to think away pain? Results from a 2005 study conducted by a cross-discipline group of researchers from Stanford and Harvard (deCharms) indicate that in fact it might be. The study got significant media attention when the researchers reported that they were able to use real-time functional MRI to help people control pain. The team's idea was to use MRI to provide real-time feedback to people in order to train them to consciously increase and decrease activity in a specific brain region thought to influence how pain is perceived.

It has been documented that people can consciously control bodily functions which are normally in the realm of the unconscious (or subconscious), such as heart rate, skin conduction, and EEG rhythms. In addition, research has shown that people can be trained to use real-time functional MRI - which produces images of brain activity in specific parts of the brain - to consciously control brain activities. deCharms' team decided to take this a step further and see if people could be taught to control brain activity in a way that would have a clinical impact.

To do this, the researchers recruited 36 healthy subjects and 12 chronic pain patients. All the participants were told they were going to try to learn how to control activity in a localized brain region associated with pain by using feedback from the MRI they would be placed in. In addition the subjects received written instructions on strategies to accomplish this (note, this is taken directly from the research publication):

1. **Attention.** Attend toward the painful stimulus vs. away from it (to the other side of the body).
2. **Stimulus quality.** Attempt to perceive the stimulus as a neutral sensory experience vs. a tissue-damaging, frightening, or overwhelming experience.
3. **Stimulus severity.** Attempt to perceive the stimulus as either low or high intensity.
4. **Control.** Attempt to control the painful experience, or allow the stimulus to control the percept.

Next, the healthy subjects were divided into an experimental group and 4 control groups. People in the experimental group were given a pre-test, a series of training sessions, and a post-test inside the MRI. During the MRI sessions feedback from the images - which showed activity in the rostral anterior congulate cortex - was provided in both line form and in video form. The subjects cycled through periods where they were supposed to increase activity in the brain region, decrease activity in the brain region, or rest. During each phase, a painful stimulus was applied to their hand with a temperature probe and they were told to rate both the intensity and unpleasantness of this on a scale of 1-10 (a computer mouse was provided in the scanner to do this).

The control groups - all healthy volunteers - underwent variations in this routine designed to eliminate factors that could confuse the results. The result of this rigorous experimental design was that the researchers found that not only were the people in the first group able to learn to control the activity in the selected brain region, but that it significantly influenced how they rated the painful stimulus. Specifically they exhibited a greater ability to increase and decrease brain activity with each practice session. Then during periods of increased activity in the rostral anterior cingulate cortex, pain was perceived as more intense and unpleasant. Similarly, and perhaps more importantly, during periods where they were decreasing activity in this brain region, the painful stimulus was rated as significantly less intense and unpleasant. Overall, the group was able to influence the pain intensity by 23% and the pain unpleasantness by 38% compared to the initial pain ratings.

Having established that healthy people can control brain activity using the MRI, and that this leads to significant changes in pain perception, the team also wanted to determine whether the technique worked for people already in pain. The chronic pain patients went through similar training sessions in the MRI, however no pain stimulus was given, rather they were asked to rate their existing pain after the session using both a simple 1-10 scale and a pain questionnaire.

Just as with the healthy subjects, the pain subjects reported significant changes in their pain perception. On average, they experienced a 64% decrease in pain as rated by the questionnaire, and a 44% decrease as rated by the simple number scale. Also, as with the healthy groups, this change was much larger - three times - than that reported by a control group of pain patients who did not receive MRI feedback.

This research has shown that given the proper training and feedback, people are not only able to control the activity of a specific brain region, but that this can translate to real changes, such as pain reduction.

Acceptance

While the Harvard study generated a good deal of buzz with its high tech methods of pain control, psychologists have been working for some time on a decidedly more low tech approach to using the mind for pain control, a concept known as acceptance.

It is human nature to avoid things which are unpleasant. Unpleasant situations, unpleasant people, unpleasant weather, it doesn't matter; we are programmed to seek out comfort. This is even truer when it comes to pain.

Anyone living with residual pain due to Chiari or syringomyelia knows the feeling. You are asked to go somewhere or do something that you know will cause a great deal of pain and discomfort. The dread starts to build. Do you find an excuse, or do you force yourself to go through with it, anxious about how it will affect you?

Obviously, avoiding pain is not a behavior limited to Chiari patients. It may, in some cases however, actually be counterproductive. In the field of pain research, there is a body of thought that, one way in which regular, short-lasting pain becomes chronic, is through avoidance. The avoidance theory states that when people are in pain, and they avoid doing activities because they are anxious or afraid of making things worse, they are in fact making things worse. The resulting inactivity leads to muscle atrophy, feelings of depression, and more.

Based on this theory, some psychologists have begun to develop treatments based on acceptance of things that can't be changed rather than avoidance. For example, people with obsessive personalities may not be able to control negative thoughts they have, but they may be able to learn to not let the negative thoughts influence their actions. Such acceptance based treatments have shown promise in helping people with borderline personality disorders and even schizophrenia.

Dealing with chronic pain may be a similar situation. It can be difficult to avoid or even control chronic pain. Trying to control something which can't be controlled can actually make things worse, by increasing anxiety and distress. As mentioned earlier, trying to avoid activities which increase pain often backfires and can increase disability.

There is however, an alternative, namely acceptance. For example (this is taken from a published research article) someone with severe chronic pain when presented with a social invitation may turn it down, think I can't go because I'm in too much pain, and feel anxiety about the whole situation. Traditional therapy would focus on identifying these thoughts as faulty and reframing them into a more positive light. An acceptance approach, on the other hand, recognizes that these thoughts happen. The pain will be there; but says, so what,. go to the party anyway. Recognize the pain, but don't let it control you.

A 2005 study (McCracken) out of the UK, showcased the potential of the acceptance based approach to dealing with chronic pain. In the research, McCracken and his colleagues evaluated the effectiveness of an acceptance based treatment program on the quality of life of 108 chronic pain patients.

The study involved patients in a pain management unit in the UK who had been in pain for at least 3 months, reported pain related stress and disability, were not eligible for any more tests or procedures, and had no psychiatric conditions which would interfere with the proposed treatment.

About half of the group suffered from low back pain, with an average duration of 10 years. As those with Chiari can relate to, they had seen an average of 6 doctors related to their pain, and most had tried opioids and antidepressants without success. More than 40% had even had some type of surgical treatment for pain.

All the patients were given a fairly intensive, multi-disciplinary, acceptance based treatment. The program lasted for 3 or 4 weeks depending on the need, and included physical therapists, occupational therapists, nurses, doctors, and clinical psychologists. The program was five days a week for six hours a day and was designed to focus on improving function.

The treatment included exercises designed to activate the whole body, programs to develop healthy habits and provide a meaningful direction in life, and an extensive psychological focus. The psychological component included reversing habits, being aware of avoidance thoughts, meditation exercises, relaxation techniques, body awareness to improve functioning, and raising awareness of the social effects of pain displays.

The team found that the acceptance based intervention resulted in a significant improvement across nine measures, including two tests of physical function. Levels of depression dropped dramatically, as did psychosocial disability, and the amount of pain-related rest needed on a daily basis. Three months later, while the improvement wasn't quite as strong, it was still significant compared to before the treatment. Interestingly, the patients also showed a greater level of acceptance and a willingness to engage in activities despite the pain. And that is the key, learning to do things even though there is pain. Overcoming the natural tendency to avoid activities – which can lead to depression and social withdrawal – and forcing yourself to engage in life despite the pain.

A 2005 study (Lame) which examined the role that beliefs about pain plays in quality of life, supports the acceptance approach. Specifically, the study surveyed more than 1,200 pain patients in Norway about their pain intensity and beliefs about pain and quality of life. Surprisingly, the research found that how people respond to pain had a bigger influence on quality of life than the pain intensity itself.

They found that people who had an exaggerated, negative response to pain score significantly lower on every quality of life aspect measured. In other words, these results stress the importance of a person's psychological response to chronic pain, and demonstrate the positive effect that acceptance can have.

Personal Experience: A short time before I came across the research on acceptance, I had pretty much reached the same conclusion on my own. I remember making a New Years resolution one year that I would try to be more active and if I was presented with a choice of doing something or not, that I would force myself to do it. I stuck with the resolution and made great strides in improving my overall quality of life. I don't think my level of pain changed, it's just that I learned to ignore it, and one of the best ways to do that is be engaging in interesting things. I strongly recommend to anyone with chronic pain to try an acceptance based approach. Yes, the pain will be there, but does that really mean you can't do things? You might be surprised.

Family Impact

"Acknowledge that your family member is having pain and is suffering. Help them build upon and expand their coping strengths, rather than solely focusing on coping limitations."~Dr. Keefe, Health Psychologist~

Spouses

Naturally, the impact of living with chronic pain and disability is not limited to just the person in pain, but extends to their family as well, especially spouses. It is reasonable to assume that many partners become a caregiver to some degree, whether it is taking on extra chores around the house, assisting with medical issues directly, or going to work to make up for lost income. Research has shown that this burden can take a heavy toll.

A 2001 review of the impact of chronic illness on a partner's quality of life (Rees) actually demonstrated that many partners/caregivers report a lower quality of life than the patients themselves. This is not surprising given that research focused on the care of the elderly has clearly shown that caregivers suffer from increased stress, anxiety, depression, decreased social life, and even worsening physical health. A study by Kornblith found that the wives of prostate cancer patients reported greater psychological distress than their husbands. A study by Weitzenkamp showed that the spouses of spinal cord injured persons had higher levels of depression than the patients themselves. The burden of care is not just psychological either. Research has shown that the added stress and anxiety can lead to loss of appetite, disrupted sleep, and generally, a lower level of overall health.

In general, caregivers are faced with many challenges and difficulties. These include everything from extreme financial difficulties, to dealing with the changed relationship with their spouse, to the physical toll the added burden can bring. In addition to the extra work that a partner may be doing, the psychological stress of worrying about the future and whether their loved one is hurting and in pain can be difficult to handle. Adding to the problem is a sense of social isolation that overcomes many partners. Even if they have the time and energy to go to social functions - such as a neighborhood gathering - they may not want to go alone. This can lead to withdrawal and social isolation, increased feelings of having to do everything themselves and increase the psychological burden.

While the effect can be large on a caregiver/partner, research has also shown that a number of factors can influence how severe that impact is, including factors involving the caregiver, the patient, and the situation itself. For example, some research has shown that women suffer more of an impact than men, and younger women in particular. Also caregivers who live alone with their partners and families with lower incomes are especially susceptible to the burden of a chronic illness.

In looking at the patient, somewhat surprisingly, it is not clear if there is a link between the severity of the illness and the impact it has on the partner. Some research has found such a link, while other research has reported the opposite. There is also research suggesting that the mental health of the patient may be more important than their physical health in predicting how much of an impact it will have on the partner.

Finally, it appears that the type of care required also influences the impact on the partner. Extra, impersonal chores, such as shopping, are often perceived as less of a burden than if the care required is personal in nature, such as feeding or bathing. In addition, restrictions brought on by the situation, such as needing to be home most of the time, can increase the negative impact on the partner.

Given all the negatives discussed so far, it may be hard to believe, but many partner/caregivers actually report positive aspects of their situation. Some people report finding a new meaning to life and an increase in self-worth and self-esteem. In addition, some people report that they feel closer to their spouses as a result of the situation and that the situation has made them a more caring person in general.

"Chiari has humbled me considerably. Once I let go of the control I thought I had and slowed down a bit, my husband's sensitivity shined through and the support that I would need over and again, began to grow, as did our relationship for probably the first time truly, since we had met." ~Melissa N.~

"I have a new appreciation for life and the people in my life. I am inspired to be a better person and help others with the same condition."
~ Anonymous Chiari Patient~

On the flipside, given the burden that caregivers must bear, burnout is a recognized and studied phenomenon and families should be aware of the signs:

- Withdrawing from friends and family
- No longer participating in activities you enjoy
- Feeling helpless and hopeless frequently
- Getting upset more quickly than usual
- Loss of appetite
- Altered sleep patterns
- Getting sick more often
- Feeling like you can't take it one more day
- Fantasizing about escape
- Feeling you want to hurt yourself or the person you are caring for

Sometimes the caregivers and partners need help. Two online resources for caregivers are:

www.caregiver.org and www.helpguide.org

Changing Roles

Even if a spouse doesn't have to take on the burden of being a full-fledged caregiver, the family dynamic can be disrupted by the impact Chiari can have on the role each partner plays in the family. For example, in a traditional family where the husband acted as provider and supported the family financially through work and the wife acted as the nurturer and cared for the family, if either one gets sick, then their roles can change. If the husband is no longer able to work, then not only does the wife have to work (which can cause resentment), but the husband must deal with not being able to provide for his family. Conversely, if the wife is no longer able to care for her family like she used to, not only does the husband have to take on that role, but the wife must deal with the emotions of not being able to do what she wants to do for her family.

Obviously, the roles described above can be switched or shared in a different way, but the point is that families tend to develop routines around specific roles that each partner plays. Family counselors focus on the importance of these roles and the impact that a disruption to these roles can have on the family dynamic. Chronic pain and illness can be a disruption to a stable family dynamic and it can take time, work and open communication to achieve a new level of stability for the family.

Spouses Have Different Views

Anyone who has been married can tell you that spouses often view things differently, so perhaps it's no surprise that the same is true for how spouses view pain and disability. A 2004 study (Cano) of 110 couples where one spouse suffered from chronic musculoskeletal pain found through interviews that spouses tend to rate their partner's pain as more severe than the patients themselves. In other words, there is a tendency for people to think their spouse is suffering from more pain than they are.

Conversely, the pain patients tended to rate their level of disability (physical, psychosocial and recreational) higher than their spouses did. So even though they were in less pain than their spouses thought, patients felt like they had more restrictions in what they were able to do. Interestingly, the amount of disagreement between spouses over levels of pain and disability was higher when the person in pain was the woman.

Pain is inherently subjective, so even for married couples it can be difficult to tell how much pain the other person is in. The key to minimizing the effect that this disparity can have is to develop ways to communicate levels of pain and disability without it sounding like complaining or blowing it out of proportion.

Children

The family impact of Chiari is not limited to spouses, as of course children are also affected. There are really two different situations, the impact on children when a parent has Chiari and the impact on the family when a child has Chiari.

Being a Chiari Parent

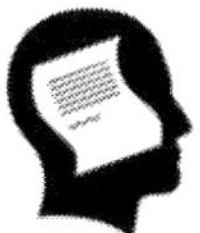

Personal Experience: I am a Chiari parent. With three kids, I know what it's like to tell them I can't do things, to say my neck hurts too much, to feel like my head is going to explode when they're running around like crazy. I know these things and I live them every day. While this is difficult, and I know that parents with Chiari struggle with feelings of not being able to do everything they want to do regarding their children, over the years I have come to realize that the parent is affected much more than the children are in this situation. I honestly believe that many Chiari parents beat themselves up needlessly for their limitations and that from the child's point of view it is no big deal.

Children are incredibly adaptable and resilient and, in my experience, very accepting of the way things are. While I understand, and share in, the frustration of not being able to do certain things that many parents take for granted, it is important to keep in mind our number one job as a parent. That is to provide our children with a safe, loving, structured environment where they can grow. In my mind, beyond that everything else is gravy. And that is the best way to approach it.

You can still fulfill your basic duties as a parent even with physical limitations, and rather than focus on what you can't do, take joy in what you can do with your children. Like the Woody Allen quote, "Eighty percent of success is showing up", I believe that 80% of parenting is just being there.

I don't mean to minimize in any way the struggles of a Chiari parent. I know how difficult it can be, especially with young children who require a lot of physical work. When my children were younger it seemed like everyday something happened involving them that hurt my neck. But I worked through it and as they've gotten older and those demands lessen it has become easier. My point is that it is hard enough being a parent, and harder enough still with

Chiari, so don't take on any burdens, such as guilt over not being able to do what the super-parent down the street does, that you don't need to bear. Find things you can do with your children which don't cause too much pain and focus your energy on those things.

I would also suggest not making a big deal of the things you can't do, but just be matter of fact about it. Over time, children learn what you can and can't do and you may find they are the most empathetic people around.

It's also important to be careful about venting your frustrations with doctors, or work, or your health in general in front of your children. Children will pick up on the tension and fears you have and may become anxious themselves about the situation.

Finally, for me personally, Chiari has been a mixed bag when it comes to being a parent. While I do resent my physical limitations at times, I also realize that if I didn't have Chiari, I probably wouldn't have spent anywhere near the time I have with my kids or had the relationship with them that I do.

When Your Child Has Chiari

Is there a parent out there who wouldn't gladly trade places with their child who has Chiari? Probably not. Hearing the stories of parents dealing with children going through multiple surgeries is incredibly heartbreaking. Between the day to day logistics of caring for a child who does not feel well and the emotional impact it has on parents and siblings, the issues parents must face could probably fill a book on its own (which Conquer Chiari hopes to publish in the future) and is not covered in-depth in this book. However as stated previously, the vast majority of the science and medical issues covered in this book do apply to both adults and children. Beyond that, it is worth touching on two of the most common issues parents face after a child has Chiari surgery, school and sports.

No matter the outcome from surgery, good or bad, parents must face the task of educating their child. Conquer Chiari has heard from quite a few teachers, principals and school nurses eager to learn more about Chiari so that they can help a child in every way possible. Unfortunately, Conquer Chiari has also heard from parents who have struggled to get teachers and school administrators to understand their child's situation.

For these situations, many parents have found the Conquer Chiari Education & Awareness Sheets to be helpful in explaining Chiari and their child's needs to teachers. The sheets can be found at:

http://www.conquerchiari.org/Patient%20Literature.htm

When dealing with public schools, parents should also be aware of what their legal rights are when it comes to the school educating their child.

Although it varies state by state, many states have laws governing what schools must do to accommodate children and the process parents can go through to exercise their rights. This topic is well documented on the internet and there are many groups and message boards available.

Another significant issue parents must face after a child has had Chiari surgery is whether to allow them to participate in sports. There are many anecdotal reports, especially in local newspapers, of children not only returning to sports, but to contact sports such as football. Similarly, there are many parents who would never allow their children to participate in such activities after finding out about Chiari.

Unfortunately, currently there is no way to know who is right in this situation. There is no research to show whether children who engage in activities such as football or gymnastics after surgery are at increased risk for Chiari symptoms returning or other types of injury. When posed this question by Conquer Chiari, many pediatric neurosurgeons have told Conquer Chiari they're not in favor of sports such as football and soccer at all, which in a way is ducking the question. However, clearly some neurosurgeons are clearing children to return to such sports.

Like so much of parenting, this becomes a judgment call. Parents should of course talk with the surgeon extensively about whether they feel there are any increased risks. Common sense would say that whether a child had a complicated case with many structural abnormalities or simple tonsillar herniation should be a factor in the decision making process as well. If children do return to sports, both parents and the children should be fully educated on what to watch for so that any problems can be caught early.

Depression & Social Withdrawal

Research has shown that depression is a major problem in the Chiari community. Whether it is a function of Chiari directly or a result of living with pain is not as important as being able to distinguish between normal variations in mood and when you (or someone else) is clinically depressed and needs help.

According to the National Mental Health Association (a nonprofit organization), the symptoms of clinical depression include:

- Persistent sad, anxious or "empty" mood
- Sleeping too much or too little, middle of the night or early morning waking
- Reduced appetite and weight loss, or increased appetite and weight gain
- Loss of pleasure and interest in activities once enjoyed, including sex
- Restlessness, irritability

- Persistent physical symptoms that do not respond to treatment (such as chronic pain or digestive disorders)
- Difficulty concentrating, remembering or making decisions
- Fatigue or loss of energy
- Feeling guilty, hopeless or worthless
- Thoughts of suicide or death

If you think you are depressed, it is important to seek professional help. Research has shown that many cases of depression respond well to treatment with medication, counseling or both. There is no need to suffer needlessly.

Ray D'Alonzo, a patient advocate, wrote a tremendous book chronicling his struggle with and eventual triumph over Chiari and Chiari related depression. The book, *"Contents Under Pressure"*, is very moving and many people have found it to be an uplifting and positive read.

Work

Chiari can have a varying impact on a person's ability to work, ranging anywhere from making it difficult to perform certain tasks, to forcing someone to go on disability. This section discusses three aspects of Chiari and employment: the Americans with Disabilities Act, deciding what to tell your employer about Chiari, and deciding whether to go on disability.

What is the ADA?

The following is excerpted from an article Jill Hess wrote for Chiari & Syringomyelia News. Jill is a Chiari patient who is also a practicing counselor with experience in many areas of disability service:

> Often, people with Chiari Malformations may encounter limitations at work as a result of their condition. The Americans with Disabilities Act (ADA) provides people with disabilities certain rights, and may make working with Chiari easier if you are aware of what it is.
>
> According to the Job Accommodation Network (2007), "The Americans with Disabilities Act of 1990 (ADA) requires employers to provide reasonable accommodation to qualified employees and applicants with disabilities, unless such accommodations would pose an undue hardship (e.g. too costly, too extensive, too substantial, too disruptive). In general, the applicant or employee with a disability is responsible for letting the employer know that an accommodation is needed to participate in the application process, to perform essential job functions, or to receive equal

benefits and privileges of employment. Employers are not required to provide accommodations if they are not aware of the need."

"The Americans with Disabilities Act of 1990 (ADA) makes it unlawful to discriminate in employment against a qualified individual with a disability. The ADA also outlaws discrimination against individuals with disabilities in State and local government services, public accommodations, transportation and telecommunications. This part of the law is enforced by the US. Equal Employment Opportunity Commission (EEOC) and State and local civil rights enforcement agencies that work with the Commission."

What conditions are covered by the ADA?

There is not a list of conditions that are considered disabilities under the ADA. Rather, the ADA recognizes a person with a disability as someone having a significant limitation in one or more daily life activities. The US Equal Employment Opportunity Commission (EEOC) states "that with respect to an individual, the term "disability" means:

- a physical or mental impairment that substantially limits one or more of the major life activities of such individual;
- a record of such impairment; or (C) being regarded as having such an impairment.

What Is A Reasonable Accommodation?

The EEOC states that "a reasonable accommodation is any change in the work environment or in the way things are usually done that results in equal employment opportunity for an individual with a disability. An employer must make a reasonable accommodation to the known physical or mental limitations of a qualified applicant or employee with a disability unless it can show that the accommodation would cause an undue hardship on the operation of its business."

Requesting an Accommodation?

Although the EEOC does not specify that accommodation requests must be made in writing, it is in the employees' best interest to write an accommodation request letter to their employer. This will help in initiating the accommodation process, and record keeping for the employee and employer.

The link below will direct you to the Job Accommodation Network's publication IDEAS FOR WRITING AN ACCOMMODATION REQUEST LETTER at

http://www.jan.wvu.edu/media/accommrequestltr.html.

This will help you format a letter that discusses your limitations and the requested accommodations.

Deciding What to Tell Your Employer

Revealing a chronic illness to an employer is a complicated decision and should be undertaken with considerable thought and deliberation. Although certain legal protections are in place as discussed above, it is natural for people to be concerned that they will be treated differently if an illness is revealed.

There is no right or wrong answer as to whether, when, or how much information to disclose to an employer, although sometimes it is driven by necessity. If a person has to undergo surgery and requires short-term disability, obviously they must tell their employer. However, even in this case, it is important to think about whether to tell just those who need to know or whether to tell colleagues as well.

A 2005 study of employees at a university in the United Kingdom (Munir) found that most people only reveal an illness if they have to do so and in general share information on a need to know basis. The study, which used surveys, found that more than 700 people out of 5,000 were managing a chronic illness while continuing to work. Of the 700, only half had told their bosses about their illness, and even among that group there was a tendency to only reveal a small level of information.

Factors that influenced people to fully divulge their health situation included the perceived importance of workplace support and whether some colleagues were already aware of the situation. In other words, people who wanted support from their workplace tended to share fully. Also, if people told some colleagues, presumably friends, they tended to fully disclose, probably in anticipation of the news spreading anyway.

Again, it's not clear whether there is a right or wrong answer in regards to what to tell an employer, but it is something many people with Chiari must deal with.

Disability

While precise data is not available, anecdotally it is clear that many people with Chiari and/or syringomyelia decide to go on disability. As with many aspects of Chiari, this is one area where there is virtually no research to speak of, but the decision to stop working should not be taken lightly. Studies involving other medical conditions have found that fatigue plays an important role in people deciding to stop working, and obviously functional limitations do as well.

The ins and outs of the disability process are beyond the scope of this book, but Conquer Chiari has heard from many people on this subject. Some report that the process was quite easy, while others report it was lengthy and difficult with no one truly understanding the impact Chiari can have.

Although it has not been studied, one has to wonder if there is a downside, psychologically, to going on disability for a person who was used to working every day. Given the tendency for depression among Chiari patients, it seems reasonable to think that not working could make that problem worse.

Pregnancy

Because Chiari is often diagnosed when people are in their late 20s or early 30s, pregnancy is a big concern for women with Chiari. Although research is limited, several publications do seem to indicate that pregnancy can be successfully managed in regards to the mother's Chiari.

Concerns regarding pregnancy for Chiari women are very valid as in fact some women have reported that labor and delivery have triggered Chiari symptoms. Obviously, if the Chiari is undiagnosed prior to the pregnancy nothing can be done, but for women with Chiari who are planning on becoming pregnant, issues such as whether a C-section is necessary and whether an epidural can be used are important to consider.

In a 2005 study, Dr. Diane Mueller, a neurosurgical nurse doctorate and a Conquer Chiari Director, published seven cases of Chiari and pregnancy. In looking at the subject, Dr. Mueller wanted to answer three questions:

1. Is there a change or worsening of Chiari related symptoms during pregnancy, delivery, or post-partum?
2. Does epidural or intrathecal anesthesia change or worsen symptoms?
3. Are there any Chiari related complications during delivery or post-partum?

To answer these questions, Dr. Mueller asked 7 women who were diagnosed with Chiari and were pregnant either at the time they were evaluated or some time afterward to answer a questionnaire. The questionnaire asked about symptoms experienced during the pregnancy, the type of delivery, anesthesia used, symptoms after delivery, and whether there were any complications.

The average age of the women was 29, while the average size of their Chiari malformations was 9mm. Most of the women got pregnant after undergoing decompression surgery, but two of the women were pregnant before surgery.

Overall, the group fared very well. For most of the women, some symptoms got slightly worse during pregnancy but resolved fairly quickly. Interestingly, in some cases, symptoms - mostly headaches - actually got better at times during the pregnancy. Labor and delivery didn't aggravate symptoms at all, and only one woman had a slight problem post-partum which resolved in the near-term. Anesthesia did not seem to be an issue as well, with several women receiving epidurals with no problems. Overall there were no Chiari related complications during delivery.

While this is good news for Chiari women, for those planning on becoming pregnant (or who are pregnant) it is still important to discuss these issues with your doctors and make sure they understand the concerns regarding straining during labor.

Living with Chiari

"[Chiari patients should] develop a variety of active coping strategies that enable them to deal with the challenges of the disease. Avoid relying solely on passive coping methods such as bedrest or avoiding daily situations that might be challenging. Find ways around obstacles so that you are able to remain involved in a varied lifestyle."~Dr. Keefe, Health Psychologist~

Living with Chiari can be challenging, to say the least. Pain, depression, financial hardships, strained relationships can all be part of the Chiari package. However, it is not all gloom and doom. Many people live normal (if there is such a thing), or near normal lives after surgery, and even people with pain and disability find ways to adapt and carry on.

While this chapter presented the harsh reality of the impact Chiari can have, the next two chapters present reasons why the future may be better and tips for how individuals can Conquer Chiari on a personal level.

8

Looking to the Future

"Hope is the thing with feathers that perches in the soul"

~Emily Dickinson, Poet~
(1830-1886)

One Day in the (hopefully) Not Too Distant Future...

"Keith Shuler!"

The nurse held the door open as Keith tossed the magazine he was reading onto a table and walked towards her. "Good morning," he said.

She gave him a half-smile, half-nod, and half-grunt and lead him down a hallway decorated with holly and Christmas lights and into an exam room. She asked him to step on the scale and dutifully noted his weight along with his blood pressure, pulse, and temperature, all without saying a word. "Now," she said, looking up at last. "How old are you?"

"I'm thirty-two."

"And what brings you here today?"

"I've been getting headaches when I play basketball," Keith replied.

"How would you describe the headaches?"

"I get an intense pain back here," Keith pointed to the back of his head. "It's like there's a fist inside my skull squeezing my brain. Then, if I lie down for a few minutes it just goes away. At first I didn't think it was any big deal, but now I'm not sure. I think they might be getting worse."

"And how long have you been having these headaches?"

"About two to three months. They just started getting really bad the last couple of weeks. I had one two days ago that didn't go away for almost half an hour. That's when I called."

"Any other problems...colds, congestion, fever...anything like that?"

"No, not really."

"OK. Are you on any medications?"

"No, I don't like taking medicines."

The nurse finished writing, gathered her paperwork and started to leave, "Dr. Hennigan will be with you shortly."

A few moments after the nurse left, Keith started to fidget on the exam table and got up to look around the room. There were the usual posters of body parts and explanations of diseases. There was a small desk with a stool and another chair beside it. Keith decided to sit in the chair. He didn't feel sick and sitting on the exam table made him uncomfortable.

There was a sharp knock on the door and Dr. Hennigan came into the room. A compact man in his late forties, his energy immediately filled the room. He shook Keith's hand, sat on the stool next to Keith, and said, "Good morning Mr. Shuler. Good to see you again. What seems to be the problem?"

Keith repeated his story of the headaches adding that he knew it was probably nothing, but they were getting very painful.

"No, you were right to come in," Dr. Hennigan said. "Headaches are often a sign that something might be wrong. Have you noticed any other activities that give you headaches? Do you jog? When you sneeze? When you cough?"

"Now that you mention it, I had a cold a couple of weeks ago, and when I coughed it would kind of hurt in the same spot. I haven't really jogged lately. Oh, I almost forgot, sometimes if I bend over for more than a few seconds I'll start to feel the pressure building."

"What about your balance, any problems there? Do you find yourself unsteady, or falling down?"

"Maybe a little. Sometimes I walk into doorways. I never paid it much attention."

"OK, let's have a look at you." Dr. Hennigan asked Keith to sit on the exam table and proceeded to look into his ears, throat, and up his nose. Next he had Keith squeeze his fingers and checked the strength in Keith's arms and legs. He got out a reflex hammer and spent some time tapping Keith in various spots. Next, he spent quite a bit of time looking into Keith's eyes. at which point he got out a small device and said, "I'm going to put this up against your eye. It will measure what is called your intracranial pressure, which is basically the pressure of the fluid inside your head." Keith felt a small push against his eye as the doctor took the reading.

When he was finished, Dr. Hennigan smiled at Keith, "Well, there are a couple of possibilities. Before we go into details, the best thing to do with headaches like this is to get an MRI of the area to see what that shows us. Lucky for you, we have a portable one here in the office. Based on what that shows, we may send you for a follow-up at a regular MRI facility. We'll also take some blood to see if that's normal."

Dr. Hennigan excused himself for a minute to get the portable MRI device. When he returned he was carrying a small lap-top computer in one hand while wheeling some type of screen attached to a tripod and connected to the computer with a cord. He asked Keith to sit very still and adjusted the tripod so that the screen was positioned to the side of Keith's head. The screen came to life and over the next few minutes, Dr.

Hennigan carefully positioned the device at various spots around Keith's head.

Dr. Hennigan turned off the portable MRI and turned to Keith with a smile, "Look, I don't want you to worry, but I do think you should get a regular MRI in a full-strength machine. When we get that report and your blood work, we should know what we're dealing with, OK? The front-desk will set up the MRI appointment for you."

Keith thanked the doctor, set up a time for his MRI, and left wondering if there was more to the headaches than he had suspected.

Three days after his doctor's visit, Keith arrived at the MRI center fifteen minutes before his appointment. After filling out the requisite paperwork, a technician escorted him to a second waiting room and reviewed his medical history and asked a thousand questions about metal implants. Keith changed into a gown and was led into the actual MRI room.

The room was cold and stark, dominated by the big MRI machine. The technician, a young guy with a pony tail, situated him on his back and placed a Hannibal Lechter looking device on his head.

"Now," the technician said, "we'll slide you into the machine. I'll be able to talk to you and you'll be able to talk to me. If you start freaking out, just squeeze this. How long you're in there will depend on what we see, but the whole test should take less than fifteen minutes. You ready?"

Keith gave him a thumbs up and the tech pushed a button and guided Keith into the machine. It was bright inside and crowded, but not claustrophobic.

"Can you hear me?" The tech's voice was coming through a microphone. Keith said he could.

"OK. The first scan will only take a minute and then once the computer looks at that, we'll know what else we need to do. Try not to move."

The machine banged, popped, and whirred for about a minute and then stopped. A short time after that, Keith heard the tech's voice again. "We're going to go ahead and do some more tests. Nothing to worry about, we just want to check some things out. You'll hear a series of noises for about 5 minutes."

Keith tried to stay calm and lie as still as possible, but inside he knew something was wrong. They would only do more tests if they found something bad.

He wondered if it was a tumor.

"One more test Keith, you're doing great. This time, when I say go, I want you to cough as hard as you can without moving too much at least five times."

Keith complied and then the test was over. The technician said he'd hear from his doctor in a couple of days.

Dr. Hennigan called Keith the next night. "The MRI did find something, but it's not that serious and it's very treatable. It's called a Chiari malformation. I'd like you to see a neurosurgeon. His name is Dr. Bellow. He's very good, he actually operated on my back."

"A neurosurgeon?" Keith asked, his voice cracking from nervousness.

"Please trust me, it's not very bad. Dr. Bellow will explain everything to you. Believe me, in the scale of things that can be wrong, this one is barely on the charts. But it does involve the brain, so the neurosurgeons are the ones who handle it. I think you already got all the tests you need, we'll forward all your information and my people will set up the appointment for you. I'll check in with you after you speak to Dr. Bellow."

Dr. Hennigan was very reassuring, but when Keith hung up the phone, a kernel of doubt remained. He wondered what a Chiari malformation was and decided to do some research on his own.

Keith had found a lot of good information about Chiari on the web, and he was feeling pretty good about things as he waited for Dr. Bellow in the exam room. Everything he read said the condition, if caught fairly early, was treatable with no lasting effects. It was the treatment he was still a little worried about, it sounded like brain surgery was the main option.

Dr. Bellow broke his reverie with a brief knock and a quick entrance. Keith placed him in his fifties with a Caribbean winter vacation type tan and a confidence that immediately put Keith at ease. He introduced himself and asked Keith some questions about his headaches. He then proceeded to repeat the strength tests and reflex check that Dr. Hennigan had performed in his office.

When he was done he sat down and looked Keith in the eye, "I know Dr. Hennigan informed you that you have a Chiari malformation. Do you know what that is?"

"Yes, I've done some research."

"Good, we'll skip the basics. Basically, you have a mild case that is starting to become symptomatic. Because of the headaches, and the risk of letting it go, I recommend we go ahead and treat it. There are a number of underlying reasons why people have Chiari malformations, such as chronically elevated pressure in their head, or an abnormality at the base of the spinal cord which puts the whole cord in traction. In your case, you were born with the back part of your skull being too small for your brain, so when it developed, it grew out of your skull. The MRI you had done created a mathematical model of the anatomy of your skull and spinal area and also how the fluid in the area moves from your brain into your spine and back. From this information, we can model how you will respond to different treatments - meaning surgeries - so we know pretty much exactly what we have to do to correct the situation. When you coughed in the MRI, it showed us how your brain/spinal system responds to abrupt pressure changes. Are you with me so far?"

"I think so. Like I said, I did a bunch of reading. Can we talk about the actual surgery?"

"Sure. In your case, it will not take much to correct the situation. Basically we need to reshape the back of your skull. To do this, we will take stem cells from your own body to grow a piece of skull to the exact shape we need. Then, for the actual surgery, we will remove a section of your skull and replace it with the one we grew. Since the bone is grown from your own cells, there are no rejection issues. We will also inject a drug which will make your dura - the covering of your brain - more flexible. For reasons we don't quite understand yet, the dura in some people gets too stiff as they reach your age and that causes a problem. Keeping the dura flexible lets us make a minimal structural change and not worry about problems down the road. In addition, your genetic screen shows that you are susceptible to developing a syrinx in the spinal cord if the problem were left untreated. We will inject another substance which should help your body resist that just in case. We'll harvest your stem cells today, but growing the new bone will take a couple of weeks. The whole surgery itself will take less than an hour. You'll spend one night in the hospital. Rest a week or two at home just to make sure everything is ok. Then it's back to normal. What do you think?"

"Wow. You make it sound so straightforward. What's the success rate?"

"Greater than 95%. For you, since there aren't other related problems, the chances of success are even higher, more like 99%. I do about 5-10 of these a year and in the last 5 years, I only had one patient that we had to go back in for. And she did fine after the second surgery."

"How do you define success?" Keith asked.

"Complete recovery. No symptoms. No restriction on activities. Like there was never anything wrong."

Keith let out a big sigh of relief, "Can anything go wrong during surgery?"

"There are always risks, but the complication rate is less than 1%, and serious complications are very rare. The biggest risk is probably if you have a bad reaction to the anesthesia." Dr. Bellow glanced at his watch, "So what do you think, should we do it?"

"Yeah, let's do it."

"Good. My people will set it up." Dr. Bellow started to leave and then turned back, "You know you're lucky. When I started my career, things were much different for people with Chiari. We were barely scratching the surface of understanding it. People went years before being diagnosed - some were even told they were crazy. Most primary care docs didn't know anything about it, and even some neurosurgeons. About 50% of the time, a cyst would develop in the spine, very painful, and would result in permanent nerve damage. And the surgery... it was black magic. Every surgeon did it different. It was very traumatic and failed as much as 30% of the time. We'd take out a big chunk of your skull, some of your spine, cut the dura wide open. Anyway, you're lucky."

Keith didn't know what to say.

A few weeks later Keith was at home watching TV when Dr. Hennigan called. "How are you feeling Keith?"

"I feel great. I'm going back to work tomorrow. I shot some baskets today no problem. No headaches, nothing. It's like there was never anything wrong. I guess I feel like I dodged a bullet."

"Good. Barring any bad luck, I guess I won't see you for awhile then, right?" Dr. Hennigan asked.

"I don't think you will be seeing me. I feel lucky."

~Rick Labuda~

Obviously, the story you just read was fictional, but it doesn't have to be. Every aspect of diagnosis and treatment described in this story is based on active, on-going research. From the concept of a portable MRI which could revolutionize the diagnosis of Chiari, to the futuristic notion of growing your own skull piece, researchers and scientists around the world are making progress on amazing technologies which may one day benefit Chiari patients.

Every week it seems the news carries a story which is truly remarkable. For example, recently a 56-year old German man who had lost his jaw to cancer was given a new one. Not a synthetic one, a real one; and not from an animal, it was custom grown from his own body.

The man's surgeon used computer imaging software to build a titanium mesh mold which precisely matched the jaw he had lost. Stem cells were then taken from the man's bone marrow and placed onto the mold. The entire thing was inserted into the man just below his shoulder blade. Several weeks later, the stem cells had grown into a full jaw, which was removed from his back and attached to its proper place. Four weeks after the operation, the man ate solid foods for the first time in 9 years.

Based on this, is it unreasonable to hope that one day a Chiari patient's skull could be reformed in a similar way, based upon computer modeling from an advanced MRI?

While it can be difficult for someone struggling with Chiari on a daily basis to believe there is a bright future (or any future for that matter), a survey of the promising research, both specific to Chiari and in general, shows without a doubt that there are indeed many reasons for hope.

Active Areas of Research

Chiari/Syringomyelia Specific

The latest research on Chiari is spread throughout this book, from potential new diagnostic criteria, to minimally invasive surgeries, to truly understanding the underlying cause or causes of Chiari and syrinx formation. Nowhere does this more directly affect patients than in the areas of diagnosis and surgery. The following sections highlight some of the more exciting avenues of research, which when taken together show that progress is indeed being made.

Diagnosis

Currently, many Chiari patients suffer with symptoms for years before being accurately diagnosed. During that time, their health can deteriorate and permanent deficits can develop. Improving the diagnosis of Chiari would have a dramatic impact on the outcomes and quality of life of Chiari patients.

As discussed previously, one reason which diagnosing Chiari is difficult is because there is not a single, objective test to say whether someone has symptomatic Chiari. However, there are several promising lines of research in this area, including geometric skull analysis, CSF flow pattern analysis, compliance, and advanced engineering calculations based on fluid dynamics theory.

If one or more of these techniques can be developed into a simple Chiari test, it would revolutionize the diagnosis of Chiari.

Surgery

Decompression surgery and its many variations is probably the most published and researched aspect of Chiari, because it is part of the clinical care of so many patients. Nonetheless, there remains a frustrating lack of agreement on which specific surgical techniques are best for which patients.

However, few (if any) would argue that surgical outcomes are improving and are likely better than 10 – 20 years ago. Some of this is driven by more surgeons gaining experience with the procedure, but this is not the only factor. As more surgeries are performed, more variations are tried and those that help in some way are kept, while older techniques, such as plugging the obex, are dropped.

Many surgical variations are tried in an attempt to reduce the trauma of a complete decompression. Indeed, techniques which don't open the dura completely have been shown to shorten hospital stays, cut down on complications, and cause less pain. Now, actual minimally invasive procedures, which only entail small incisions and utilize special instruments, are being developed. Over the next five to ten years, while there still will likely be many variations to the surgery, it is also likely that the success rate will continue to improve while the trauma of the surgery itself is reduced.

On another front, technology continues to advance and many surgeons today are using devices and equipment that weren't available several years ago. A new generation of dural patches, which reduce CSF leaks and scarring, are gaining acceptance in the surgical community. Similarly, medical companies are developing Chiari plates to replace the skull piece which is removed during decompression. The plate gives the muscles of the neck a place to attach and should reduce post-operative headaches and neck pain. To determine the extent of surgery necessary, some surgeons now use ultrasound during the surgery itself to ensure that CSF flow is adequate.

In the future, detailed computer modeling built from MRI data may allow surgeons to know exactly how much bone to remove and whether/or how much to open the dura. Operating room based MRIs may be able to verify in a quantifiable way that CSF flow has been properly restored.

While it is impossible to predict what Chiari surgery (or treatment) will be like in the future, there are good indications that it will be more successful and less traumatic.

Other Research

Interestingly, some of the most promising advances come not from research on Chiari itself, but from other areas, such as advanced imaging, nerve regeneration, and stem cells. Unlike Chiari, these endeavors attract attention from researchers all over the world and millions of dollars, even billions, are spent pursuing them. Because of their potential to impact so many people, commercial interests come into play as well, which bring a level of resources and focus that Chiari will likely never see.

However, that does not mean that Chiari and syringomyelia patients can't benefit from this work. While it may cost $50 million to design and build a new type of MRI machine, it may cost only thousands of dollars to apply the new technology to Chiari patients in a beneficial way. In this way, the Chiari community can leverage the massive resources being applied to these research areas and piggyback on their successes.

Below are some the most promising avenues of research with the potential to have a major impact on Chiari patients. While these specific items are exciting in their own right, the most exciting and revolutionary developments are often impossible to predict.

Advanced Imaging

As discussed previously in this book, the introduction and widespread adoption of MRI technology has revolutionized the diagnosis, understanding, and treatment of Chiari. What was not discussed, however, is that MRI technology, and other types of imaging such as ultrasound, have revolutionized a lot more than Chiari. Orthopedic medicine, cardiac care, and maternal/fetal monitoring all have benefited dramatically from MRI and ultrasound. In fact, one could say that the non-invasive imaging technologies have revolutionized medicine by allowing doctors to see what is going on inside the body.

It is not surprising then that non-invasive imaging is big business, and with money to be made companies large and small are continuing to push technological advances in MRI magnet strength and data acquisition. Like any hi-tech product, MRIs become more accurate and faster with each generation, and much like how computers have rapidly evolved, in ten to twenty years, the capabilities of MRIs will be far beyond what exists today.

In addition to advancing the basic technology, new types of MRIs are continuously being developed which enable new applications on what seems like a daily basis. Diffusion-tensor MRIs, for example, are able to create images of, and map, individual nerve fibers with stunning clarity. Phase-contrast MRI has been used to not only measure the flow of CSF, but to calculate physical parameters such as compliance as well. As MRIs continue to advance and provide more information, researchers will be able to use that information in creative ways to open up new avenues of research and further advance our understanding of Chiari (and other diseases).

One of the most promising potential MRI advances for Chiari patients would be the development of a portable MRI. While MRIs did open the door to diagnosing Chiari, currently the bar is often set too high for people to get an MRI. Whether its cost, or some other factor, many doctors are reluctant to order MRIs for the often vague and common symptoms associated with Chiari.

A portable MRI, which could be used in a doctor's office like a stethoscope, would have a huge impact on the early diagnosis of Chiari. Imagine, as the story above does, if anyone with frequent headaches gets some type of cheap scan in the doctor's office to help in the diagnosis. Is it fantasy that one day portable MRIs will be used by front-line doctors? Maybe not, recently a research team from Princeton University announced the results of an experiment which showed that they could detect the same thing that a large MRI detects (specifically the spin of hydrogen atoms) with a small device. While it is not certain that this technique will lead to hand-held imaging machines, it is a promising start and the Princeton scientists are not the only ones pursuing it.

Non-invasive ICP Measurement

In our story, the doctor (who obviously suspects Chiari because he is aware of it) looks into Keith's eyes for a long time. He is looking to see if Keith shows any signs of elevated intracranial pressure. In most people, certain veins in the eye pulsate with the heartbeat; this is known as spontaneous venous pulsation (SVP). When the pressure inside someone's skull is elevated however the veins are not able to pulsate. Thus the absence of SVPs can be a sign of elevated ICP. When Dr. Hennigan notes that Keith does not have SVPs, he next uses a non-invasive ICP measuring device to check his intracranial pressure.

Intracranial pressure is a critical parameter for a number of medical conditions, perhaps none more so than trauma. A traumatic head injury can lead to internal bleeding and swelling of the brain which elevates ICP to dangerous levels. Thus, monitoring and managing ICP is an integral part of treating head trauma. Today, measuring ICP is an invasive process, accomplished by either drilling a hole in the skull to insert a device, or via a lumbar puncture at the base of the spine. While with head trauma opening the skull is often necessary anyway, for a non-traumatic disease such as Chiari, the inherent risks of an invasive procedure are too much, so doctors often do not have actual ICP measurements when working with Chiari patients.

Because of the value of ICP as a medical data point, researchers have been working for years to find a way to measure it non-invasively. Various groups have tried techniques involving a wide range of approaches, such as measuring minor skull fluctuations and cerebral blood flow using ultrasound. Two of the more promising approaches are an MRI based technique and an ocular device from a small company called NeuroLife.

The MRI technique uses phase-contrast MRI to measure blood and CSF flow into and out of the brain during the cardiac cycle, and from that can calculate ICP. While this has proven useful from a research point of view, it is still an MRI and thus entails all the obstacles of a regular MRI, meaning cost and inconvenience.

NeuroLife's product is what is described in our tale of the future. It is a device which measures a person's ICP by using the eye. If and when it is shown to work, approved for use, and comes to market, it would provide a cheap, portable, readily-available method for measuring ICP.

What does this mean for Chiari patients? Since Chiari blocks the natural flow of CSF, it often results in an elevated ICP. A portable ICP device, much like a portable MRI, would be a valuable tool in diagnosis. There are many, many causes of headaches, but a headache with elevated ICP is clearly an indication something is wrong. An ICP device would also be useful after surgery to see if it successfully relieved the pressure, and to help determine if post-surgery headaches are an indication that the surgery failed. Also, for patients who end up getting shunts inserted to divert CSF, a non-invasive device could help identify if a shunt is clogged or malfunctioning, a major problem with such devices.

While it may not directly relieve suffering, a non-invasive ICP measuring device would be a welcome addition to the Chiari community.

Nerve Regeneration

The power of celebrity is truly phenomenal. Nowhere is this more evident than in what Christopher Reeve accomplished after he was paralyzed due to a spinal cord injury from a horse riding accident. Reeve was able to leverage his celebrity status to bring national attention and awareness to the devastating effects of spinal cord injuries.

Through his foundation (which has awarded millions in research grants), public appearances, and lobbying efforts, Reeve energized the scientific community into taking a hard look at how to repair the damage done by spinal cord injuries. Why does this matter for the Chiari community. The effects of syringomyelia, which often stretches and damages the nerves of the spine, may be similar to that of a traumatic injury, only to a lesser degree. If doctors can one day cure paralysis by enabling the nerves of the spine to regenerate, it seems reasonable to think that the same types of treatments would be able to fix the nerve damage caused by a syrinx, which often results in pain and debilitation.

With the attention Reeve has brought to the subject, scientists from around the world are attacking the problem from all angles. Some are looking at how the body responds to damage in the spine and at amplifying its own ability to heal. Others are studying novel materials which can act as a platform for nerves to grow on and reconnect. Still others are turning to the promise of stem cells (cells which can become other types of cells) to regenerate and repair damaged nerves.

While the capability to fully repair damaged nerves in the spine may be years (or decades) away, researchers are making progress. Reports come out on a regular basis about techniques which can restore some function to rats with damaged spinal cords.

For example, consider this press release from the Massachusetts Institute of Technology in March, 2006:

> *Rodents blinded by a severed tract in their brains' visual system had their sight partially restored within weeks, thanks to a tiny biodegradable scaffold invented by MIT bioengineers and neuroscientists.*
>
> *This technique, which involves giving brain cells an internal matrix on which to regrow, just as ivy grows on a trellis, may one day help patients with traumatic brain injuries, spinal cord injuries and stroke.*
>
> *The study, which will appear in the online early edition of the Proceedings of the National Academy of Sciences (PNAS) the week of March 13-17, is the first that uses nanotechnology to repair and heal the brain and restore function of a damaged brain region.*
>
> *"If we can reconnect parts of the brain that were disconnected by a stroke, then we may be able to restore speech to an individual who is able to understand what is said but has lost the ability to speak," said co-author Rutledge G. Ellis-Behnke, research scientist in the MIT Department of Brain and Cognitive Sciences. "This is not about restoring 100 percent of damaged brain cells, but 20 percent or even less may be enough to restore function, and that is our goal."*
>
> *Spinal cord injuries, serious stroke and severe traumatic brain injuries affect more than 5 million Americans at a total cost of $65 billion a year in treatment.*
>
> *"If you can return a certain quality of life, if you can get some critical functions back, you have accomplished a lot for a victim of brain injury," said study co-author Gerald E. Schneider, professor of brain and cognitive sciences at MIT. Ellis-Behnke and Schneider worked with*

colleagues from the MIT Center for Biomedical Engineering (CBE) and medical schools in Hong Kong and China.

In the experiment on young and adult hamsters with severed neural pathways, the researchers injected the animals' brains with a clear solution containing a self-assembling material made of fragments of proteins, the building blocks of the human body. These protein fragments are called peptides.

Shuguang Zhang, associate director of the CBE and one of the study's co-authors, has been working on self-assembling peptides for a variety of applications since he discovered them by accident in 1991. Zhang found that placing certain peptides in a salt solution causes them to assemble into thin sheets of 99 percent water and 1 percent peptides. These sheets form a mesh or scaffold of tiny interwoven fibers. Neurons are able to grow through the nanofiber mesh, which is similar to that which normally exists in the extracellular space that holds tissues together.

The process does not involve growing new neurons, but creates an environment conducive for existing cells to regrow their long branchlike projections called axons, through which neurons form synaptic connections to communicate with other neurons. These projections were able to bridge the gap created when the neural pathway was cut and restore enough communication among cells to give the animals back useful vision within around six weeks. The researchers were surprised to find that adult brains responded as robustly as the younger animals' brains, which typically are more adaptable.

"Our designed self-assembling peptide nanofiber scaffold created a good environment not only for axons to regenerate through the site of an acute injury but also to knit the brain tissue together," said Zhang. The technique may be useful for helping close cuts in the brain made during surgery to remove tumors.

Doctors treating traumatic brain injury are confronted with a number of obstacles. When brain tissue is injured, the tissue closes itself like a skin wound. When this happens, scar tissue forms around the injury and large gaps appear where there was once continuous gray matter.

When the clear fluid containing the self-assembling peptides is injected into the area of the cut, it flows into gaps and starts to work as soon as it comes into contact with the fluid that bathes the brain. After serving as a matrix for new cell growth, the peptides' nanofibers break down into harmless products that are eventually excreted in urine or used for tissue repair.

The MIT researchers' synthetic biological material is better than currently available biomaterials because it forms a network of nanofibers similar in scale to the brain's own matrix for cell growth; it can be broken down into natural amino acids that may even be beneficial to surrounding tissue; it is free of chemical and biological contaminants that may show up in animal-derived products such as collagen; and it appears to be immunologically inert, avoiding the problem of rejection by surrounding tissue, the authors wrote.

The researchers are testing the self-assembling peptides on spinal cord injuries and hope to launch trials in primates and eventually humans.

Exciting stuff, especially since the researchers already have a plan to apply the technology to spinal cord injuries. While research into nerve repair doesn't represent a cure for Chiari and syringomyelia, it does hold out the promise of limiting, or even eliminating, their most troublesome and damaging long-term effects.

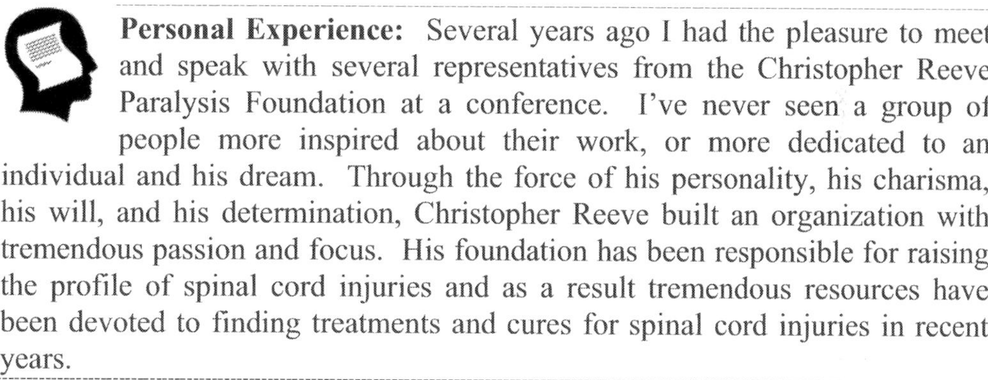

Personal Experience: Several years ago I had the pleasure to meet and speak with several representatives from the Christopher Reeve Paralysis Foundation at a conference. I've never seen a group of people more inspired about their work, or more dedicated to an individual and his dream. Through the force of his personality, his charisma, his will, and his determination, Christopher Reeve built an organization with tremendous passion and focus. His foundation has been responsible for raising the profile of spinal cord injuries and as a result tremendous resources have been devoted to finding treatments and cures for spinal cord injuries in recent years.

Stem Cells

Stem cells, young cells which can be coaxed to become other types of cells such as muscle, heart, and nerve, have generated an incredible amount of promise, controversy, political debate, and hyperbole in recent years.

The promise is that they represent a way to replenish damaged cells and thus hold out the hope of curing debilitating diseases such as Parkinson's, diabetes, Alzheimer's, and even spinal cord injuries.

The controversy stems from (pun intended) the fact that one of the main sources of potential stem cells is from embryos and that embryos may be destroyed in the process of collecting the valuable cells.

From this, there erupted an intense political debate surrounding the ethics of stem cell research which culminated, but did not end, with the decision by President Bush to restrict federal funding of stem cell research to work involving stem cell lines that already exist. This did not end the debate however, as scientists set up private labs and individual states debated issuing bonds to fund research at the state level.

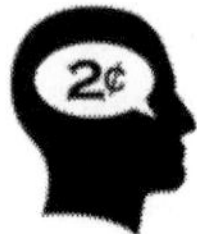

Editor's Note: Conquer Chiari has not taken a position regarding the use of embryonic stem cells for research and does not advocate for or against such use. However, our newsletter, Chiari & Syringomyelia News, has and will continue to report on news and advances from stem cell researchers which are relevant to the Chiari community.

The hyperbole, to no great surprise, came from the mainstream media, who insisted on including phrases such as 'which may cure diabetes, heart disease, spinal cord injury, etc.' any time they wrote about stem cells (which was and is often). With celebrities taking strong positions on the stem cell issue, the hype has continued unchecked and shows no signs of slowing down.

Scientifically, stem cells do have a lot of potential, but most reputable scientists would agree that their reputation is fast getting ahead of their capabilities. The truth is we are in the early stages of researching stem cells and well proven therapeutics based upon them are years, if not decades, away.

Nonetheless, underneath all the controversy and hype researchers are making progress on a number of fronts. Scientists are working on methods to efficiently entice stem cells to become specific cells (this is known as differentiation) and are exploring what happens to these cells when they are transferred to animals. Other researchers are working on techniques which may bypass the ethical issues of using embryonic stem cells, either by developing methods which do not harm the embryo, or by showing that stem cells taken from adults can be just as effective. The most promising of these techniques involve stem cells taken from patients themselves as this would eliminate any potential rejection issues.

To get a picture of where the research is at regarding stem cells, consider these **two** recent press releases, one from the National Institutes of Health, and one from the University College of London, both of which involve stem cells to treat paralysis.

From the NIH:

> June 20, 2006 -- *For the first time, researchers have enticed transplants of embryonic stem cell-derived motor neurons in the spinal cord to connect with muscles and partially restore function in paralyzed animals. The study suggests that similar techniques may be useful for treating such disorders as spinal cord injury, transverse myelitis, amyotrophic lateral sclerosis (ALS), and spinal muscular atrophy. The study was funded in part by the NIH's National Institute of Neurological Disorders and Stroke (NINDS).*
>
> *The researchers, led by Douglas Kerr, M.D., Ph.D., of The Johns Hopkins University School of Medicine, used a combination of transplanted motor neurons, chemicals capable of overcoming signals*

that inhibit axon growth, and a nerve growth factor to attract axons to muscles. The report is published in the July 2006 issue of Annals of Neurology.

"This work is a remarkable advance that can help us understand how stem cells might be used to treat injuries and disease and begin to fulfill their great promise. The successful demonstration of functional restoration is proof of the principle and an important step forward. We must remember, however, that we still have a great distance to go," says Elias A. Zerhouni, Director of the National Institutes of Health.

"This study provides a 'recipe' for using stem cells to reconnect the nervous system," says Dr. Kerr. "It raises the notion that we can eventually achieve this in humans, although we have a long way to go."

In the study, Dr. Kerr and his colleagues cultured embryonic stem cells from mice with chemicals that caused them to differentiate into motor neurons. Just before transplantation, they added three nerve growth factors to the culture medium. Most of the cells were also cultured with a substance called dibutyrl cAMP (dbcAMP) that helps to overcome axon-inhibiting signals from myelin, the substance that insulates nerve fibers in the spinal cord.

The cells were transplanted into eight groups of paralyzed rats. Each group received a different combination of treatments. Some groups received injections of a drug called rolipram under the skin before and after the transplants. Rolipram, a drug approved to treat depression, helps to counteract axon-inhibiting signals from myelin. Some animals also received transplants of neural stem cells that secreted the nerve growth factor GDNF into the sciatic nerve (the sciatic nerve extends from the spine down the back of the hind leg). GDNF causes axons to grow toward it.

Three months after the transplants, the investigators examined the rats for signs that the stem cell-derived neurons had survived and integrated with the nervous system. The rats that had received the full cocktail of treatments — transplanted motor neurons, rolipram, dbcAMP, and GDNF-secreting neural stem cells in the sciatic nerve — had several hundred transplant-derived axons extending into the peripheral nervous system, more than in any other group. The axons in these animals reached all the way to the gastrocnemius muscle in the lower leg and formed functional connections, called synapses, with the muscle. The rats showed an increase in the number of functioning motor neurons and an approximately 50 percent improvement in hind limb grip strength by 4 months after transplantation. In contrast, none of the rats given other combinations of treatments recovered lost function.

"We found that we needed a combination of all of the treatments in order to restore function," Dr. Kerr says.

Follow-up experiments with GDNF treatment on only one side of the body showed that, by 6 months after treatment, 75 percent of rats given the full combination of treatments regained the ability to bear weight on the GDNF-treated limbs and to take steps and push away with the foot on that side of the body.

"This research represents significant progress," says David Owens, Ph.D., the NINDS program director for the grant that funded the work. "It is a convergence of embryonic stem cell research with other areas of research that we've funded, including work that uses combination therapies such as rolipram and dbcAMP, growth factors, and cells to facilitate the repair of the injured spinal cord."

Previous studies have shown that stem cells can halt spinal motor neuron degeneration and restore function in animals with spinal cord injury or ALS. However, this study is the first to show that transplanted neurons can form functional connections with the adult mammalian nervous system, the researchers say. They used both electrophysiological and behavioral studies to verify that the recovery was due to connections between the peripheral nervous system and the transplanted neurons.

"We've previously shown that stem cells can protect at-risk neurons, but in ongoing neurodegenerative diseases, there is a very small window of time to do so. After that, there is nothing left to protect," says Dr. Kerr. "To overcome the loss of function, we need to actually replace lost neurons."

While these results are promising, much work remains before a similar strategy could be tried in humans, Dr. Kerr says. The therapy must first be tested in larger animals to determine if the nerves can reconnect over longer distances and to make sure the treatments are safe. There currently is no large-animal model for motor neuron degeneration, so Dr. Kerr's group is working to develop a pig model. Researchers also need to test human embryonic stem cells to learn if they will work in the same way as the mouse cells. It has only recently become possible to grow motor neurons from human embryonic stem cells, Dr. Kerr adds. However, if the future studies go well, this type of therapy might eventually be useful for spinal muscular atrophy, ALS, and other motor neuron diseases.

From University College, London:

November 30, 2005-- *British scientists say they have, for the first time, attempted to treat paralyzed spinal cord injury patients with the patients' own stem cells.*

University College London researchers said although it is not the first time such a transplant has been attempted, the event is remarkable because, unlike earlier efforts, it rests on a 40-year program of animal research and has an established scientific pedigree, The London Telegraph reported.

Scientists say the outlook for such procedures has brightened since they discovered there is only one part of the nervous system in which nerve fibers are in a state of continuous growth. The nerves are at the top of the nose and are concerned with the sense of smell.

The director of the Spinal Repair Unit at UCL, Dr. Geoffrey Raisman, announced Tuesday his team will harvest nasal cells to treat at least 10 patients in a pilot study early next year at London's National Hospital for Neurology and Neurosurgery, the Telegraph said.

"I have spent my research career in trying to find a treatment for spinal cord injury, and I never anticipated that we would get this far when I started out," he said

With billions of dollars being spent, scientists will continue to make progress on the stem cell front and with time, hard work, and a little luck, the stem cell promise may win out over the hype.

Until that time however, patients need to be careful about seeking out stem cell treatments. All the media hype, money, and desperation which comes from living with terrible diseases has led to an inordinate amount of fraud. From a formerly well respected South Korean scientist who faked results of a significant breakthrough, to supposed miracle treatments in second and third world countries which may in fact be outright scams, care must be taken in evaluating and especially participating in any stem cell treatments.

Neuropathic Pain

As discussed in-depth in the previous chapter neuropathic pain can be very difficult to treat. However, Chiari patients are not alone in their suffering; millions of Americans struggle to cope with neuropathic pain due to diabetes, post-herpetic neuralgia, and other causes.

The good news is that pain in general, and neuropathic pain in particular, are widely studied and researched around the world. Doctors and scientists are using a variety of approaches to unravel the riddle of what pain really is in the physical sense of nerves, brain cells, and molecular messengers, and are working to understand why some types of pain become chronic and disabling. While there are still more questions than answers, progress is being made.

Consider the following announcement from researchers at the University of Bristol in the UK:

January 24, 2006 -- *New research shows that it is undamaged nerve fibres that cause ongoing spontaneous pain, not those that are injured.*

These unexpected findings, by Dr Laiche Djouhri, Professor Sally Lawson and colleagues from the University of Bristol, UK, are reported in the " Journal of Neuroscience Today" [25 January, 2006].

Previous research into ongoing chronic pain has tended to focus on the damaged nerve fibres after injury or disease and overlooked the intact fibres. This new understanding may help pharmaceutical companies formulate novel pain killers.

Professor Lawson said: "The cause of this ongoing pain and why it arises spontaneously was not understood before. Now that we know the type of nerve fibres involved, and especially that it is the undamaged fibres that cause this pain, we can examine them to find out what causes them to continually send impulses to the brain. This should help in the search for new analgesics that are effective for controlling ongoing pain."

"Chronic pain is a devastating and widespread problem, affecting one in five adults across Europe." Professor Sally Lawson.

Ongoing pain is a burning or sharp stabbing/shooting pain that can occur spontaneously after nerve injury. Unlike 'evoked' pain caused, for example, by hitting your thumb with a hammer, ongoing pain is particularly difficult to live with because it is often impossible to treat with currently available pain killers.

Djouhri and Lawson show that the nerve cells responsible are 'nociceptors' or damage detectors. There are thousands of these nerves cells, each of which has a very long, fine nerve fibre emerging from it. These fibres run within nerves and connect the skin or other tissues to the spinal cord.

When activated through damage or disease, these nerve fibres fire electrical impulses that travel along the fibre from the site of injury to the spinal cord, from where information is sent to the brain. The faster the undamaged fine fibres fire, the stronger the ongoing pain becomes.

Dr Djouhri added: "The cause of this firing appears to be inflammation within the nerves or tissues, caused by dying or degeneration of the injured nerve fibres within the same nerve."

The mechanism described by Djouhri and Lawson occurs following nerve injury and in nerve and tissue inflammation. Further research is now needed to establish how generally this mechanism may contribute to ongoing pain associated with a wide variety of diseases such as back pain or shingles.

Or the following announcement from the University of Virginia Health System:

> September 21, 2005 -- *We all know that if you put your hand over an open flame it's very painful. What you may not know is that, for some people, just lying under a blanket is painful as well. They have neuropathic pain--annoying, chronic pain that comes from a diseased nerve cell rather than a specific stimulus. Feeling phantom pain in a missing limb is another, more famous, example.*
>
> *Experts say up to two percent of the U.S. population suffers from neuropathic pain. But this pain generally responds poorly to analgesics and other standard treatment and get worse over time, causing permanent disability in some people. Now there may be new hope for these pain sufferers.*
>
> *Scientists at the University of Virginia Health System have identified a new type of pain-sensing neuron in rats, which are unusually dense in a subtype of calcium channels called T-type channels. It is possible that these "T-rich cells" could be targets for future therapies to treat neuropathic pain as well as acute onset pain, which can happen after invasive surgery or inflammation.*
>
> *A UVa anesthesiologist, Dr. Slobodan Todorovic, and his colleagues identified these novel cells and believe that the T-type calcium channels in them may serve as a volume control for pain impulses. "We hope that this new type of neuron will be amenable to new therapies. The next step will be to find a drug to block the action of these calcium channels," Todorovic said.*
>
> *It was once thought that calcium channels were only important for brain function. But, Todorovic and his team show that the T-type channels are important to the functioning of peripheral nerves, especially when the nerves are injured.*
>
> *A PhD student in UVa's neuroscience graduate program, Mike Nelson, discovered these T-rich nerve cells in Todorovic' lab. "It's very exciting to make an initial observation like this," Nelson said. "It's one reason we go to grad school in the first place." There are no drugs now that effectively treat neuropathic pain, Nelson added. "Hopefully, observations like this will lead to new and more efficacious drugs in the future. Our findings are another piece of evidence that these calcium channels are excellent targets for new analgesic development."*

In addition, because the millions of people who suffer from neuropathic pain represent a large commercial market, pharmaceutical companies have spent, and continue to spend, millions of dollars researching and developing potential pain drugs. In fact, new neuropathic drugs are working their way through clinical trials and the regulatory process, and will hit the market in the near future. It is likely that as scientists learn more about what causes neuropathic pain, that more effective treatments will follow, and hopefully relief is not too far down the road.

A Reason for Concern – Lack of Research Funds

While there are many reasons for hope on the research front, there continues to be one very large reason for concern. Namely, the lack of research funds focused directly on Chiari. The National Institutes of Health is a collection of 27 institutes and centers organized under the US Department of Health & Human Services whose mission is to uncover new knowledge that will lead to better health for everyone. With a budget of more than $28 billion dollars to pursue its mission through internal and external research, the NIH is in a unique position to influence the activities of the medical research community. If the NIH decides to fund a certain disease or topic, it is essentially guaranteed to attract top-level researchers.

Unfortunately, Chiari is not even on the map when it comes to NIH funding. For certain conditions, the NIH spends enough money on them that they track and report the spending by disease. For example, in 2007 the NIH spent $207 million researching Parkinson's disease (Figure 8-1). This is not surprising given that as many as a million people in the US may suffer from Parkinson's. Similarly, the NIH spent $47 million and $44 million on Huntington's and ALS respectively. Although these diseases affect less people they are fatal diseases. Multiple Sclerosis, which affects about the same number of people as Chiari, and often in similar ways, benefited from the NIH to the order of $109 million in research spending in 2007. These numbers are staggering, and support numerous research projects across a wide variety of subtopics.

Figure 8-1: 2007 NIH Funding By Disease

Disease	$ Millions
Parkinson's	207
Multiple Sclerosis	109
Huntington's	47
ALS	44
Chiari/Syringomyelia	N/A

So where does Chiari fit into this picture? It doesn't, the NIH does not split out spending on Chiari because there isn't enough spent. However, we can get a picture of the Federal support for Chiari research by using the NIH's own research database. The NIH keeps a database of all research it funds, both internal and external. A search of this database using the term 'Chiari' for the year 2006 returns 3 studies.

One study is a multi-center trial involving fetal repair of myelomeningocele (spina bifida) where severity of Chiari is an outcome measure. One study is looking at potential genes responsible for hindbrain development problems. Interestingly, Chiari is cited even though most experts do not consider Chiari to be a problem with brain development, but bone development. Finally, one project directly focused on Chiari; the study of the clinical relevance of intracranial compliance (compliance is discussed several times in this book) as it relates to Chiari.

Despite the fact that Chiari potentially affects more than 300,000 Americans, it is barely acknowledged in terms of federal funding.

The effect of this lack of funding becomes all to clear when looking at Chiari research publications in a given year.

Figure 8-2: PubMed CM/SM Citations By Year

	'07	'06	'05	'04
Total English Language Citations	161	131	137	122
Adjusted Total	72	52	39	53

Note: Adjusted Total refers to the Total Number of Citations minus the Incidental and Case Study citations

In 2007, the same year the NIH spent over $100 million on MS, there were 161 publications which mentioned Chiari and/or syringomyelia (Figure 8-2), which made 2007 a fairly typical year in Chiari research. Compare this to Multiple Sclerosis, which had more than 2,000 publications in the medical literature in 2007 (Figure 8-3). Similarly, diseases which affect fewer people but with more serious consequences, such as ALS and Huntington's, saw 3-5 times as much research activity as Chiari.

It's not just quantity either. While a quick survey of MS research shows a wide variety of rigorous, controlled studies, whereas the Chiari literature is dominated by incidental research and Case Reports. Of the 161 publications, 18 were focused on other topics and only incidentally referred to CM/SM. Setting these aside, a whopping 71 of the remaining publications were Case Reports. This means that 44% of all publications where Chiari and/or SM was the main subject were actually just descriptions of one or two patients. Unfortunately, Case Reports do little to advance the scientific knowledge of the disease, because one or two patients is not enough to draw any conclusions from. Historically, there has been, and continues to be, a conspicuous absence of the most rigorous types of scientific studies and randomized controlled trials.

Figure 8-3: Number of 2007 Citations for Various Diseases

Disease	# of Citations
Mutliple Sclerosis	2,221
Parkinson's	>2,000
Hydrocephalus	704
ALS	667
Huntington's	486
Spinal Stenosis	205
Chiari/SM	161

Source: PubMed search with limit of publication date between 1/1/07 and 12/31/07. Foreign language publications were excluded.

While it is not entirely clear why Chiari continues to essentially be ignored year after year, several factors may play a role. Clearly, awareness and advocacy are a big part of the equation. Multiple Sclerosis has a long history of successful advocacy groups who have funneled enormous amounts of money towards their cause.

Another issue may be the fact that there are no beneficial estimates of how many people suffer from Chiari and how it impacts them. Without this basic information, it is difficult for many people to place Chiari in the spectrum of disease. Is it rare? Is it common? Does it affect a person's lifespan? Is it severe? Is it no big deal? Until these questions are answered scientifically, with quantifiable data, it will be challenging to raise awareness of Chiari and its impact.

Finally, the fact that Chiari is corrected surgically may play a role in the lack of research. Any disease which can potentially be treated medically with a drug, carries with it an inherent economic incentive. As discussed above, millions of dollars are spent looking for neuropathic pain drugs (which is a side effect of Chiari) because the company which develops an effective one will make many times more than what they have spent on research. There is literally no economic incentive for a company to spend money researching Chiari.

A second aspect to the possible surgical limitations of Chiari is the fact that neurosurgeons are a relatively small group who spend most of their time in surgery. A disease like MS attracts neuroscientists, neurologists, and other types of physicians and researchers, and studies are published in a range of medical journals. Conversely, there are very few Chiari publications outside of the neurosurgical arena.

No matter what the current state of research is, it is clear that only with more money, awareness, and advocacy will Chiari research rise to the level where it should be, and until that occurs, it will remain an area of concern for the Chiari community.

Other Reasons for Hope

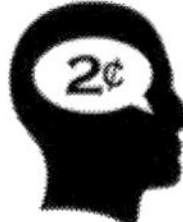

Editorial Opinion: This entire section should be considered my personal opinion and is based solely on my recent, non-scientific, anecdotal observations. I have been involved with Chiari for more than eight years as a patient and advocate. I clearly remember what it was like when I was diagnosed, and I strongly believe that things are getting better in a number of ways and there are many reasons for hope:

1. **More and earlier diagnoses**. In the past few months, I have bumped into several people (not in the course of my Conquer Chiari work) for whom Chiari had affected them or their direct families. While it may just be a statistical fluke, I don't think it is. Eight years ago when I was diagnosed, it seemed like there were very few Chiari people out there. Now, when I talk to people who are newly diagnosed, I hear things like, "I had never heard of it, but when I started asking around I found several friends or family members who knew someone." I also think Chiari is being diagnosed earlier. Lately, I have heard what once I would have considered amazing stories. Pediatricians identifying Chiari from unusual scoliosis. Primary care doctors realizing something is wrong and starting patients on the path to an accurate diagnosis. While much work remains, I think there is definitely a positive trend in the area of diagnosis.
2. **More awareness**. Again, it’s not scientific, but it's my impression that Chiari is getting a lot more attention from the media than it used to. While the stories are not always accurate (in fact rarely so), I do track when Chiari and syringomyelia are mentioned in newspapers, etc., and it is definitely getting more press.

3. **Better outcomes**. In talking with neurosurgeons, I hear that many are seeing better outcomes as the operative techniques become more refined and more surgeons gain experience. This is not to minimize the work that remains in this area, many patients end up with permanent deficits and multiple surgeries, but at the same time, it is important to balance this with a recognition of successful outcomes.
4. **Research continues to advance**. While the amount of Chiari research continues to lag far behind other comparable diseases, advances in understanding continue nonetheless. It appears that we are on the verge of redefining what Chiari really is, and with that, hopefully will come improved treatments.
5. **More information is available.** I saw a great post on a non-Chiari message board a couple of weeks ago. A newly diagnosed patient was told by someone else that while Chiari was serious, there was a lot of information about it available on the web. This was definitely not the case 5 years ago, and represents a significant advance in our fight against Chiari.

I believe that things are getting better largely because of the hard work of people in the Chiari community who are spreading the word, raising our profile, and demanding better care, and if we continue to advocate for ourselves, the situation will improve even more.

9

Conquering Chiari

*"It's not whether you get knocked down;
it's whether you get back up"*

~Vince Lombardi~

This entire chapter should be considered my personal, editorial opinion (thus the extensive use of the first person). While it is not based on published medical and scientific research like the rest of the book, it is based upon my own experience as a patient, and my personal interactions – at times quite in depth – with literally hundreds of patients and professionals. You may agree with what I have to say or you may disagree. You may think I'm putting too much of a burden on patients themselves, after all they've been afflicted with this terrible disease, but that is at the core of what I am trying to say. Despite what has happened, perhaps even because of what has happened, we have to take responsibility for ourselves.

When the C&S Patient Education Foundation Board of Directors decided we needed a catchier name, naturally we brainstormed many, many ideas. After a while, two quickly rose to the top: Cure Chiari and Conquer Chiari. The discussion and debate that ensued among our Board of Directors, advisors, and other key stakeholders was interesting not only in that it resulted in a clear winner, but that in the end we were discussing much more than a name or catchphrase. As we thought about what Chiari is and how it impacts people, it became clear that we were actually further clarifying our mission, our overarching goal, and even how we were to go about accomplishing it.

Despite the background and expertise of many of the participants, the debate between the two words, cure and conquer, went way beyond marketing to the heart of what Chiari is. In the end, we decided that Chiari needs to be conquered not cured. Because of its inherent nature, it is difficult to envision a cure for Chiari in the traditional sense (at least at this time), such as one could cure cancer or eradicate smallpox, but it can beaten. It can be conquered. And thus, Conquer Chiari was born, with a simple name, a simple goal, and the recognition that achieving that goal would not come from a single, silver bullet.

Chiari is a very complex condition, and to defeat it will require many people working on many fronts, both as individuals and as a community. To Conquer Chiari will require each and every patient to stand up and say I will not be beaten. It will take a community to come together in a call for action; to provide support where needed; to raise our voices and spread awareness; to advocate when necessary, and yes, to raise money so that we may understand the enemy and develop new weapons for the battle.

I truly believe that it is the responsibility of each person affected by Chiari to not let it win. How to do this? Below are what I consider to be the keys for an individual to Conquer Chiari. Note, that these steps are intended for patients for whom dealing with Chiari will be a long-term struggle. For those who have become symptom free after surgery, congratulations, you've already won.

10 Steps to Conquering Chiari as an Individual

1. Move Past the Anger to Acceptance

Anger is a very powerful emotion, and when confronted with what seems like a gross injustice, a very understandable one. While anger is a very natural, and probably necessary part of coping with the shock of dealing with a disease like Chiari, it should also be a temporary one.

Many people are familiar with the five stages of grief: denial, anger, bargaining, depression, and acceptance. Interestingly, the five stages of grief were originally the five stages of receiving catastrophic news. One would have to consider being diagnosed with Chiari as catastrophic news, so the five stages definitely apply. It is important not to get caught up in the details and order of the stages, grief (for lack of a better word) is complicated and everyone reacts differently. Human emotions don't always fit easily into well-defined categories. However, it is also important to note that anger is a transitional phase and not the end goal. Someone who works through their emotions in a healthy way will in the end reach some level of acceptance.

Unfortunately, far too often I have seen people stuck in anger. The power of anger becomes all consuming and they are never able to accept the situation and take positive steps to improve their health and lives. This is a terrible situation, with patients feeling they have been hurt and treated unfairly by life. While in one sense this is true, it is also extremely counterproductive to dwell on it.

As patients, at some point we must accept the situation and move on with our lives. I think that after a normal period of adjustment, we must let go of the anger, recognize that our lives have changed, and move forward as best we know how. Does this mean we should never think about the way our lives used to be or the dreams we had? No, I think it's healthy to work through those thoughts and emotions when they come up, as long as they don't become overwhelming.

Anger can be a problem for many people outside of the Chiari community as well, but if you listen to angry people who have let go, they speak of a feeling of liberation and as if a great weight has been lifted from them. This is because anger is such a strong emotion, and if we hold on to it for too long, it becomes destructive.

Research supports that acceptance can be critical in dealing with a chronic disease or disability. In fact studies have shown that whether someone with a chronic disease or disability has accepted their situation has a strong influence on both their quality of life and overall health in general.

Letting go of the anger and accepting the situation at hand is the first step in dealing with, and overcoming, Chiari on a long-term basis.

2. Prioritize & Focus

Once you have moved past the anger and accepted the situation for what it is, it is much easier to take positive, productive steps to building a good quality of life. One of the most important early steps you can take is to prioritize what is important in your life. If you have real limitations, whether they involve pain, mobility, or something else, they will have an impact on your life. The key is to manage their impact, and maximize your capabilities and resources. In order to do this, you need to decide what is important in life and focus on that.

Depending on your individual situation, this could range from making minor modifications in your daily routine, such as lying down for 20 minutes in the afternoon to rest your neck and back, to making major lifestyle changes involving career and family. To accomplish this takes introspection and the ability to take a realistic view of where you are at in your life and what you hope to accomplish in the future.

Chiari strikes many people at a time in their life where they are extremely active and involved in building careers, starting families, and other activities. It can be difficult for someone who is used to being able to accomplish many things to really slow down, take a look at their life, and decide what is important. But the payoff is worth it. Focusing on fewer things and being able to do them well will lead to a better quality of life than falling short by trying to do too much.

At least that was the case with me. Four years after my surgery, I still didn't feel very good. My neck was so weak it seemed like I couldn't do anything without flaring it up. I wasn't able to be the father I wanted to be for my children and going to my job every day was an exercise in pain and frustration. It was a struggle just to get through each day and about an hour after waking up in the morning, I would look forward to the end of the day when I could collapse on the couch. My surgery was technically a success, but my quality of life was not very good.

I realized I needed to make a change. I was surviving, but that wasn't enough. I thought about what was important to me and quickly realized I needed to put my family first. I wanted to have the energy to be with my kids in a positive way, to play outside and go to fun places. Also, I was tired of wasting time and energy in the job I was in. Boring meetings which used to be a minor irritation had become intolerable. My time and energy were precious and I didn't want to waste any of it. Finally, I realized that I needed to put a lot more effort into getting stronger and recovering. I needed to work as hard on recovering as anything else in order to do the things I wanted to do.

Needless to say, I left my job and career and started what would become Conquer Chiari, working out of my home. Over the next couple of years my strength, health, and quality of life steadily improved. Being able to rest when I needed to and control my environment was a big factor. Also, by eliminating the wasted time each day which comes with working for a company (especially a big one) I was able to be more productive work wise and still have time to focus on my family and perhaps most importantly rehabbing. As I gradually increased my level of exercise, I was able to do more and more, not only in the gym, but in life. I was able to build the kind of life I wanted, while being aware of – but not completely giving into – my physical limitations. And needless to say, Conquer Chiari is by far the most rewarding work I have ever done. Today, I'm able to do things physically that I once thought would not be possible, and I'm still getting stronger.

Everyone's situation is unique, and the point is not the specifics of what worked for me, but rather to recognize that if you do have limitations due to Chiari, a change in lifestyle, from modest to drastic, can make a big difference.

Often, it's all too easy to say, "Oh, well, this is the way it is," and just try to get through each day. But if you take the time to take stock of your resources, reflect on what is important, and be creative, good things can happen.

I realize that economic factors are an overriding concern for most people, but there are many ways to make money and for people with disabilities to be productive. With modern communications technology, this is more true today than it ever has been before. Millions of people across the country work out of their homes, and that is an option I would encourage any Chiari patient to explore. Today's work environment is primed for people to work at home, work varied hours, and be independent.

What is important to you? Just because some dreams may no longer be possible, doesn't mean you can't have new dreams, hopes and aspirations. It just takes the mental effort and discipline to decide what to focus on, and the creativity and willpower to make it happen. It may involve sacrifice. It will definitely involve hard work, but nothing good is easy and with some focus and effort you can find a new path.

3. Be Smart & Creative

Once priorities are established, it is important to be smart and creative both in pursuing those priorities and in the mundane activities of everyday life. Many Chiari patients have limited physical resources, but by being smart and creative these resources can go a long way.

It's important to not hold onto the old ways of doing things if they aren't working for you. Don't waste time and energy bemoaning what you can't do. Instead, use your mind to compensate for what your body is not able to do. Be creative in how you approach your daily life and find ways to modify your activities to fit your situation. Just because you can't do something the way you used to doesn't mean you can't find a new approach or a whole new solution altogether.

In other words, maximize your brain and minimize the pain.

Be Smart In Everyday Life

For people with Chiari, the mundane tasks of daily life can be anything but. What was once routine and simple can quickly become painful, frustrating, and overwhelming. Cleaning house, driving to work and taking care of kids can pose a new set of challenges to those dealing with the lingering effects of Chiari and syringomyelia.

The stakes go beyond the specific task at hand as well. Repeated failure and frustration in daily living can lead to depression, a loss of identity and an attitude of giving up. That is why it is so important to be smart in approaching the tasks of daily life. For every activity, large or small, which causes pain and frustration, think hard about different ways to make it easier and take less of a toll.

Obviously, everyone is different, but here are some examples of ways to approach "problems" in daily living:

- Does standing in the kitchen cause pain? Try orthopedic shoes and get some carpet squares to stand on.
- Does holding a phone lock up your neck? Use a speakerphone and just explain briefly to people that you have to use a speakerphone because you have a bad neck.
- Is typing at the computer difficult? Try voice activated software. It's even built into many Microsoft products.
- For me, wearing a tie is near impossible as I immediately get a headache. However, if needed I just wear a collar-less shirt and sport coat. If a restaurant requires a tie, I call ahead and tell them I can't due to a medical condition.
- Travel can be particularly exhausting and challenging, so it is extra important to think creatively. For example, I have trouble carrying something hanging straight down at my side because it pulls at my neck and shoulder muscles. Even pulling a roll-along bag over the long distances will inevitably flare up my neck. So, unless I'm with someone who can haul my carry-on (see Know When to Ask tor Help below), I only take a very small bag as a carry-on and check everything else curbside.
- Is vacuuming too challenging? Look into getting a small robo-vac which will vacuum automatically.

The specifics of what works for me (or others) are not important. What works for one person may not work for someone else. This is why when you see good ideas on message boards about tips for daily living, you should not assume that it applies to everyone, but rather should evaluate each piece of advice against your own situation. Everyone's situation is unique and should be treated as such.

What is important is to be proactive in trying to make your life easier. Be relentless in finding ways to ease the burden of Chiari. Use technology to your advantage. New products are coming out all the time which can make life easier and many old products are still around which were developed for people with spinal injuries or the elderly.

Instead of saying 'I can't do this; I can't do that', think 'How can I do this, how can I do that.' The benefits of this approach are tremendous. Not only will you get more done day in and day out which is good for mental attitude, but by reworking taxing activities, more energy will be left to focus beyond the basics of daily living. You will stop feeling like you are drowning and instead can being swimming to a better quality of life.

Use Your Brain to Get Stronger

Once daily living is under control, you can turn some attention to getting physically stronger. As discussed previously, Chiari patients may suffer from weakness due directly to nerve compression, but also may be weak and physically out of shape due to an overall lower level of activity. While the earlier chapter talked about rehabbing after the surgery, it is also important to continue to work at getting stronger day after day and year after year.

My surgery was in January, 1999 and I'm still getting stronger. However, the road was not easy and one of the most frustrating aspects has been trying to find ways to exercise and physically rehab. Time and again it seemed like I was just getting on track and able to do things when invariably I would suffer from some sort of set back. As I have explained elsewhere in the book, my main residual problem is neck pain and the fact that the muscles in my neck, shoulders and upper back get very tight and go into spasm easily.

Because of this limitation, I have tried many different ways to exercise. From walking to swimming to playing with the kids to lifting very light weights, I do whatever I'm capable of doing at a given point in time. If one activity starts causing me pain, I switch to something else. The key is to find what works and when it stops working find something else.

Chiari patients can become very sedentary, which of course not only can lead to further health problems but can limit capabilities as strength is lost and general energy levels decline. I believe most Chiari people don't work hard enough at recovering physical strength and stamina because it can seem impossible at times. When you hit the wall and are thinking there's no way to do this type of exercise or that type of exercise, that's when you have to use your brain to come up with new ideas. Even a modest amount of physical activity during the day can have a very positive effect.

Try to do something physical each day, even if it's just a short walk, and then build from there, slowly. Once you've done an activity for a few weeks try something new so that your body is working in a different way. Continue to build up slowly and change things on a regular basis.

Once you become used to a certain level of physical activity you will likely find that you can begin to do things that you thought you weren't going to be able to do again and your quality of life will improve dramatically.

Ray D'Alonzo is a great example of this. Ray is a Chiari advocate who went from being barely able to get out of bed to running marathons for Conquer Chiari. Of course it took a large physical effort for Ray to do this, but he also had to be smart in his approach. Intellectually he had to figure out he could slowly build up to the marathon level of performance and set up the training regimen to accomplish it.

I'm not saying that every Chiari patient should try to run a marathon, but I am saying that to truly beat Chiari, you have to be smart in finding ways to be physically active.

Don't Do Stupid Things

Part of being smart is not doing stupid things. While this sounds trite, it's actually more difficult than you might think; at least it has been for me. Like many of you, before my Chiari symptoms became serious I was an extremely active person and physically very fit. When it came to doing something physical, such as picking something up or carrying something, I could either do it or I couldn't. However, after my Chiari surgery all of a sudden there was a third possible outcome which was brand new. Namely, try to do something and hurt my neck/shoulders/back.

The muscles in this area had changed so much over time that now if I tried to pick something up or carry something, there was a good chance I would flare up my neck and be sidelined for days or weeks. It was not just lifting things that I had to be careful of either. If I used the computer for too long, or my head was bent over for a period of time, bad things would happen.

What made it especially difficult was that by the time I would realize that something might be wrong, it was too late. The end result was me saying way too many times, "I can't believe I did that. That was so stupid!"

What I had to learn, and what many Chiari patients have to learn, is to use the conscious part of the brain to monitor what might normally be subconscious activities. Basically you have to unlearn patterns of behavior that might result in flaring up symptoms. Trust me this is not easy and it takes time. One thing that helps is to have another person point out to you when you're doing something (like changing a light bulb with your head tilted back) that you should be careful about. My wife has become very good over the years at recognizing – often before I do – activities which I may come to regret.

This isn't to say that you shouldn't try things, but rather that it should be a conscious decision, with close monitoring, rather than a Homer Simpson moment, "DOH!"

4. Live A Healthy Lifestyle

Obviously it's a good idea to live a healthy lifestyle, but for Chiari patients, I believe it becomes more than a good idea. In fact, to Conquer Chiari and have a good quality of life it becomes absolutely necessary. When you are struggling with a chronic disease like Chiari, the body's natural ability to respond to different stressors is reduced and the margin for error becomes razor thin and the cost of making mistakes increases dramatically.

As discussed previously, chronic disease and pain take a high toll on the body and often lead to other health problems. Thus it is critical to minimize this impact. Also, if you want any chance of feeling good again, you have to be as healthy as you possibly can. For Chiari patients it goes beyond the general benefits of being healthy, as I strongly believe that the impact of Chiari can be mitigated directly through healthy living.

What does this mean? First and foremost in my mind is that it means no alcohol or nicotine. While you might think this is draconian and unnecessary, consider that both alcohol and nicotine have a direct effect not only on the neurotransmitters in the brain, but on blood flow as well. As I have said repeatedly in this book, the natural flow of CSF in the brain/spine is intimately linked to blood flow in the same area. So it would seem natural to assume that ingesting something that affects blood flow may in fact have an impact on CSF flow. I don't know about you, but I'd rather not mess with my CSF flow anymore than it already has been.

A close second (more like tied for first) is that it means you have to achieve and maintain a good weight. In my personal experience with Chiari, the lighter I have been the better I have felt. I think there are a number of reasons for this. Going back to the heart, the heavier you are the harder your heart has to work to pump blood which of course can influence the CSF system. Recall that there appears to be some kind of link between obesity and chronically elevated CSF pressure in the brain. Elevated CSF pressure can obviously aggravate Chiari-type symptoms and may even increase the risk for developing a syrinx.

Beyond the heart, Chiari and SM tend to weaken muscles and make them prone to tightness and spasm. So if you're lighter the muscles don't have to work as hard and will likely feel better. Also, if you weigh less the general impact that comes with each step of walking will be reduced, which is obviously a good thing.

Naturally the best way to maintain a good weight is to eat a healthy, balanced diet and get plenty of exercise. While this is easier said than done if you want to Conquer Chiari you have to develop the discipline to eat well and exercise.

** Talk with your doctor(s) about developing a nutritional diet and exercise plan and to make sure there aren't activities you should avoid **

No drinking, no smoking, eat well, get plenty of exercise and keep the weight off. Those are the biggies, but of course it's also important to drink plenty of fluids and get plenty of regular rest. Many people have told me that their symptoms get much worse when they're tired and run down, so turn off the TV, put away the book and get to bed at a decent time each night.

I would also encourage people to think about ways to minimize the mental stress in their lives. This goes back to prioritizing and focusing. If you have limited resources, don't try to do so many things that nothing gets done well (which of course leads to stress), but rather focus on what is really important and enjoy the positive feelings that result.

5. Stay Active (Don't Give in to Fear)

"The only thing we have to fear is fear itself"
~President Franklin D. Roosevelt in his first inaugural address~

Fear is a big problem for people with Chiari. Many of us start to believe that if we try to do certain things we will fall apart. Fear and anxiety lead to inactivity which almost inevitably leads to depression. Which is better, to sit around doing nothing and feeling bad, or to fill your days even though you may still be in pain and feel bad? I choose the latter and try to fill my days with as much as I possibly can. If you go a mile a minute, the pain doesn't have as much time to catch up. Invariably, it is the days when I decide I must rest which are the hardest, because then the pain comes to the surface and the negative thoughts creep in. Staying active keeps it in the background; I know it's there but I don't have time to focus on it.

We have already talked quite a bit about staying physically active, but it is just as important to be active in other ways as well. At times when you're resting physically, stretch your mind by engaging in something stimulating.

Studying a new subject, reading an interesting book and working on a crossword puzzle are all simple ways to keep the mind active. When the mind is engaged in something it has less time to focus on pain and negative thoughts, and the long-term benefits of stimulating the brain are well established.

It's also important to stay active with family and friends from a social point of view. Many Chiari and syringomyelia patients, because of fear of pain, end up avoiding social situations and become isolated. This too leads to depression and requires a conscious effort to overcome. Maybe going to the neighborhood party will cause some pain and make you tired, but it might just be worth it. Connecting with people is an integral part of life and I think Chiari people give this up too easily. It's too easy to say no one understands so I'll just stay home.

Well I understand. It causes me great discomfort to sit in most chairs, stand for more than a couple of minutes, drive anywhere, and even wear most shirts, but I force myself to do things. Am I in pain? Yes, but usually it's worth it up to a point. If I go to a party, I may only stay for an hour, but at least I got out of the house and usually the sense of accomplishment outweighs the pain and fatigue. When we go to restaurants, we try to go where we know the service will be quick because sitting in their chairs usually becomes intolerable after a period of time. But we do go to restaurants.

A couple of years ago, my New Year's resolution was that if I was thinking about whether to do something or not, I would just do it. I've stuck with this resolution better than most resolutions and it has been well worth it. Sometimes I overdo it and regret it, but that just comes with the territory. More often, after the event or activity I think to myself, that was really great and I'm glad I pushed myself to do it.

And by the way, I just got back from lunch with one of our board members. He called right as I was about to start eating and it would have been easy to say no, not today. But I didn't and as usual was glad that I didn't. This individual has a tremendous ability to make people feel better about themselves and the lunch was well worth it.

Being active is a great way to keep Chiari at bay.

6. Know When to Push & When to Ask for Help

Just as important as staying active however is understanding what your limits are, knowing when to push them and realizing when you should ask for help. At the risk of venturing into politically incorrect territory, research (or at least general wisdom) in exercise physiology shows that women tend to not push themselves hard enough when they exercise but are good at doing them correctly. Men, on the other hand, tend to push too hard, use too much weight and work out too fast resulting in poor form, reduced benefit and injuries.

I don't know if this observation applies to the Chiari population in general, but I do know that it applied to me. I pushed too hard and too fast many times and suffered the consequences. My thinking was that dealing with Chiari and the surgery would be just like recovering from a sports injury (I have heard this from other people as well). Of course I was wrong and it took a long time for me to change my thinking and my approach.

Living with Chiari is a balance of give and take; two steps forward, one step back, three steps forward, three steps back, one step forward. While I could probably write pages about navigating the hills, valleys and plateaus of the Chiari terrain, in the end there is no substitute for experience. Over time, and if you work at it, you will learn to listen to your body and will develop a feel for when to push and reach for something new; when to pull back and rest; and when to ask for help.

I'm not sure I believe 100% in the gender split cited above, but I will say to those with driven personalities, who are used to accomplishing things and being independent, temper your natural personality and learn when to ask for help. For some people it becomes a matter of pride, and I completely understand this. But there are situations where it's just not worth it and asking for help is the right thing to do. Think about going up a flight of stairs. Normally you'd take the steps one at a time. If you're in a hurry, you might go two at a time, or maybe even three at a time, but you probably wouldn't try to go up 5 steps at a time. It's just not possible. Learn to overcome your natural tendency to try things and if the job is too big, ask for help.

One time, I was at the pet store picking up food for our dog (a beautiful black Lab mix). I knew going in that this was a risky situation for me, as the bags of food weigh 40 pound each. Luckily, when I asked one of the clerks where the specific brand was I was looking for, he led me to it and threw two bags in the cart.

When I checked out, the cashier asked me if I would like help taking them to my car. I hesitated for a moment and then did the smart thing and told her that would be great. Now, I do not look like someone who needs help loading dog food. In fact, people are often shocked when I tell them about Chiari and how it has affected me. However, I knew from the painful lessons of past experience that lifting something heavy out of a shopping cart was not a good move for me.

A young kid pushed the cart out to my car and threw the bags in the back. Did I feel a little strange watching him do this? Yes, I did. But on the way home I wasn't rubbing my neck and cursing myself for doing something foolish (which I have done more times than I care to admit).

When I got home, I then faced another decision. Obviously I couldn't leave the food in the car, so I had to decide whether to ask my wife for help or move it myself. I looked at the situation and realized I could slide the bags out of the back (we have a wagon) without really lifting them and then kind of carry them resting on my legs. I decided to take a chance and push my limits and did just that. It worked out well as I got the bags put away with no problems, and in fact they didn't really feel all that heavy. I went two for two that day; it was a good day.

It's harder for me to speak to those of you who need to learn to push yourselves, that is just not who I am. However, I would say just start with small steps and work from there. Try to do more each week or month, but keep moving forward and making progress. Once you realize that you can in fact do certain things, life will become easier and much more fulfilling. When you're feeling good, try taking the steps two at a time.

7. Pursue Your Dreams

At this point, daily living is now not such a burden and you're living an active, healthy life with plenty of physical activity. You've learned to understand your body and know when to push and when to back off. Now it's time to become proactive in living your life and pursuing your dreams. You've prioritized your life so that you have the energy to focus on what is most important, but now it's time to move beyond just getting through each day and it's time to start living life again.

Many self-help books talk about living with a purpose and pursuing dreams and goals. Just because you have Chiari, doesn't change the fact that working towards a dream can be incredibly rewarding. In fact, you will likely find that as you focus on a dream that you actually begin to feel better. Focusing your mind on achieving something means that your mind will not be focused on the pain you are in or thinking about how life used to be.

Obviously some dreams may no longer be possible, but the human imagination has a near limitless capacity to conceive of what might be. Use your imagination and stretch your mind to think about what you want to accomplish.

The importance of this step can not be overstated. It is essentially the difference between trying to make it through the day and living life. Believe me, I've had plenty of days when a short time after waking up I couldn't wait for the day to be over in the hope that I would feel better the next day (the joke in my household is, 'Is it 8:00 yet?'; this is when the kids go to bed and I can collapse on the couch). However, it's easier to get through those days if there is something to focus on during the day, if there is something that can be accomplished, even if it's just something small, that will make me feel like I'm moving forward in life and not drifting along with the flow of time.

Also, since reprioritizing my life and creating new dreams, I have had many days where I felt like I've lived the day to the fullest. Pursuing dreams is a way to Conquer Chiari on a personal level and affirm that your are more than your disease. This thought came to light in an interview with Dr. Carol Greco, a psychologist who specializes in using mind-body therapies such as biofeedback and meditation to help chronic disease and pain patients. Dr. Greco said,

> *"Probably most important is - the person needs to keep in mind that they are more than their disease, and realize that there is always more that is right with them than wrong with them!"*

We are all more than our diseases, we just need to prove it to ourselves by not letting Chiari control our lives and by pursuing our dreams.

8. Have Faith, Stay Positive & Find Laughter Where You Can

To Conquer Chiari you must have faith. Whether it's faith in the traditional religious sense, faith in yourself or faith in some higher purpose, Chiari will always bring times that test your strength and faith. For most people with Chiari, it is inevitable that they will experience down times. Times when they feel miserable physically and feel like giving up. It is during these rough patches that it is important to have faith, to truly believe that things will get better.

You have to find a way, either through faith in God or a deep belief in yourself, to convince yourself that you will feel better one day, that things will improve. During these times it is easy to give up hope and fall into despair, but you must fight it at all costs. Do whatever you can to maintain a positive mental attitude. Chiari can be test of wills, and you must have faith to win it.

When dealing with Chiari it can be a struggle to maintain a positive attitude. I don't claim to have the secret, but I do know it's possible. In an early issue of the newsletter, I posed a very controversial question, "Has anything positive come from having Chiari?"

Naturally, I got many replies questioning my sanity in thinking that anything positive could possibly come from such a terrible affliction. However, it turned out I was not misguided. For some, the experience with Chiari had become a positive, transforming event.

Consider the following feedback from three different people:

"Chiari has opened my eyes to a level of physical suffering I did not know was possible. Though I disdain my current situation, I have to say that to live in a world oblivious to what others may go through would be worse than suffering along side of them. Love is what is most important to me and what better way to love than to truly understand another's pain."

"I have a new appreciation for life and the people in my life. I am inspired to be a better person and help others with the same condition."

"I have to tell you that the positives that have come from this for myself is that I now know who my friends are and that true love can get through anything."

These sentiments were just a sampling of the feedback received from people who were able to find something positive in their situation. I don't know exactly why some people are able to achieve (or maintain) a positive outlook through their battle with Chiari, but I think letting go of the anger (Step 1) plays a big role. I also think that consciously looking for and identifying any positive changes that have occurred in your life can be part of the process. Do you get to spend more time with your children? Do you appreciate certain sights, sounds and sensations more than before? If some things are taken away, do you get angry or appreciate what you do have even more?

Although, I haven't figured out all the details, I am not surprised that many people have found something positive in their experience; it is very human. Like tempering steel, tragedy and hardship can bring out the best in people and make them and the relationships around them incredibly strong. While I am not yet ready to say that I'm glad to have Chiari and that I wouldn't change things if I could, I can say with certainty that I am a much better person because of it.

I also know that laughter can play a role and help during the rough times. Some people are shocked and outraged that we run a piece in the newsletter called, 'You Gotta Laugh!' They say things like, how can you laugh about something so serious, or you belittle the suffering of people with Chiari by doing this. While I respect their views, I also fundamentally disagree with them.

Laughter has tremendous healing qualities, both emotionally, and some research suggests, even physically. Personally, I can't understand how some people could choose to shut off that part of their lives; I can find humor in almost any situation.

Faith, positive attitude and laughter are all valuable weapons in the fight against Chiari.

9. Look to Yourself, Not Others

Many people with Chiari tell me that no one seems to understand what they are going through. I tell them they're right. As I've said elsewhere in this book, I believe everyone's Chiari experience is unique and while some people will be more empathetic and understanding than others, no one can truly understand how another person feels pain or deals with physical limitations. It is inherently a subjective experience.

Because of this, I encourage people to not look to others for validation of what they are experiencing. If you are experiencing it, it is real. I can understand why people look to others for validation, especially when they are feeling overwhelmed, but by doing so they give up control over a very important aspect of their life and set themselves up for disappointment.

This is because sometimes looking to others for validation can have very negative consequences. For example, research has shown that an amazing number of Chiari patients are told at one time by a doctor that there is nothing wrong with them, that it is all in their head. If a person is looking for validation from a doctor and that doctor does not provide it (and many don't), it just makes a bad situation worse. While some people will dismiss what the doctor says and go to someone else, others will begin to question themselves, disengage and give up hope.

A doctor is just a person like everyone else. What they say should be evaluated in the context of everything else that is going on. Have the strength and confidence to believe in yourself and make your own decisions.

For similar reasons, I also discourage people from asking their doctor if every little ache and pain they feel is related to Chiari. In the totality of the situation, it just doesn't matter. The real question is, are the symptoms in total bad enough to warrant surgery? If you feel a symptom, it is real whether it is due to compression of brain tissue, spine tissue or something altogether different.

Finally, I think it is important not to place the burden of expectations on our friends, family and loved ones. I get emails and see message board postings from people who are extremely bitter about how their family members don't understand what it is like. They're right, how can someone who doesn't have Chiari understand what it is like? But does that make them a bad person? I don't think so.

Maybe some of these people are justified in their criticisms, but what does it accomplish? One post in particular sticks out in my mind. A person was saying how angry they were at their spouse because they didn't acknowledge how much pain they were in on a particular day. This person went on to say that while the spouse took care of the kids and the house (and probably worked as well) they were really hurt that their spouse didn't seem to understand and wasn't sympathetic enough. I felt really bad for the spouse who was working hard every day to take care of things, but failed in the expectations department by not tending properly to emotional needs.

Rather than be angry and bitter about how people react to our situation, why not look inside for validation of how we are feeling and spare our loved ones the extra burden of our expectations? From a selfish point of view, it means never being disappointed, and from a selfless point of view, it seems like the least we can do in an effort to Conquer Chiari.

10. Never Give Up, Never Give In

In the end, Conquering Chiari is more mental than it is physical. It's about discipline, mental toughness, inner strength, willpower and making the decision that you are not going to be controlled by the disease. It's about saying that no matter how many times you get knocked down you are going to pick yourself back up and keep trying. It's about never giving up and never giving in. It's about not surrendering to despair. It's about being more than a disease.

Once you have made that decision at a deep level, at the very core of your being, you have already won. It doesn't matter what you can or can't do physically. It doesn't matter how much pain you're in or how Chiari has affected your life. If you've made the decision to not let Chiari control you then it won't.

I'm not saying it is easy - it may be the hardest thing you have ever done - but I am saying that it is your choice. Don't be afraid of it and don't shy away from it. Face it head on and believe in yourself. And most of all, never give up and never give in. Keep putting one foot in front of the other as you walk the Chiari tightrope.

That is how you Conquer Chiari!

Conquering Chiari as A Community

While it is important for each and every person to Conquer Chiari on their own terms, it is just as important that the Chiari community come together to truly conquer this disease. Chiari is very complex and it will take a sustained effort by many people on many fronts to defeat it, and Conquer Chiari is trying to do just that.

In order to maximize our resources and chances of success, we have devoted a good deal of time developing a long-term strategy to guide our efforts. I thought it would be useful to share parts of our 5-year strategic plan with you, the Chiari community, so that you can get a better feel for what we are doing, where we are going, and how you can help.

The C&S Patient Education Foundation Five-Year Strategy is a living document which we revisit and update regularly. It is not meant to limit our efforts by forcing us to stick within a given plan, but rather to guide us and provide a backdrop against which to evaluate new ideas and opportunities.

Everything the Foundation does, from programs to budgeting to evaluating new ideas, flows from our mission statement.

Mission Statement

The C&S Patient Education Foundation is dedicated to improving the experiences and outcomes of Chiari & syringomyelia patients by:

1) Providing accurate, up-to-date, and easy to understand information to patients so that they can take control of their health care and make intelligent, informed decisions
2) Raising awareness among family, friends, and the general public so that they can understand what patients are going through and are better able to provide support
3) Raising awareness among, and providing accurate, up-to-date information to, the medical community, so that errors in diagnosis and treatment are reduced
4) Providing support services to mitigate the overwhelming experience that coping with Chiari can be, and to reduce the rate of and level of depression and anxiety among patients
5) Sponsoring research to advance the understanding of these conditions and to, in the end, Conquer Chiari

From the individual elements of our Mission Statement, and by taking into account the needs of the Chiari community, we developed specific goals to strive for. The goals have been categorized according to the major items of the mission statement. Specifically, for each of the areas of education, general awareness, medical awareness, support, and research two goals were developed; one relating to the Patient Experiences and one relating to Patient Outcomes.

Conquer Chiari Goals

Education

- *Patient Experiences:* If a question has an answer, it is available, easy to access, and easy to understand.
- *Patient Outcomes:* Patients have the knowledge they need to make informed, intelligent decisions about their care.

General Awareness

- *Patient Experiences:* Chiari goes from being something that no one has heard of, to something that a significant percentage of people have a rudimentary understanding of; in addition, enable friends, families, and co-workers to better understand the experience and eliminate the "you don't look sick" problem.
- *Patient Outcomes:* Reduce the average time between first-symptoms and accurate diagnosis to less than 2 years.

Medical Awareness

- *Patient Experiences:* Improve the patient-doctor relationship to the point where, on average, patients report a positive experience with their doctors.
- *Patient Outcomes:* Reduce the average time between first-symptoms and accurate diagnosis to less than 2 years.

Support Services

- *Patient Experiences:* Being diagnosed with Chiari moves from an overwhelming experience to one which people feel well-equipped to handle.
- *Patient Outcomes:* Significantly reduce depression and anxiety among both newly diagnosed and existing patients.

Research

- *Patient Experiences:* Currently, the Chiari experience is a life-altering event for at least 50% of the population. The goal is to change Chiari from life-altering to a bump in the road type of experience for 100% of patients.
- *Patient Outcomes:* 100% of patients are fully functional after medical intervention, with a minimal amount of trauma.

Needs Analysis

In order to develop the goals and the programs to accomplish them, Conquer Chiari analyzed the needs of the Chiari community based upon personal experience and talking with hundreds of patients, family members, and medical professionals.

For the purposes of analysis, the Chiari community was segmented as follows, with the corresponding sizes in the US:

Figure 9-1: US Chiari Community

Patients	
Newly Diagnosed Surgical	3,000
Newly Diagnosed Non-surgical	9,000
Existing	300,000
Friends And Family	954,000
Medical Professionals	
Neurosurgeons	4,000
Pediatricians	22,000
Primary Care Providers	100,000
Registered Nurses	1,850,000
Other	10,000
Community Total	3,252,000

Notes:

- 3,000 surgical cases/year based on AANS survey and published estimates
- Assume 3:1 non-surgical/surgical ratio; based on correspondence with neurosurgeons
- Existing assumes prevalence of 1 in 1,000 and a 300 million US population
- Assume 6 FF/new surgical case, 4 FF/new non-surgical case, 3 FF/existing patient
- Parents of pediatric patients are included in FF, but will be split out in needs analysis
- Interested public is not sized, but will be addressed in needs analysis

The Chiari community was segmented into newly diagnosed patients, existing patients, friends and family, parents of pediatric patients, medical professionals, interested public, and the research community. For each segment, needs were assessed as follows:

Newly Diagnosed Patients

In general the needs of newly diagnosed patients can be described as: What is wrong with me? What can I expect? What do I do about it?

- Come up to speed quickly
- Understand basic terminology/concepts
- Understand what the key issues are and decisions they will have to make (or abdicate)
- Get a feel for what to expect, what the process will be like, how they will end up
- Validation for what they are feeling and going through
- Are their symptoms normal
- Practical issues for navigating the healthcare system (keep MRIs)
- Meet and talk with others in a similar situation
- General emotional support – everything will be ok, vent, run the gamut of emotions
- Find a qualified doctor(s)
- Financial assistance
- Detailed information on specific topics, such as will my children get it, can I have more kids, etc.

Existing Patients

- Stay in touch with medical advances
- Will my symptoms come back
- Detailed information on specific topics, such as labor and delivery issues with Chiari
- How to deal with residual symptoms, e.g. pain
- Practical issues of living with CM/SM: work, family, activities, etc.
- On-going support and sense of community, especially for people on disability
- Validation of their overall experience
- Opportunity to do something proactive against the disease, volunteering
- Financial assistance

Friends & Family

- Understand, in broad terms, what is wrong with their loved one
- Understand, in broad terms, what will happen
- How can they best help, and provide support to the patient
- Opportunity to do something on behalf of patient

Parents of Pediatric Patients

- What is wrong with my child
- What will happen to my child, will he/she be alright
- What symptoms are related
- What activities will my child be able to participate in
- Deal with the emotional impact on family
- Connect with other families in similar situations

Medical Professionals

- Quickly understand basics
- Stay in touch with important advances
- Understand the patient's point of view

Interested Public

- General sense of what CM/SM are
- Understand how it impacts patient functionally at work, school, etc.

Research – In A Better World

- Earlier, accurate diagnosis without being told your crazy
- Consensus in treatment philosophy
- Don't have to seek out a Chiari specialist
- Less, or non-traumatic, highly successful treatments
- Understand where you fit in the spectrum of Chiari
- Understand how to recover and deal with any residual problems
- Minimize emotional and family impact

Corporate Tenets

As part of the strategy discussions, we also decided how we wanted to run the Foundation; in other words, what type of organization we would be. These thoughts were then captured in ten corporate tenets which articulate our philosophy:

The Foundation will operate under the following tenets:

1. We will always remember that patients come first.
2. We will recognize that each person's Chiari/syringomyelia experience is unique, and be cognizant of the physical, mental, emotional, financial, and spiritual challenges that shape their experience.
3. We will serve the majority and engage in activities which produce the most benefit for the least amount of resources.
4. We will leverage technology to maximize the impact of our activities, while realizing that this may pass over some people.
5. We expect patients to take responsibility for themselves, and as such will provide tools for people to use whenever possible.
6. We will focus on solving real problems of the patient community, not on building an organization.
7. We will be aggressive and proactive in our business practices.
8. We will avoid duplication of services and will try not to compete with existing organizations.
9. We will not align ourselves with any specific doctor, hospital, medical provider, or vendor.
10. We will avoid taking sides on controversial issues, while recognizing the importance of providing people with enough information to make informed decisions.

Accomplishments So Far

Using our Mission Statement, Goals, and Corporate Tenets to guide us, we believe Conquer Chiari (along with the help of you, the community) has made significant progress in just a short period of time.

Web Site

The Conquer Chiari website has become widely recognized as the single most comprehensive source of information about Chiari and related topics. We are especially proud of the fact that the site is utilized by such a broad array of people, from patients to family members to medical professionals from all over the world. In fact, recently Conquer Chiari has received requests to translate the website materials into several foreign languages.

We are also proud of the feedback we get which acknowledges our efforts to present an objective, balanced view of the subject matter. This is especially important in becoming a trusted source of information in the eyes of the medical community.

A quick way to assess the impact of the website is by looking at the number of people who use it. The Conquer Chiari site now averages nearly 500 visits each day (a visit is when a person enters the site, as opposed to hits which counts each and every page that someone looks at) which of course translates to well more than 100,000 visits each year.

In fact, the numbers since the sites inception are astronomical:

- Nearly 400,000 individuals have visited the site
- The site averages over 500 visits per day
- Over 4,500,000 pages of information have been viewed
- The Overview Presentation and FAQ have each been viewed more than 90,000 times
- The Chiari Education and Awareness Sheets have been downloaded more than 50,000 times

Interestingly, traffic to the website is still growing. So while we have not yet reached everyone we want to reach, we are well on our way to doing so.

Newsletter

Chiari & Syringomyelia News is the flagship program of the Foundation. Since its launch in August of 2003, literally hundreds of research articles, interviews, and personal stories have been published (which are all available in the Newsletter Archives). Thousands of people in the Chiari community look to the newsletter as their main source of information about Chiari and related topics.

But more important than quantity is quality. Since the beginning, Chiari & Syringomyelia News has strived to bring accurate, objective, and timely information to the Chiari community. With scientific articles clearly differentiated from personal and opinion pieces, the newsletter does not engage in scare tactics or hysteria and does not favor or endorse any specific doctors or hospitals.

This approach has been validated daily by the feedback we receive from patients and medical professionals alike. In fact, there has not been a single complaint from a medical professional or researcher regarding the content of the newsletter articles. To the contrary, many surgeons and researchers have sent in feedback saying how impressed they are with the accuracy of the articles and coverage of their specific research. Some doctors now even refer their patients to the site to learn more. In addition, we have not heard from a single patient who had a bad experience taking a Chiari & Syringomyelia News article to a doctor to discuss.

Our approach to the newsletter will not change. We will continue to maintain the highest level of scientific and journalistic integrity in serving the Chiari community.

Answer Questions

As the reach of organization grows, naturally we come into contact with more and more members of the Chiari community. Conquer Chiari averages about 100 inquiries, questions, and comments per month via phone and email. I personally respond to each and every one. While I am able to reply to many in the same day, our stated goal is to reply no later than one week from receiving the email or call.

If you, or someone you know, does not get an answer within a week, please try again. It could be there was a problem with the contact information (for example some people forget to include their email address when submitting a question through the website).

On-Line Meeting Place

One of our Corporate Tenets is to utilize technology to leverage our limited resources and create high-impact programs. When the social networking sites like MySpace started to explode, it became clear that a Chiari based social networking site could provide a valuable tool to help Chiari people connect.

The On-Line Meeting Place has accomplished just that. With over 1,000 users, hundreds of people have been able to connect with one another, share stories, and find support.

Research Grants

In 2006, Conquer Chiari issued a joint call for research proposals with Column of Hope and the response was tremendous. More than 20 researchers and surgeons from around the world submitted exciting proposals on a wide variety of topics. After a methodical review by a highly qualified committee, Conquer Chiai awarded a $50,000 research grant to study what genes are active during a critical time of embryological development. Column of Hope also awarded a $50,000 research grant.

In 2007, Conquer Chiari asked a group of researchers to form a collaboration in order to develop a new, objective Chiari test. The group was awarded a $75,000 research grant to do just that.

Clearly to improve the outcomes of Chiari patients more research is required and Conquer Chiari intends to continue awarding grants in order to push the limits of knowledge and develop new treatments.

Research Symposium

In June, 2007 the University of Illinois-Chicago and Conquer Chiari held a one-day professional research symposium at the Neurosurgery Department of UIC. The event was a tremendous success with over 40 surgeons, engineers, and other interested professionals in attendance. Conquer Chiari is planning an even larger professional research conference for 2008.

Research Agenda

In order to make the most of our limited resources, and in an attempt to focus the research community on common goals, Conquer Chiari has developed a Research Agenda. The Agenda was presented at the Research Symposium in 2007 and was enthusiastically received by the surgeons and researchers in attendance.

In fact, working groups – comprised of a small number of surgeons and scientists - are in the process of being created to address the specific goals and objectives laid out in the Agenda.

Goal #1: Reduce the average time to an accurate diagnosis to less than 2 years from time of first symptoms.

Objectives:

- Develop a standard, simple, objective definition and test of symptomatic Chiari
- Enable the introduction of new technologies, such as inexpensive, portable imaging, which will reduce the barriers to diagnosis

Goal #2: Develop an effective, widely adopted, and minimally traumatic standard of care.

Objectives:

- Design, and encourage the adoption of, a standard outcome measure, such that the results from different studies can be compared and combined
- Establish whether the surgical variations that currently exist have a significant effect on long-term patient outcomes, and further develop a standardized surgical approach
- Encourage the development of minimally invasive surgical techniques
- Pursue non-surgical treatment approaches which don't just address symptoms, but are targeted at the core problem(s)

Goal #3: Minimize the impact that Chiari has on the quality of life of patients.

Objectives:

- Develop, and encourage the adoption of, a Chiari Impact Measure, which takes into account patient focused issues such as career, family, economics, recreation, and socialization
- Understand, and develop treatments for, the neuropsychological effects of Chiari, including both cognitive and emotional manifestations
- Develop widely accepted protocols for physical, occupational, and other types of therapies designed to maximize functional capabilities
- Enable the development of innovative technologies and treatments targeted at the neuropathic pain and loss of function associated with Chiari

Goal #4: Understand the pathophysiology, natural history, and epidemiological characteristics of Chiari.

Objectives:

- Establish, with reasonable accuracy, the incidence and prevalence of Chiari and Chiari related syringomyelia

- Characterize, and quantify, the Chiari experience, such as average age of diagnosis, time to diagnosis, number of doctors seen, major symptoms, etc.
- Develop a sound theoretical model for the pathophsyiology of Chiari, which explains how symptoms develop, and will enable predictions about who needs surgery, who will develop syringomyelia, etc.
- Identify and characterize the genetic basis of Chiari

Together We Can Make A Difference

Chiari can be conquered, but the C&S Patient Education Foundation can not do it alone. Everyone in the community must pull together, stand up and make a difference. Whether it's raising awareness, distributing information, or raising money for research, everyone can make a difference. Conquer Chiari is committed, I am committed, to making it happen, and together we will.

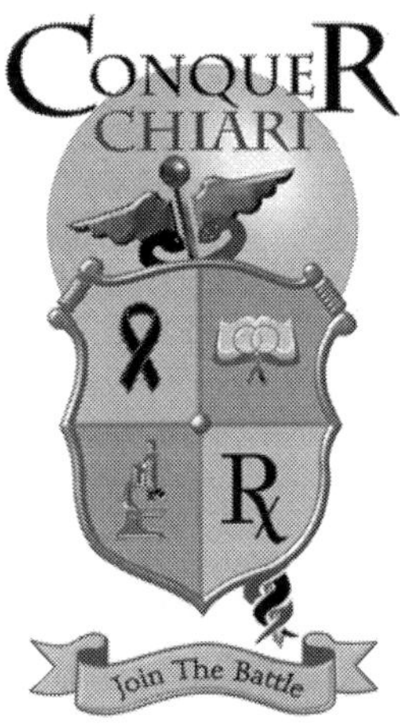

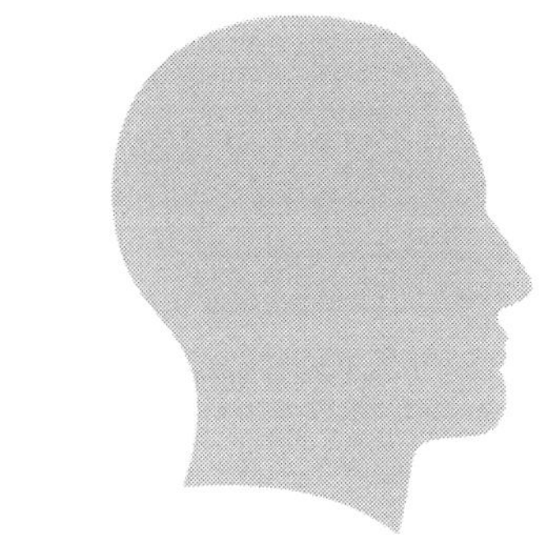

-Appendix-

- List of Figures -

Chapter 1 - Figures

Chapter 2 - Figures

Chapter 3 - Figures

Chapter 4 - Figures

Chapter 5 - Figures

Chapter 7 - Figures

Chapter 8 - Figures

Chapter 9 - Figures

Conquer Chiari
www.conquerchiari.org

American Syringomyelia Alliance Project
www.asap.org

Arnold Chiari Malformation Message Board
http://groups.msn.com/arnoldchiarimalformation

Australian Syringomyelia Network
www.tvnmc.com/asn

Carrie's Chiari Connection
http://www.freewebs.com/carrieschiariconnection/index.htm

Chiari Awareness
http://chiariawareness.com/

Chiari & Syringomyelia In Canada
http://www.chiariandsyringomyeliaincanada.blogspot.com/

Chiari Connection International
http://www.chiariconnectioninternational.com/

Devin's Diary
www.devinsdiary.com

Our Chiari Kids
www.communityzero.com/ock

The Chiari Times (Dr. John Oro)
www.chiaritimes.com

United Kingdom Arnold Chiari and Syringomyelia Association
www.domus.plus.com

World Arnold Chiari Malformation Association
www.pressenter.com/~wacma

Abel TJ, Chowdhary A, Gabikian P, Ellenbogen RG, Avellino AM. Acquired chiari malformation type I associated with a fatty terminal filum. Case report. Journal of Neurosurgery. 2006 Oct; 105(4 Suppl):329-32.

Agosta F, Rovaris M, Benedetti B, Valsasina P, Filippi M, Comi G. Diffusion tensor MRI of the cervical cord in a patient with syringomyelia and multiple sclerosis. Journal of Neurology Neurosurgery Psychiatry. 2004 Nov;75(11):1647

Agustí M, Adàlia R, Fernández C, Gomar C. Anaesthesia for caesarean section in a patient with syringomyelia and Arnold-Chiari type I malformation. International Journal of Obstetrics and Anesthesia. 2004 Apr; 13(2):114-6.

Alperin N, Kulkarni K, Loth F, Roitberg B, Foroohar M, Mafee MF, Lichtor T. Analysis of magnetic resonance imaging-based blood and cerebrospinal fluid flow measurements in patients with Chiari I malformation: a system approach. Neurosurgical Focus. 2001 Jul 15; 11(1):E6.

Alperin N, Sivaramakrishnan A, Lichtor T. Magnetic resonance imaging-based measurements of cerebrospinal fluid and blood flow as indicators of intracranial compliance in patients with Chiari malformation. Journal of Neurosurgery. 2005 Jul 103(1):46-52.

Alzate JC, Kothbauer KF, Jallo GI, Epstein FJ. Treatment of Chiari I malformation in patients with and without syringomyelia: a consecutive series of 66 cases. Neurosurgical Focus. 2001 Jul 15; 11(1):E3.

Anderson RC, Dowling KC, Feldstein NA, Emerson RG. Chiari I malformation: potential role for intraoperative electrophysiologic monitoring. Journal of Clinical Neurophysiology. 2003 Feb; 20(1):65-72.

Anderson RC, Emerson RG, Dowling KC, Feldstein NA. Improvement in brainstem auditory evoked potentials after suboccipital decompression in patients with chiari I malformations. Journal of Neurosurgery. 2003 Mar; 98(3):459-64.

Ang BT, Steinbok P, Cochrane DD. Etiological differences between the isolated lateral ventricle and the isolated fourth ventricle. Childs Nervous System. 2006 Sep; 22(9):1080-5.

Arora P, Behari S, Banerji D, Chhabra DK, Jain VK. Factors influencing the outcome in symptomatic Chiari I malformation. Neurology India. 2004 Dec; 52(4):470-4.

Arora P, Pradhan PK, Behari S, Banerji D, Das BK, Chhabra DK, Jain VK. Chiari I malformation related syringomyelia: radionuclide cisternography as a predictor of outcome. Acta Neurochirurgica (Wien). 2004 Feb 146(2):119-30.

Asgari S, Engelhorn T, Bschor M, Sandalcioglu IE, Stolke D. Surgical prognosis in hindbrain related syringomyelia. Acta Neurology Scandinavia. 2003 Jan; 107(1):12-21.

Apkarian AV, Sosa Y, Sonty S, Levy RM, Harden RN, Parrish TB, Gitelman DR.Chronic back pain is associated with decreased prefrontal and thalamic gray matter density. Journal of Neuroscience. 2004 Nov 17;24(46):10410-5.

Attal N, Parker F, Tadié M, Aghakani N, Bouhassira D. Effects of surgery on the sensory deficits of syringomyelia and predictors of outcome: a long term prospective study. Journal of Neurology Neurosurgery Psychiatry. 2004 Jul;75(7):1025-30.

Aydin S, Hanimoglu H, Tanriverdi T, Yentur E, Kaynar MY. Chiari type I malformations in adults: a morphometric analysis of the posterior cranial fossa. Surgical Neurology. 2005 Sep; 64(3):237-41 discussion 241.

Banik R, Lin D, Miller NR. Prevalence of Chiari I malformation and cerebellar ectopia in patients with pseudotumor cerebri. Journal of Neurological Science. 2006 Aug 15; 247(1):71-5.

Bateman GA. The role of altered impedance in the pathophysiology of normal pressure hydrocephalus, Alzheimer's disease and syringomyelia. Medical Hypotheses. 2004;63(6):980-5.

Batzdorf U, Khoo LT, McArthur DL. Observations on spine deformity and syringomyelia. Neurosurgery. 2007 Aug;61(2):370-7.

Batzdorf U. Primary spinal syringomyelia. Invited submission from the joint section meeting on disorders of the spine and peripheral nerves, March 2005. Journal of Neurosurgery Spine. 2005 Dec;3(6):429-35.

Batzdorf U. Primary spinal syringomyelia: a personal perspective. Neurosurgical Focus. 2000 Mar 15;8(3).

Bejjani GK, Cockerham KP, Rothfus WE, Maroon JC, Maddock M. Treatment of failed Adult Chiari Malformation decompression with CSF drainage: observations in six patients. Acta Neurochirurgica (Wien). 2003 Feb 145(2):107-16discussion 116.

Bejjani GK, Zabramski JDurasis Study Group. Safety and efficacy of the porcine small intestinal submucosa dural substitute: results of a prospective multicenter study and literature review. Journal of Neurosurgery. 2007 Jun; 106(6):1028-33.

Bejjani GK. Association of the Adult Chiari Malformation and Idiopathic Intracranial Hypertension: more than a coincidence. Medical Hypotheses. 2003 Jun; 60(6):859-63.

Bejjani GK. Definition of the adult Chiari malformation: a brief historical overview. Neurosurgical Focus. 2001 Jul 15; 11(1):E1.

Berger A, Dukes EM, Oster G., Clinical characteristics and economic costs of patients with painful neuropathic disorders. Journal of Pain. 2004 Apr;5(3):143-9.

Berkouk K, Carpenter PW, Lucey AD. Pressure wave propagation in fluid-filled co-axial elastic tubes. Part 1: Basic theory. Journal Biomechanical Engineering. 2003 Dec;125(6):852-6.

Bertram CD, Brodbelt AR, Stoodley MA. The origins of syringomyelia: numerical models of fluid/structure interactions in the spinal cord. Journal of Biomechanical Engineering. 2005 Dec;127(7):1099-109.

Bhangoo R, Sgouros S. Scoliosis in children with Chiari I-related syringomyelia. Childs Nervous System. 2006 Sep 22(9):1154-7.

Bogdanov EI, Heiss JD, Mendelevich EG, Mikhaylov IM, Haass A. Clinical and neuroimaging features of "idiopathic" syringomyelia. Neurology. 2004 Mar 9;62(5):791-4.

Bogdanov EI, Heiss JD, Mendelevich EG. The post-syrinx syndrome: stable central myelopathy and collapsed or absent syrinx. Journal of Neurology. 2006 Jun 253(6):707-13.

Bogdanov EI, Mendelevich EG. Syrinx size and duration of symptoms predict the pace of progressive myelopathy: retrospective analysis of 103 unoperated cases with craniocervical junction malformations and syringomyelia. Clinical Neurology Neurosurgery. 2002 May; 104(2):90-7.

Botelho RV, Bittencourt LR, Rotta JM, Tufik S. A prospective controlled study of sleep respiratory events in patients with craniovertebral junction malformation. Journal of Neurosurgery. 2003 Dec; 99(6):1004-9.

Botelho RV, Bittencourt LR, Rotta JM, Tufik S. Adult Chiari malformation and sleep apnoea. Neurosurgery Review. 2005 Jul; 28(3):169-76.

Boyles AL, Enterline DS, Hammock PH, Siegel DG, Slifer SH, Mehltretter L, Gilbert JR, Hu-Lince D, Stephan D, Batzdorf U, Benzel E, Ellenbogen R, Green BA, Kula R, Menezes A, Mueller D, Oro' JJ, Iskandar BJ, George TM, Milhorat TH, Speer MC. Phenotypic definition of Chiari type I malformation coupled with high-density SNP genome screen shows significant evidence for linkage to regions on chromosomes 9 and 15. American Journal of Medical Genetics. 2006 Dec 15; 140(24):2776-85.

Bradley LJ, Ratahi ED, Crawford HA, Barnes MJ. The outcomes of scoliosis surgery in patients with syringomyelia. Spine. 2007 Oct 1;32(21):2327-33.

Brickell KL, Anderson NE, Charleston AJ, Hope JK, Bok AP, Barber PA. Ethnic differences in syringomyelia in New Zealand. Journal of Neurology Neurosurgery Psychiatry. 2006 Aug;77(8):989-91.

Brockmeyer D, Gollogly S, Smith JT. Scoliosis associated with Chiari 1 malformations: the effect of suboccipital decompression on scoliosis curve progression: a preliminary study. Spine. 2003 Nov 15; 28(22):2505-9.

Brodbelt AR, Stoodley MA, Watling AM, Tu J, Burke S, Jones NR. Altered subarachnoid space compliance and fluid flow in an animal model of posttraumatic syringomyelia. Spine. 2003 Oct 15;28(20):E413-9.

Brodbelt AR, Stoodley MA, Watling AM, Tu J, Jones NR. Fluid flow in an animal model of posttraumatic syringomyelia. European Spine Journal. 2003 Jun;12(3):300-6. Epub 2002 Dec 6.

Brodbelt AR, Stoodley MA. Syringomyelia and the arachnoid web. Acta Neurochirurgica (Wien). 2003 Aug;145(8):707-11.

Bruehl S, Chung OY, Jirjis JN, Biridepalli S. Prevalence of clinical hypertension in patients with chronic pain compared to nonpain general medical patients. Clinical Journal of Pain. 2005 Mar-Apr;21(2):147-53.

Buoni S, Zannolli R, di Bartolo RM, Donati PA, Mussa F, Giordano F, Genitori L. Surgery removes EEG abnormalities in patients with Chiari type I malformation and poor CSF flow. Clinical Neurophysiology. 2006 May 117(5):959-63.

Cakmakkaya OS, Kaya G, Altintas F, Bakan M, Yildirim A. Anesthetic management of a child with Arnold-Chiari malformation and Klippel-Feil syndrome. Paediatric Anaesthesia. 2006 Mar; 16(3):355-6.

Caldarelli M, Novegno F, Vassimi L, Romani R, Tamburrini G, Di Rocco C. The role of limited posterior fossa craniectomy in the surgical treatment of Chiari malformation Type I: experience with a pediatric series. Journal of Neurosurgery. 2007 Mar; 106(3 Suppl):187-95.

Cano A, Johansen AB, Geisser M. Spousal congruence on disability, pain, and spouse responses to pain. Pain. 2004 Jun;109(3):258-65.

Carpenter PW, Berkouk K, Lucey AD. Pressure wave propagation in fluid-filled co-axial elastic tubes. Part 2: Mechanisms for the pathogenesis of syringomyelia. Journal of Biomechanical Engineering. 2003 Dec;125(6):857-63.

Chang HS, Nakagawa H. Hypothesis on the pathophysiology of syringomyelia based on simulation of cerebrospinal fluid dynamics. Journal of Neurology Neurosurgery Psychiatry. 2003 Mar;74(3):344-7.

Chang HS, Nakagawa H. Theoretical analysis of the pathophysiology of syringomyelia associated with adhesive arachnoiditis. Journal of Neurology Neurosurgery Psychiatry. 2004 May;75(5):754-7.

Chantigian RC, Koehn MA, Ramin KD, Warner MA. Chiari I malformation in parturients. Journal of Clinical Anesthesia. 2002 May; 14(3):201-5.

Cheng JC, Chau WW, Guo X, Chan YL. Redefining the magnetic resonance imaging reference level for the cerebellar tonsil: a study of 170 adolescents with normal versus idiopathic scoliosis. Spine. 2003 Apr 15; 28(8):815-8.

Chow RT, Barnsley L. Systematic review of the literature of low-level laser therapy (LLLT) in the management of neck pain. Lasers and Surgical Medicine. 2005 Jul;37(1):46-52.

Chu WC, Man GC, Lam WW, Yeung BH, Chau WW, Ng BK, Lam TP, Lee KM, Cheng JC. A detailed morphologic and functional magnetic resonance imaging study of the craniocervical junction in adolescent idiopathic scoliosis. Spine. 2007 Jul 1; 32(15):1667-74.

da Silva JA, Holanda MM. Basilar impression, Chiari malformation and syringomyelia: a retrospective study of 53 surgically treated patients. Arq Neuropsiquiatr. 2003 Jun 61(2B):368-75.

Daffner SD et al.; Impact of Neck and Arm Pain on Overall Health Status. Spine, Sep 1; 28(17):2030-5.

Danish SF, Samdani A, Hanna A, Storm P, Sutton L. Experience with acellular human dura and bovine collagen matrix for duraplasty after posterior fossa decompression for Chiari malformations. Journal of Neurosurgery. 2006 Jan; 104(1 Suppl):16-20.

Dauvilliers Y, Stal V, Abril B, Coubes P, Bobin S, Touchon J, Escourrou P, Parker F, Bourgin P. Chiari malformation and sleep related breathing disorders. Journal of Neurology Neurosurgery Psychiatry. 2007 Dec; 78(12):1344-8.

Decharms RC, Maeda F, Glover GH, Ludlow D, Pauly JM, Soneji D, Gabrieli JD, Mackey SC. Control over brain activation and pain learned by using real-time functional MRI. Proceedings of the National Academies of Science U S A. 2005 Dec 20;102(51):18626-31.

Defoort-Dhellemmes S, Denion E, Arndt CF, Bouvet-Drumare I, Hache JC, Dhellemmes P. Resolution of acute acquired comitant esotropia after suboccipital decompression for Chiari I malformation. American Journal of Ophthalmology. 2002 May; 133(5):723-5.

Dersh J, Gatchel RJ, Mayer T, Polatin P, Temple OR. Prevalence of psychiatric disorders in patients with chronic disabling occupational spinal disorders. Spine. 2006 May 1;31(10):1156-62.

Di Lorenzo N, Cacciola F. Adult syringomielia. Classification, pathogenesis and therapeutic approaches. Journal of Neurosurgical Science. 2005 Sep;49(3):65-72.

Dolar MT, Haughton VM, Iskandar BJ, Quigley M. Effect of craniocervical decompression on peak CSF velocities in symptomatic patients with Chiari I malformation. AJNR American Journal of Neuroradiology. 2004 Jan; 25(1):142-5.

Dones J, De Jesús O, Colen CB, Toledo MM, Delgado M. Clinical outcomes in patients with Chiari I malformation: a review of 27 cases. Surgical Neurology. 2003 Aug; 60(2):142-7.

Drake JM. Occult tethered cord syndrome: not an indication for surgery. Journal of Neurosurgery. 2006 May;104(5 Suppl):305-8.

Ducreux D, Attal N, Parker F, Bouhassira D. Mechanisms of central neuropathic pain: a combined psychophysical and fMRI study in syringomyelia. Brain. 2006 Apr;129(Pt 4):963-76. Effects of surgery on the sensory deficits of syringomyelia and predictors of outcome: a long term prospective study. Journal of Neurology Neurosurgery Psychiatry. 2004 Jul; 75(7):1025-30.

Ellenbogen RG, Armonda RA, Shaw DW, Winn HR. Toward a rational treatment of Chiari I malformation and syringomyelia. Neurosurgical Focus. 2000 Mar 15; 8(3):E6.

Eule JM, Erickson MA, O'Brien MF, Handler M. Chiari I malformation associated with syringomyelia and scoliosis: a twenty-year review of surgical and nonsurgical treatment in a pediatric population. Spine. 2002 Jul 1; 27(13):1451-5.

Fagan LH, Ferguson S, Yassari R, Frim DM. The Chiari pseudotumor cerebri syndrome: symptom recurrence after decompressive surgery for Chiari malformation type I. Pediatric Neurosurgery. 2006; 42(1):14-9.

Farley FA, Puryear A, Hall JM, Muraszko K. Curve progression in scoliosis associated with Chiari I malformation following suboccipital decompression. Journal of Spinal Disorders Technique. 2002 Oct; 15(5):410-4.

Fischbein NJ, Dillon WP, Cobbs C, Weinstein PR. The "presyrinx" state: is there a reversible myelopathic condition that may precede syringomyelia? Neurosurgical Focus. 2000 Mar 15;8(3):E4.

Flynn JM, Sodha S, Lou JE, Adams SB Jr, Whitfield B, Ecker ML, Sutton L, Dormans JP, Drummond DS. Predictors of progression of scoliosis after decompression of an Arnold Chiari I malformation. Spine. 2004 Feb 1; 29(3):286-92.

Gagnadoux F, Meslier N, Svab I, Menei P, Racineux JL. Sleep-disordered breathing in patients with Chiari malformation: improvement after surgery. Neurology. 2006 Jan 10; 66(1):136-8.

Galarza M, Sood S, Ham S. Relevance of surgical strategies for the management of pediatric Chiari type I malformation. Childs Nervous System. 2007 Jun 23(6):691-6.

García-Real I, Kass PH, Sturges BK, Wisner ER. Morphometric analysis of the cranial cavity and caudal cranial fossa in the dog: a computerized tomographic study. Veterinary Radiology and Ultrasound. 2004 Jan-Feb 45(1):38-45.

Gezen F, Kahraman S, Ziyal IM, Canakçi Z, Bakir A. Application of syringosubarachnoid shunt through key-hole laminectomy. Technical note. Neurosurgical Focus. 2000 Mar 15;8(3):E10.

Green C, Martin CW, Bassett K, Kazanjian A. A systematic review of craniosacral therapy: biological plausibility, assessment reliability and clinical effectiveness. Complementary Therapies in Medicine. 1999 Dec;7(4):201-7.

Greenlee J, Garell PC, Stence N, Menezes AH. Comprehensive approach to Chiari malformation in pediatric patients. Neurosurgical Focus. 1999 Jun 15; 6(6):e4.

Greenlee JD, Donovan KA, Hasan DM, Menezes AH. Chiari I malformation in the very young child: the spectrum of presentations and experience in 31 children under age 6 years. Pediatrics. 2002 Dec; 110(6):1212-9.

Greitz D. Unraveling the riddle of syringomyelia. Neurosurgery Review. 2006 Oct;29(4):251-63.

Guillen A, Costa JM. Spontaneous resolution of a Chiari I malformation associated syringomyelia in one child. Acta Neurochirurgica (Wien). 2004 Feb 146(2):187-91.

Guo F, Wang M, Long J, Wang H, Sun H, Yang B, Song L. Surgical management of Chiari malformation: analysis of 128 cases. Pediatric Neurosurgery. 2007; 43(5):375-81.

Haughton VM, Korosec FR, Medow JE, Dolar MT, Iskandar BJ. Peak systolic and diastolic CSF velocity in the foramen magnum in adult patients with Chiari I malformations and in normal control participants. AJNR American Journal of Neuroradiology. 2003 Feb 24(2):169-76.

Heller JB, Lazareff J, Gabbay JS, Lam S, Kawamoto HK, Bradley JP. Posterior cranial fossa box expansion leads to resolution of symptomatic cerebellar ptosis following Chiari I malformation repair. Journal of Craniofacial Surgery. 2007 Mar; 18(2):274-80.

Hentschel SJ, Yen KG, Lang FF. Chiari I malformation and acute acquired comitant esotropia: case report and review of the literature. Journal of Neurosurgery. 2005 May; 102(4 Suppl):407-12.

Hilton EL, Henderson LJ. The nature, meanings, and dynamics of lived experiences of a person with syringomyelia: a phenomenological study. SCI Nursing. 2003 Spring;20(1):10-7.

Himmelstein DU, Warren E, Thorne D, Woolhandler S. MarketWatch: Illness And Injury As Contributors To Bankruptcy. Health Affairs (Millwood). 2005 Feb 2;

Hofkes SK, Iskandar BJ, Turski PA, Gentry LR, McCue JB, Haughton VM. Differentiation between symptomatic Chiari I malformation and asymptomatic tonsilar ectopia by using cerebrospinal fluid flow imaging: initial estimate of imaging accuracy. Radiology. 2007 Nov 245(2):532-40.

Holly LT, Batzdorf U. Slitlike syrinx cavities: a persistent central canal. Journal of Neurosurgery. 2002 Sep;97(2 Suppl):161-5.

Inoue M, Nakata Y, Minami S, Kitahara H, Otsuka Y, Isobe K, Takaso M, Tokunaga M, Itabashi T, Nishikawa S, Moriya H. Idiopathic scoliosis as a presenting sign of familial Neurologyogic abnormalities. Spine. 2003 Jan 1; 28(1):40-5.

Iskandar BJ, Haughton V. Age-related variations in peak cerebrospinal fluid velocities in the foramen magnum. Journal of Neurosurgery. 2005 Dec; 103(6 Suppl):508-11.

Iskandar BJ, Quigley M, Haughton VM. Foramen magnum cerebrospinal fluid flow characteristics in children with Chiari I malformation before and after craniocervical decompression. Journal of Neurosurgery. 2004 Nov; 101(2 Suppl):169-78.

James HE, Brant A. Treatment of the Chiari malformation with bone decompression without durotomy in children and young adults. Childs Nervous System. 2002 May; 18(5):202-6.

Jatavallabhula NS, Armstrong J, Sgouros S, Whitehouse W. Spontaneous resolution of isolated Chiari I malformation. Childs Nervous System. 2006 Feb 22(2):201-3.

Joseph V, Rajshekhar V. Resolution of syringomyelia and basilar invagination after traction. Journal of Neurosurgery. 2003 Apr;98(3 Suppl):298.

Klekamp J, Iaconetta G, Batzdorf U, Samii M. Syringomyelia associated with foramen magnum arachnoiditis. Journal of Neurosurgery. 2002 Oct; 97(3 Suppl):317-22.

Klekamp J. The pathophysiology of syringomyelia - historical overview and current concept. Acta Neurochirurgica (Wien). 2002 Jul;144(7):649-64.

Kontio K, Davidson D, Letts M. Management of scoliosis and syringomyelia in children. Journal of Pediatric Orthopedics. 2002 Nov-Dec;22(6):771-9.

Kowal L, Yahalom C, Shuey NH. Chiari 1 malformation presenting as strabismus. Binocular Vision Strabismus Quarterly. 2006; 21(1):18-26.

Kuczkowski KM. Spinal anesthesia for Cesarean delivery in a parturient with Arnold-Chiari type I malformation. Canadian Journal of Anaesthesia. 2004 Jun-Jul; 51(6):639.

Kumar A, Patni AH, Charbel F. The Chiari I malformation and the neurotologist. Otology and Neurotology. 2002 Sep; 23(5):727-35.

Kyoshima K, Bogdanov EI. Spontaneous resolution of syringomyelia: report of two cases and review of the literature. Neurosurgery. 2003 Sep;53(3):762-8.

Kyoshima K, Kuroyanagi T, Oya F, Kamijo Y, El-Noamany H, Kobayashi S. Syringomyelia without hindbrain herniation: tight cisterna magna. Report of four cases and a review of the literature. Journal of Neurosurgery. 2002 Mar;96(2 Suppl):239-49.

Kyoshima K, Kuroyanagi T, Toriyama T, Takizawa T, Hirooka Y, Miyama H, Tanabe A, Oikawa S. Surgical experience of syringomyelia with reference to the findings of magnetic resonance imaging. Journal of Clinical Neuroscience. 2004 Apr; 11(3):273-9.

Lame IE, Peters ML, Vlaeyen JW, Kleef M, Patijn J. Quality of life in chronic pain is more associated with beliefs about pain, than with pain intensity. European Journal of Pain. 2005 Feb;9(1):15-24.

Landau R, Giraud R, Delrue V, Kern C. Spinal anesthesia for cesarean delivery in a woman with a surgically corrected type I Arnold Chiari malformation. Anesthesia & Analgesia. 2003 Jul; 97(1):253-5.

Lazareff JA, Galarza M, Gravori T, Spinks TJ. Tonsillectomy without craniectomy for the management of infantile Chiari I malformation. Journal of Neurosurgery. 2002 Nov; 97(5):1018-22.

Lee GY, Jones NR, Mayrhofer G, Brown C, Cleland L. Origin of macrophages in a kaolin-induced model of rat syringomyelia: a studyusing radiation bone marrow chimeras. Spine. 2005 Jan 15;30(2):194-200.

Levine DN. The pathogenesis of syringomyelia associated with lesions at the foramen magnum: a critical review of existing theories and proposal of a new hypothesis. Journal of Neurological Science. 2004 May 15;220(1-2):3-21.

Levy LM. MR identification of Chiari pathophysiology by using spatial and temporal CSF flow indices and implications for syringomyelia. AJNR American Journal of Neuroradiology. 2003 Feb; 24(2):165-6.

Lichtor T, Egofske P, Alperin N. Noncommunicating cysts and cerebrospinal fluid flow dynamics in am patient with a Chiari I malformation and syringomyelia--part I. Spine. 2005 Jun 130(11):1335-40.

Lichtor T, Egofske P, Alperin N. Noncommunicating cysts and cerebrospinal fluid flow dynamics in a patient with a Chiari I malformation and syringomyelia--part II. Spine. 2005 Jun 15; 30(12):1466-72.

Limonadi FM, Selden NR. Dura-splitting decompression of the craniocervical junction: reduced operative time, hospital stay, and cost with equivalent early outcome. Journal Neurosurgery. 2004 Nov 101(2 Suppl):184-8.

Liu B, Wang ZY, Xie JC, Han HB, Pei XL. Cerebrospinal fluid dynamics in Chiari malformation associated with syringomyelia. Chinese Medical Journal (Engl). 2007 Feb 5; 120(3):219-23.

Lollis SS, Hug EB, Gladstone DJ, Chaffee S, Duhaime AC. Acquired Chiari malformation type I following fractionated radiation therapy to the anterior skull base in a 20-month-old boy. Journal of Neurosurgery. 2006 Feb;104(2 Suppl):133-7.

Maroon JC, Bost JW. Omega-3 fatty acids (fish oil) as an anti-inflammatory: an alternative to nonsteroidal anti-inflammatory drugs for discogenic pain. Surgical Neurology. 2006 Apr;65(4):326-31.

Martin BA, Kalata W, Loth F, Royston TJ, Oshinski JN. Syringomyelia hydrodynamics: an in vitro study based on in vivo measurements. Journal of Biomechanical Engineering. 2005 Dec;127(7):1110-20.

Martínez-Lage JF, Rábano A, Bermejo J, Martínez Pérez M, Guerrero MC,Contreras MA, Lunar A. Creutzfeldt-Jakob disease acquired via a dural graft: failure of therapy with quinacrine and chlorpromazine. Surgical Neurology. 2005 Dec;64(6):542-5.

Matsuoka T, Ahlberg PE, Kessaris N, Iannarelli P, Dennehy U, Richardson WD, McMahon AP, Koentges G. Neural crest origins of the neck and shoulder. Nature. 2005 Jul 21; 436(7049):347-55.

Mazzola CA, Fried AH. Revision surgery for Chiari malformation decompression. Neurosurgical Focus. 2003 Sep 15; 15(3):E3.

McCracken LM, Vowles KE, Eccleston C. Acceptance-based treatment for persons with complex, long standing chronic pain: a preliminary analysis of treatment outcome in comparison to a waiting phase. Behavior Research & Therapy. 2005 Oct;43(10):1335-46.

McGirt MJ, Nimjee SM, Floyd J, Bulsara KR, George TM. Correlation of cerebrospinal fluid flow dynamics and headache in Chiari I malformation. Neurosurgery. 2005 Apr; 56(4):716-21discussion 716-21.

McGirt MJ, Nimjee SM, Fuchs HE, George TM. Relationship of cine phase-contrast magnetic resonance imaging with outcome after decompression for Chiari I malformations. Neurosurgery. 2006 Jul; 59(1):140-6discussion 140-6.

McLone DG, Dias MS. The Chiari II malformation: cause and impact. Childs Nervous System. 2003 Aug 19(7-8):540-50.

Menick BJ. Phase-contrast magnetic resonance imaging of cerebrospinal fluid flow in the evaluation of patients with Chiari I malformation. Neurosurgical Focus. 2001 Jul 15; 11(1):E5.

Messing-Jünger AM, Ibáñez J, Calbucci F, Choux M, Lena G, Mohsenipour I, Van Calenbergh F. Effectiveness and handling characteristics of a three-layer polymer dura substitute: a prospective multicenter clinical study. Journal of Neurosurgery. 2006 Dec; 105(6):853-8.

Metcalfe PD, Luerssen TG, King SJ, Kaefer M, Meldrum KK, Cain MP, Rink RC, Casale AJ. Treatment of the occult tethered spinal cord for neuropathic bladder: results of sectioning the filum terminale. Journal of Urology. 2006 Oct;176(4 Suppl):1826-30.

Milhorat TH, Bolognese PA, Black KS, Woldenberg RF. Acute syringomyelia: case report. Neurosurgery. 2003 Nov;53(5):1220-1.

Milhorat TH, Bolognese PA, Nishikawa M, McDonnell NB, Francomano CA. Syndrome of occipitoatlantoaxial hypermobility, cranial settling, and chiari malformation type I in patients with hereditary disorders of connective tissue. Journal of Neurosurgery Spine. 2007 Dec; 7(6):601-9.

Milhorat TH, Bolognese PA. Tailored operative technique for Chiari type I malformation using intraoperative color Doppler ultrasonography. Neurosurgery. 2003 Oct; 53(4):899-905discussion 905-6.

Milhorat TH. Classification of syringomyelia. Neurosurgical Focus. 2000 Mar 15;8(3):E1.

Monsivais D. Self-organization in chronic pain: a concept analysis. Rehabilitation Nursing. 2005 Jul-Aug;30(4):147-51.

Morcuende JA, Dolan LA, Vazquez JD, Jirasirakul A, Weinstein SL. A prognostic model for the presence of neurogenic lesions in atypical idiopathic scoliosis. Spine. 2004 Jan 1; 29(1):51-8.

Mueller D, Oro' JJ. Prospective analysis of self-perceived quality of life before and after posterior fossa decompression in 112 patients with Chiari malformation with or without syringomyelia. Neurosurgical Focus. 2005 Feb 15; 18(2):ECP2.

Mueller DM, Oro' J. Chiari I malformation with or without syringomyelia and pregnancy: case studies and review of the literature. American Journal of Perinatology. 2005 Feb; 22(2):67-70.

Mueller DM, Oro' JJ. Prospective analysis of presenting symptoms among 265 patients with radiographic evidence of Chiari malformation type I with or without syringomyelia. Journal of American Academy of Nurse Practitioners. 2004 Mar 16(3):134-8.

Munir F, Leka S, Griffiths A. Dealing with self-management of chronic illness at work: predictors for self-disclosure. Social Science and Medicine. 2005 Mar;60(6):1397-407.

Muraszko KM, Ellenbogen RG, Mapstone TB. Controversies in the surgical management of Chiari I malformations: what is the surgical procedure of choice? To open dura or not to open dura? Clinical Neurosurgery. 2004; 51:241-7.

Murphy RL, Tubbs RS, Grabb PA, Oakes WJ. Chiari I malformation and idiopathic growth hormone deficiency in siblings. Childs Nervous System. 2006 Jun; 22(6):632-4.

Murray C, Seton C, Prelog K, Fitzgerald DA. Arnold Chiari type 1 malformation presenting with sleep disordered breathing in well children. Archives of Diseases in Childhood. 2006 Apr; 91(4):342-3.

Nakamura M, Chiba K, Nishizawa T, Maruiwa H, Matsumoto M, Toyama Y. Retrospective study of surgery-related outcomes in patients with syringomyelia associated with Chiari I malformation: clinical significance of changes in the size and localization of syrinx on pain relief. Journal of Neurosurgery. 2004 Mar; 100(3 Suppl Spine):241-4.

Navarro R, Alonso I, Costa JM. Relevance of surgical strategies for the management of paediatric Chiari type I malformation. Childs Nervous System. 2007 Jul; 23(7):725-6.

Oldfield EH. Cerebellar tonsils and syringomyelia. Journal of Neurosurgery. 2002 Nov;97(5):1009-10.

Ono A, Suetsuna F, Ueyama K, Yokoyama T, Aburakawa S, Numasawa T, Wada K, Toh S. Surgical outcomes in adult patients with syringomyelia associated with Chiari malformation type I: the relationship between scoliosis and Neurologyogical findings. Journal of Neurosurgery Spine. 2007 Mar; 6(3):216-21.

Ozerdemoglu RA, Denis F, Transfeldt EE. Scoliosis associated with syringomyelia: clinical and radiologic correlation. Spine. 2003 Jul 1; 28(13):1410-7.

Ozerdemoglu RA, Transfeldt EE, Denis F. Value of treating primary causes of syrinx in scoliosis associated with syringomyelia. Spine. 2003 Apr 15;28(8):806-14.

Pandey A, Robinson S, Cohen AR. Cerebellar fits in children with Chiari I malformation. Neurosurgical Focus. 2001 Jul 15; 11(1):E4.

Panigrahi M, Reddy BP, Reddy AK, Reddy JJ. CSF flow study in Chiari I malformation. Childs Nervous System. 2004 May 20(5):336-40.

Parker JD, Broberg JC, Napolitano PG. Maternal Arnold-Chiari type I malformation and syringomyelia: a labor management dilemma. American Journal of Perinatology. 2002 Nov; 19(8):445-50.

Penney DJ, Smallman JM. Arnold-Chiari malformation and pregnancy. Internationa Journal of Obstetrics and Anesthesia. 2001 Apr; 10(2):139-41.

Perrini P, Benedetto N, Tenenbaum R, Di Lorenzo N. Extra-arachnoidal cranio-cervical decompression for syringomyelia associated with Chiari I malformation in adults: technique assessment. Acta Neurochirurgica (Wien). 2007 Oct; 149(10):1015-22.

Pinna G, Alessandrini F, Alfieri A, Rossi M, Bricolo A. Cerebrospinal fluid flow dynamics study in Chiari I malformation: implications for syrinx formation. Neurosurgical Focus. 2000 Mar 15; 8(3):E3.

Pirouzmand F, Tucker WS. A modification of the classic technique for expansion duroplasty of the posterior fossa. Neurosurgery. 2007 Feb; 60(2 Suppl 1.

Poca MA, Sahuquillo J, Topczewski T, Lastra R, Font ML, Corral E. Posture-induced changes in intracranial pressure: a comparative study in patients with and without a cerebrospinal fluid block at the craniovertebral junction. Neurosurgery. 2006 May; 58(5):899-906.

Povedano M, Gascon J, Galvez R, Ruiz M, Rejas J. Cognitive Function Impairment in Patients with Neuropathic Pain Under Standard Conditions of Care. Journal of Pain Symptom Management. 2007 Jan;33(1):78-89.

Proctor M, Scott RM. Redefining the magnetic resonance imaging reference level for the cerebellar tonsil: a study of 170 adolescents with normal versus idiopathic scoliosis. Spine. 2004 Jan 1; 29(1):105.

Pueyrredon F, Spaho N, Arroyave I, Vinters H, Lazareff J. Histological findings in cerebellar tonsils of patients with Chiari type I malformation. Childs Nervous System. 2007 Apr 23(4):427-9.

Quigley MF, Iskandar B, Quigley ME, Nicosia M, Haughton V. Cerebrospinal fluid flow in foramen magnum: temporal and spatial patterns at MR imaging in volunteers and in patients with Chiari I malformation. Radiology. 2004 Jul 232(1):229-36.

Raij TT, Numminen J, Narvanen S, Hiltunen J, Hari R. Brain correlates of subjective reality of physically and psychologically induced pain. Proceedings of the National Academies of Science U S A. 2005 Feb 8;102(6):2147-51.

Rees J, O'Boyle C, MacDonagh R. Quality of life: impact of chronic illness on the partner. Journal of the Royal Society of Medicine. 2001 Nov;94(11):563-6.

Rinaldi F, Cioffi FA, Columbano L, Krasagakis G, Bernini FP. Tethered cord syndrome. Journal of Neurosurgical Science. 2005 Dec; 49(4):131-5.

Rocchi L, Chiari L, Cappello A. Feature selection of stabilometric parameters based on principal component analysis. Medical and Biological Engineering and Computing. 2004 Jan; 42(1):71-9.

Rosen DS, Wollman R, Frim DM. Recurrence of symptoms after Chiari decompression and duraplasty with nonautologous graft material. Pediatric Neurosurgery. 2003 Apr; 38(4):186-90.

Royo-Salvador MB, Solé-Llenas J, Doménech JM, González-Adrio R. Results of the section of the filum terminale in 20 patients with syringomyelia, scoliosis and Chiari malformation. Acta Neurochirurgica (Wien). 2005 May; 147(5):515-23.

Rusbridge C, Knowler P, Rouleau GA, Minassian BA, Rothuizen J. Inherited occipital hypoplasia/syringomyelia in the cavalier King Charles spaniel: experiences in setting up a worldwide DNA collection. Journal of Hereditary. 2005; 96(7):745-9.

Rusbridge C, Knowler SP. Hereditary aspects of occipital bone hypoplasia and syringomyelia (Chiari type I malformation) in cavalier King Charles spaniels. Veterinary Record. 2003 Jul 26; 153(4):107-12.

Rusbridge C, Knowler SP. Inheritance of occipital bone hypoplasia (Chiari type I malformation) in Cavalier King Charles Spaniels. Journal of Veterinary Internal Medicine. 2004 Sep-Oct; 18(5):673-8.

Sacco D, Scott RM. Reoperation for Chiari malformations. Pediatric Neurosurgery. 2003 Oct; 39(4):171-8.

Sakas DE, Korfias SI, Wayte SC, Beale DJ, Papapetrou KP, Stranjalis GS, Whittaker KW, Whitwell HL. Chiari malformation: CSF flow dynamics in the craniocervical junction and syrinx. Acta Neurochirurgica (Wien). 2005 Dec 147(12):1223-33.

Sansur CA, Heiss JD, DeVroom HL, Eskioglu E, Ennis R, Oldfield EH. Pathophysiology of headache associated with cough in patients with Chiari I malformation. Journal of Neurosurgery. 2003 Mar; 98(3):453-8.

Schijman E, Steinbok P. International survey on the management of Chiari I malformation and syringomyelia. Childs Nervous System. 2004 May 20(5):341-8.

Schijman E. History, anatomic forms, and pathogenesis of Chiari I malformations. Childs Nervous System. 2004 May 20(5):323-8.

Sekula RF Jr, Jannetta PJ, Casey KF, Marchan EM, Sekula LK, McCrady CS. Dimensions of the posterior fossa in patients symptomatic for Chiari I malformation but without cerebellar tonsillar descent. Cerebrospinal Fluid Research. 2005 Dec 18; 2:11.

Selden NR. Occult tethered cord syndrome: the case for surgery. Journal of Neurosurgery. 2006 May;104(5 Suppl):302-4.

Sgouros S, Kountouri M, Natarajan K. Posterior fossa volume in children with Chiari malformation Type I. Journal of Neurosurgery. 2006 Aug; 105(2 Suppl):101-6.

Sgouros S, Kountouri M, Natarajan K. Skull base growth in children with Chiari malformation Type I. Journal of Neurosurgery. 2007 Sep; 107(3 Suppl):188-92.

Shibuya R, Yonenobu K, Koizumi T, Kato Y, Mitta M, Yoshikawa H. Pulsatile cerebrospinal fluid flow measurement using phase-contrast magnetic resonance imaging in patients with cervical myelopathy. Spine. 2002 May 15; 27(10):1087-93.

Sindou M, Chávez-Machuca J, Hashish H. Cranio-cervical decompression for Chiari type I-malformation, adding extreme lateral foramen magnum opening and expansile duroplasty with arachnoid preservation. Technique and long-term functional results in 44 consecutive adult cases -- comparison with literature data. Acta Neurochirurgica (Wien). 2002 Oct; 144(10):1005-19.

Sivaramakrishnan A, Alperin N, Surapaneni S, Lichtor T. Evaluating the effect of decompression surgery on cerebrospinal fluid flow and intracranial compliance in patients with chiari malformation with magnetic resonance imaging flow studies. Neurosurgery. 2004 Dec; 55(6):1344-50.

Skau M, Brennum J, Gjerris F, Jensen R. What is new about idiopathic intracranial hypertension? An updated review of mechanism and treatment. Cephalalgia. 2006 Apr;26(4):384-99

Smyth MD, Banks JT, Tubbs RS, Wellons JC 3rd, Oakes WJ. Efficacy of scheduled nonnarcotic analgesic medications in children after suboccipital craniectomy. Journal of Neurosurgery. 2004 Feb;100(2 Suppl):183-6.

Spiegel DA, Flynn JM, Stasikelis PJ, Dormans JP, Drummond DS, Gabriel KR, Loder RT. Scoliotic curve patterns in patients with Chiari I malformation and/or syringomyelia. Spine. 2003 Sep 15; 28(18):2139-46.

Spanos NP, Barber TX, Lang G. Cognition and self-control: cognitive control of painful sensory input. Integr Physiology and Behavioral Science. 2005 JulSep;40(3):119-28.

Steinbok P, Garton HJ, Gupta N. Occult tethered cord syndrome: a survey of practice patterns. Journal of Neurosurgery. 2006 May;104(5 Suppl):309-13.

Stoodley MA, Jones NR, Yang L, Brown CJ. Mechanisms underlying the formation and enlargement of noncommunicating syringomyelia: experimental studies. Neurosurgical Focus. 2000 Mar 15; 8(3):E2.

Sudo K, Miyazaki Y, Tajima Y, Matsumoto A, Tashiro K, Miyasaka K. Spontaneous resolution of idiopathic syringomyelia. Neurology. 2002 May 28;58(10):1576-7.

Sun X, Qiu Y, Zhu Z, Zhu F, Wang B, Yu Y, Qian B. Variations of the position of the cerebellar tonsil in idiopathic scoliotic adolescents with a cobb angle >40 degrees: a magnetic resonance imaging study. Spine. 2007 Jul 1; 32(15):1680-6.

Takayasu M, Takagi T, Hara M, Anzai M. A simple technique for expansive suboccipital cranioplasty following foramen magnum decompression for the treatment of syringomyelia associated with Chiari I malformation. Neurosurgical Review. 2004 Jul 27(3):173-7.

Takeuchi K, Yokoyama T, Ito J, Wada K, Itabashi T, Toh S. Tonsillar herniation and the cervical spine: a morphometric study of 172 patients. Journal of Orthopedic Science. 2007 Jan 12(1):55-60.

Todor DR, Mu HT, Milhorat TH. Pain and syringomyelia: a review. Neurosurgical Focus. 2000 Mar 15;8(3):E11.

Trigylidas T, Baronia B, Vassilyadi M, Ventureyra EC. Posterior fossa dimension and volume estimates in pediatric patients with Chiari I malformations. Childs Nervous System. 2007 Jul 27.

Tsara V, Serasli E, Kimiskidis V, Papagianopoulos S, Katsaridis V, Fylaktakis M, Christaki P, Kazis A. Acute respiratory failure and sleep-disordered breathing in Arnold-Chiari malformation. Clinical Neurology Neurosurgery. 2005 Oct 107(6):521-4.

Tubbs RS, Bui CJ, Rice WC, Loukas M, Naftel RP, Holcombe MP, Oakes WJ. Critical analysis of the Chiari malformation Type I found in children with lipomyelomeningocele. Journal of Neurosurgery. 2007 Mar; 106(3 Suppl):196-200.

Tubbs RS, Iskandar BJ, Bartolucci AA, Oakes WJ. A critical analysis of the Chiari 1.5 malformation. Journal of Neurosurgery. 2004 Nov 101(2 Suppl):179-83.

Tubbs RS, McGirt MJ, Oakes WJ. Surgical experience in 130 pediatric patients with Chiari I malformations. Journal of Neurosurgery. 2003 Aug; 99(2):291-6.

Tubbs RS, Oakes WJ. Treatment and management of the Chiari II malformation: an evidence-based review of the literature. Childs Nervous System. 2004 Jun 20(6):375-81.

Tubbs RS, Smyth MD, Wellons JC 3rd, Oakes WJ. Arachnoid veils and the Chiari I malformation. Journal of Neurosurgery. 2004 May; 100(5 Suppl Pediatrics):465-7.

Tubbs RS, Webb D, Abdullatif H, Conklin M, Doyle S, Oakes WJ. Posterior cranial fossa volume in patients with rickets: insights into the increased occurrence of Chiari I malformation in metabolic bone disease. Neurosurgery. 2004 Aug; 55(2):380-3.

Tubbs RS, Webb DB, Oakes WJ. Persistent syringomyelia following pediatric Chiari I decompression: radiological and surgical findings. Journal of Neurosurgery. 2004 May;100(5 Suppl Pediatrics):460-4.

Tubbs RS, Wellons JC 3rd, Blount JP, Grabb PA, Oakes WJ. Inclination of the odontoid process in the pediatric Chiari I malformation. Journal of Neurosurgery. 2003 Jan; 98(1 Suppl):43-9.

Tubbs RS, Wellons JC 3rd, Blount JP, Oakes WJ. Posterior atlantooccipital membrane for duraplasty. Technical note. Journal of Neurosurgery. 2002 Sep; 97(2 Suppl):266-8.

Tubbs RS, Wellons JC 3rd, Oakes WJ. Asymmetry of tonsillar ectopia in Chiari I malformation. Pediatric Neurosurgery. 2002 Oct; 37(4):199-202.

Tubbs RS, Wellons JC 3rd, Smyth MD, Bartolucci AA, Blount JP, Oakes WJ, Grabb PA. Children with growth hormone deficiency and Chiari I malformation: a morphometric analysis of the posterior cranial fossa. Pediatric Neurosurgery. 2003 Jun; 38(6):324-8.

Turk A, Iskandar BJ, Haughton V, Consigny D. Recording CSF pressure with a transducer-tipped wire in an animal model of Chiari I. AJNR American Journal of Neuroradiology. 2006 Feb; 27(2):354-5.

Ventureyra EC, Aziz HA, Vassilyadi M. The role of cine flow MRI in children with Chiari I malformation. Childs Nervous System. 2003 Feb; 19(2):109-13.

Vinck A, Maassen B, Mullaart R, Rotteveel J. Arnold-Chiari-II malformation and cognitive functioning in spina bifida. Journal of Neurology Neurosurgery Psychiatry. 2006 Sep77(9):1083-6.

Wehby MC, O'Hollaren PS, Abtin K, Hume JL, Richards BJ. Occult tight filum terminale syndrome: results of surgical untethering. Pediatric Neurosurgery. 2004 Mar-Apr;40(2):51-7.

Wellons JC 3rd, Tubbs RS, Bui CJ, Grabb PA, Oakes WJ. Urgent surgical intervention in pediatric patients with Chiari malformation type I. Report of two cases. Journal of Neurosurgery. 2007 Jul; 107(1 Suppl):49-52.

White A. A cumulative review of the range and incidence of significant adverse events associated with acupuncture. Acupuncture Medicine. 2004 Sep;22(3):122-33.

Widerstrom-Noga EG, Turk DC, Types and effectiveness of treatments used by people with chronic pain associated with SCI: influence of pain and psychosocial characteristics. Spinal Cord. Nov, 2003, 41(11) 600-9.

Yabe I, Kikuchi S, Tashiro K. Familial syringomyelia: the first Japanese case and review of the literature. Clinical Neurology Neurosurgery. 2002 Dec; 105(1):69-71.

Yeom JS, Lee CK, Park KW, Lee JH, Lee DH, Wang KC, Chang BS. Scoliosis associated with syringomyelia: analysis of MRI and curve progression. European Spine Journal. 2007 Oct;16(10):1629-35.

Yoshikawa H. Sudden respiratory arrest and Arnold-Chiari malformation. European Journal of Paediartic Neurology. 20037(4):191.

Zhang ZQ, Chen YQ, Chen YA, Wu X, Wang YB, Li XG. Chiari I malformation associated with syringomyelia: a retrospective study of 316 surgically treated patients. Spinal Cord. 2007 Nov 20[Epub].

Ziadeh MJ, Richardson JK. Arnold-Chiari malformation with syrinx presenting as carpal tunnel syndrome: a case report. Archive of Physical Medicine and Rehabilitation. 2004 Jan; 85(1):158-61.

Ziegler DK, Mallonee W. Chiari-1 malformation, migraine, and sudden death. Headache. 1999 Jan; 39(1):38-41.

Zileli M, Cagli S. Combined anterior and posterior approach for managing basilar invagination associated with type I Chiari malformation. Journal of Spinal Disorders Technique. 2002 Aug; 15(4):284-9.

Made in the USA
Lexington, KY
16 May 2011